EAT WELL, BE WELL

AYURVEDA COOKING FOR HEALTHY LIVING

Lois Leonhardi

Table of Contents

List of Tables iv
Dedication vii
About The Author viii
Preface ix
Introduction xiii
Chapter 1 About Ayurveda 1
Chapter 2 The Five Elements: The Key To Deciphering Your Unique Energetic Nature 3
Chapter 3 The Three Doshas 9
Vata – Air 9
Pitta – Fire 9
Kapha - Water 10
Dosha Times 12
Chapter 4 The Six Tastes 15
Sweet 15
Sour 15
Salty 16
Pungent 16
Bitter 16
Astringent 17
Exceptions To The Rules 17
Chapter 5 Food Combining – Quality And Quantity 19
Top 10 Essential Ayurvedic Tips For Wellness 22
Foods For The Doshas 26
Chapter 6 Ayurveda For The Family 29
Chapter 7 Kitchen Essentials 33
Spices 35
Organize Your Shopping 36
Tips – The Healthy Kitchen & Specialty/International Foods 37
Chapter 8 Let's Cook! 47
Chapter 9 Morning Meals 49
Chapter 10 Mid-day Main Meals 61
Tips for the aspiring vegetarian 61

Legumes: Lentils, Dals & Beans 62

Grains & Seeds 66

Animal & Dairy 87

Chapter 11 Any Time Soups & Stews 101

Chapter 12 Vegetables 117

Chapter 13 Salads & Vinaigrettes 127

Chapter 14 Sauces, Chutneys & Churnas 143

Chapter 15 Snacks and Dips 155

Chapter 16 Drinks 167

Chapter 17 Not Too Sweet Desserts & Gluten Free Options 173

Chapter 18 Leftovers 185

Appendix A Elements And The Twenty Qualities 186

Appendix B Dosha Evaluation 187

Appendix C Dosha Diet Aid For Vata 190

Appendix D Dosha Diet Aid For Pitta 192

Appendix E Dosha Diet Aid For Kapha 194

Appendix F Ama 196

LIST OF TABLES

Table 1 – Dosha Times	12
Table 2 – Food Combining	20
Table 3 – Top 10 Essential Ayurveda Tips For Wellness	24
Table 4 – Dosha Condiment Table	30
Table 5 – Pans, Utensils, Gadgets	33
Table 6 – The Pantry	34
Table 7 - Dried Spices & Fresh Herbs	35
Table 8 – Stocking the Refrigerator	36
Table 9 – Knives	38
Table 10 – Healthy Cookware	39
Table 11 – Lentils, Dals & Beans	66
Table 12 - Rice Cooking Chart	68
Twenty Qualities - Paired with Opposites	186

Legal disclaimer – the information provided herein is not intended to be medical advice and is not intended to diagnose, treat, cure, or prevent any disease. Please consult a knowledgeable health care professional before making any major dietary changes or consuming any home remedies that may interfere with medications.

Text©2013 by Lois Leonhardi
Photographs©2013 by Lois Leonhardi

Lois Leonhardi has asserted her right to be identified as the author of this work in accordance with the Copyright, Designs and Patents Act of 1988

All rights reserved. No part of this publication may be reproduced, stored in a retrieval system, or transmitted in any form or by any means, electronic, mechanical, photocopying, recording or otherwise, without the prior permission of the copyright owner.

ISBN: 978-1492942634

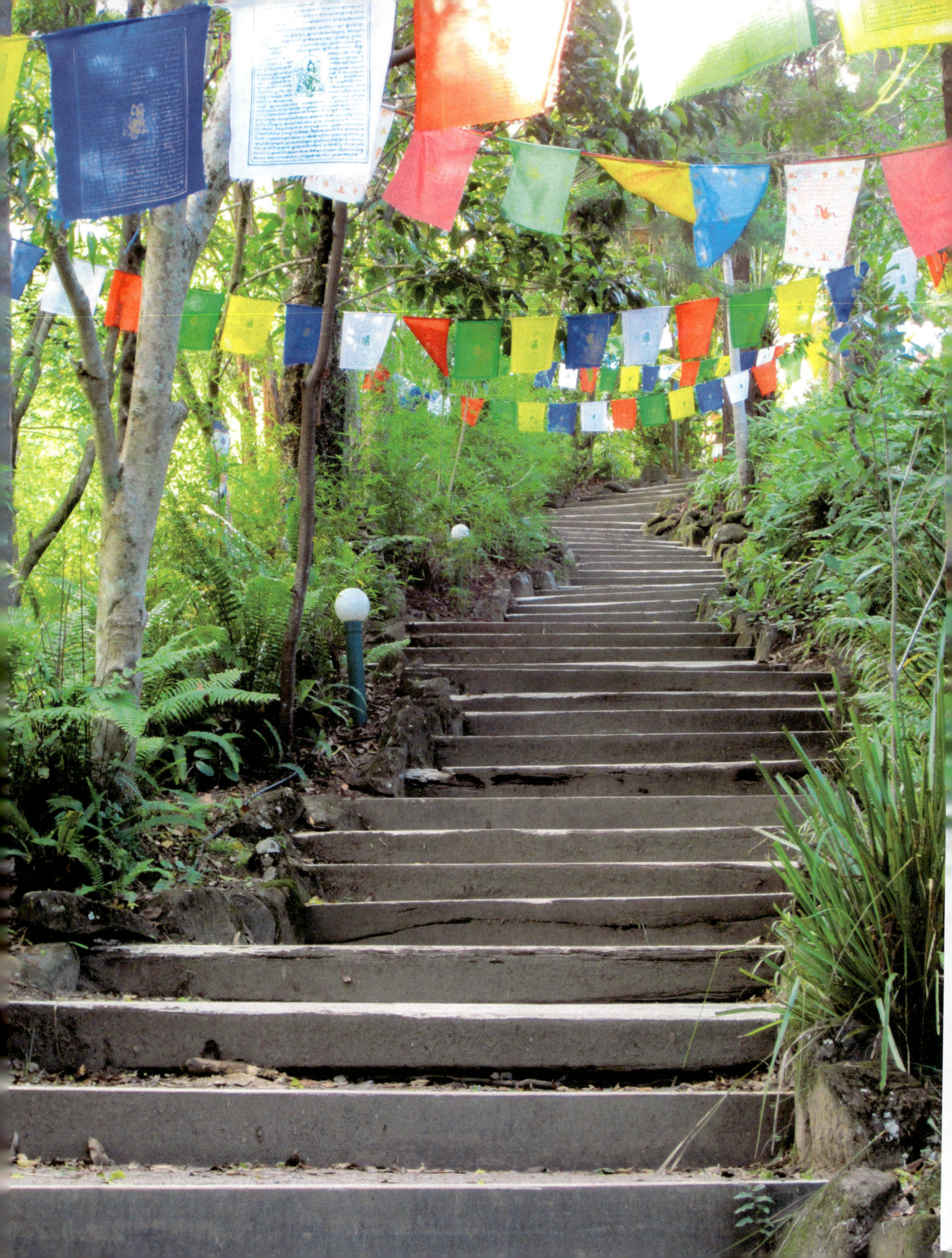

DEDICATION

This book was prepared with gratitude to Ed Danaher, my ayurvedic counselor who first introduced me to ayurveda and the healing cookbooks of Dr. Vasant Lad. Heartfelt appreciation goes to Dr. Lad, for his prolific teachings (textbooks, classroom lectures and clinics), generosity and compassion in which he has begun to reveal a glimmer of the vast wisdom of ayurveda. The recipes were created using the information from Dr. Lad's "Qualities of Food Substances" and "Food Combining" tables which are found in his book "Ayurvedic Cooking for Self-Healing". Thanks to Raj Chattergoon and the many reviewers, classmates, friends, family and taste testers who helped with candid feedback, recommendations and support. And to Jiwan Shakti Khalsa whose words of inspiration ("may your way to a smooth graceful finish be shown to you with ease") magically helped me stay focused and meet my deadlines.

It is my intention that this book be of benefit to all those seeking to make positive change in their lives. May that change bring harmony and balance to their body, mind and spirit, reverberating and reaching all sentient beings.

About the Author

Lois Leonhardi is a wellness coach specializing in creating holistic diet, exercise and anti-stress programs for time-pressed individuals. Using her knowledge of the systems of ayurveda and yoga, she creates custom-designed plans based on one's unique constitution. She has successfully worked as a private yoga instructor and personal chef in Los Angeles and on the east coast, helping clients reach their wellness goals.

Having worked in the frenetic financial industry for 20 years, she understands firsthand the challenges of maintaining balance (physically, emotionally and spiritually). This makes her uniquely qualified to create a realistic plan for her clients that they can seamlessly integrate into their life.

Whole body wellness entails putting you in control. Using time-tested techniques, you are taught to listen and observe energetic patterns to reveal the root causes of suffering; once identified, it's easy to dissolve physical and emotional hindrances (such as emotional eating, excess weight, sciatic pain, back pain and the stresses of life).

Lois enjoys facilitating the process and keeping clients motivated so they reach their goal. Ideally, she wants to empower you to tap into your inner state of peace, balance and joy.

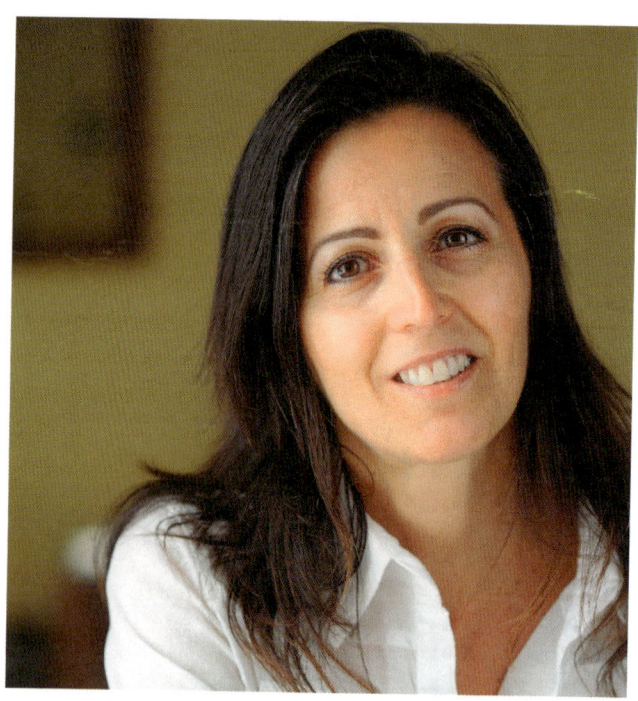

PREFACE

I was first introduced to ayurveda in 2001 while living in Portsmouth, New Hampshire. I had no idea what it was, but all my yoga friends were going to see the visiting ayurvedic practitioner from Albuquerque, New Mexico, Ed Danaher. I didn't understand why I should see a wellness practitioner if I didn't feel sick, but they persuaded me to go. We all signed up for appointments. The consultation was a leisurely half hour and included a comprehensive intake interview and pulse diagnosis. "You're vata" he said "and your vata is high". Then he proceeded to recommend herbs and dietary changes (no raw salads!) to bring things back to a state of balance; an ayurvedic wellness plan. I was intrigued and wanted to learn more, so he suggested further reading and directed me to a table of books. My eyes lit up when I saw a cookbook, "Ayurvedic Cooking for Self Healing". Always on the lookout for new recipes, I grabbed that first. Then Ed suggested the "The Science of Self-Healing" book as a good primer on ayurveda, so I selected that book too. Both were written by his teacher, Dr. Vasant Lad. That was the beginning of my ayurvedic journey. I read those books over and over; and continued to purchase more of Dr. Lad's books over the years.

Often referred to as the 'sister-science' to yoga, I found the concepts and terminology in ayurveda to be very similar and symbiotic with my yoga studies. I began to implement the prescribed lifestyle and dietary changes, gradually over time as space became available in my life. Eventually the ayurvedic way of living became my priority and I managed my career around my ayurvedic lifestyle. I started cooking ayurvedically for friends and eventually as a personal chef in Los Angeles. I began integrating the ayurvedic concepts into my yoga classes, to work more effectively with the various imbalances I observed in the students.

Curiously, the more engrossed in ayurveda I became, the more I found myself encountering people who had sworn off ayurveda! They were unsuccessful in their attempt at integrating their prescribed wellness plan into their life and quit. Their objections to ayurveda were the same: I'm not vegetarian; I don't understand the Sanskrit words; how am I supposed to cook for my family if we are all different constitutions; I don't like Indian food; I don't have time for this; no eating leftovers – are you serious?

So I would try to get them back on track. I would guide them through the maze of rules and help them prioritize and streamline the recommendations. Cooking was a major obstacle so I started creating recipes that would be balancing to their constitution. Sometimes I would be requested to teach their cooks how to shop for the food and prepare the ayurvedic meals. The food was simple and tasty. I was told I should write a book to explain all this. So I began recording my recipes with the intention of some day writing a cook book.

In 2010, I attended some of Dr. Lad's summer intensives - marma and pulse practicum - at The Ayurvedic Institute in New Mexico. That experience was life changing as it opened my eyes to the magnitude of ayurveda. I had until now, been exposed to a very small part of the vast system. I decided to take a sabbatical and study ayurveda full time. Needing confirmation from an unbiased source, I consulted with my vedic astrologer, Chakrapani. He confirmed I was predisposed to a career involving natural medicine, cooking, writing, consulting and yoga. He also mentioned investing (which explains my previous career in finance); and he mentioned I could have been a great dancer (which perhaps explains my love of salsa dancing!).

With positive reinforcement from my astrologer, I researched school options then enrolled in Dr. Lad's ASP-1 course, graduating in May 2012. From there I travelled to India to attended Dr. Lad's six-week clinical application program in Pune and travel. During the course of my five months in India, I met informally with other ayurveda doctors in Dharamsala, Pune, Varkala and Thodupuza. It was fascinating to see the regional differences, from north to south. I was able to experience first-hand the ayurvedic remedies for anemia, malnutrition, lung infections and dysentery. I noticed a direct correlation between my attitude and my health. When I was feeling healthy and energetic, I enjoyed everyone I met and laughed about communication challenges and travel disruptions; when I felt sick and exhausted I was extremely irritable and easily became impatient or angry when dealing with routine travel hassles. This made me think about all the cranky people in the world and wondered if perhaps they too were not feeling well; maybe they have underlying physical health issues related to inadequate nutrition that is keeping them from optimal wellness and a feeling of joy?

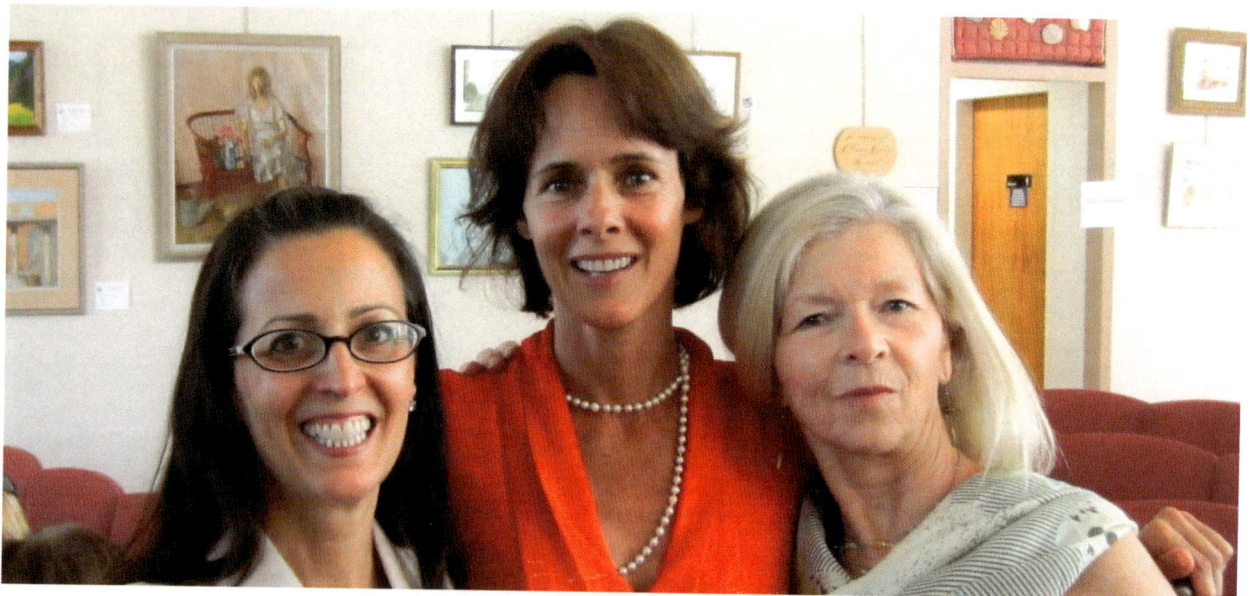

After India, I travelled to Thailand and New Zealand where I began writing this ayurveda wellness cookbook. I sought out native doctors in each country I visited, informally gathering information on the local traditions, researching online and comparing to ayurveda. From there, I went to a Buddhist monastery in Australia where I lived while studying Buddhism for 2½ months. I was fortunate to meet a Tibetan doctor there who accurately diagnosed the root cause of my "frozen shoulder" (vata in majja dhatu) as being severe anemia. Protein, iron and B12 deficiencies along with depleted reserves were confirmed with blood tests. As a yoga practitioner/instructor, I was relieved it was not arthritis. Things began to make sense as I thought back and connected this shoulder pain with my experimentation with vegetarianism during Ayurvedic School and at various other times in the past 20+ years (symptoms such as clumps of hair falling out, loose teeth, inability to focus, memory loss, deterioration in my vision, sleeping 10+ hours per day, etc.).

With my allergies to wheat, dairy, soy and nuts, a diet that is 100% vegetarian is difficult at best. I'm particular about the animal protein I ingest. At a minimum it is organic. Ideally it's from a local farm where the animals are treated humanely. For me, including meat in my diet is what brings balance.

With all this information, I returned to the U.S. to finish the book. My intention was to provide a general introduction to the principles of ayurveda in a manner that was accessible to westerners and addressed the common complaints I had heard over the years. I designed the book with the following guidelines:
- recipes suited to a western palate (i.e., minimal curry recipes)
- recipes containing animal protein are included for the carnivores
- easy to digest, tasty bean/lentil recipes for the aspiring vegetarians
- dairy-free, gluten-free and soy-free alternatives are provided with most recipes
- recipes designed to be balancing to all constitutions (i.e., "tri-doshic") to minimize guess work as to what recipe is appropriate for each individual
- dosha-specific condiment tables for those that want to target specific doshas
- well-organized charts and time-saving tips to help prioritize and implement the most important concepts in a time frame that suits busy lifestyles
- minimal use of Sanskrit language

Now the book is done and I will soon start a blog at www.yogawithlois.com. Check out the website and join my email list to be notified of new recipes and ayurvedic tips. I will be adding more gluten-free recipes that didn't make it into this book.

I encourage you to use this book as a guide to help develop an awareness of how food affects your body/mind energetics. The connection is profound.

Who will benefit from this book?
- People seeking to improve their dietary habits - This book provides an introduction to the key concepts of ayurveda. These principles have been used successfully in India for thousands of years to provide overall wellness. By adapting ancient dietary principles to suit a western lifestyle and palate, living healthy is now accessible to all.
- Clients of ayurvedic practitioners – New clients may feel overwhelmed at how to implement the food recommendations for themselves and their family; this book will provide them with answers when their practitioner is not available. The book should empower them to understand the concepts and easily assimilate them into their life.
- Ayurvedic practitioners – Practitioners will find this a valuable resource to recommend to old and new clients alike. The initial consultation can be overwhelming for a new client. This book reinforces key concepts explained during their visit, serving as a handy reference (the notes that they wished they had taken). Most importantly, it will help all clients easily implement their customized ayurvedic plan and diets, resulting in higher compliance and retention rates. The goal is to spread wellness (and happiness) to everyone.

Namaste,

Lois Leonhardi
www.yogawithlois.com

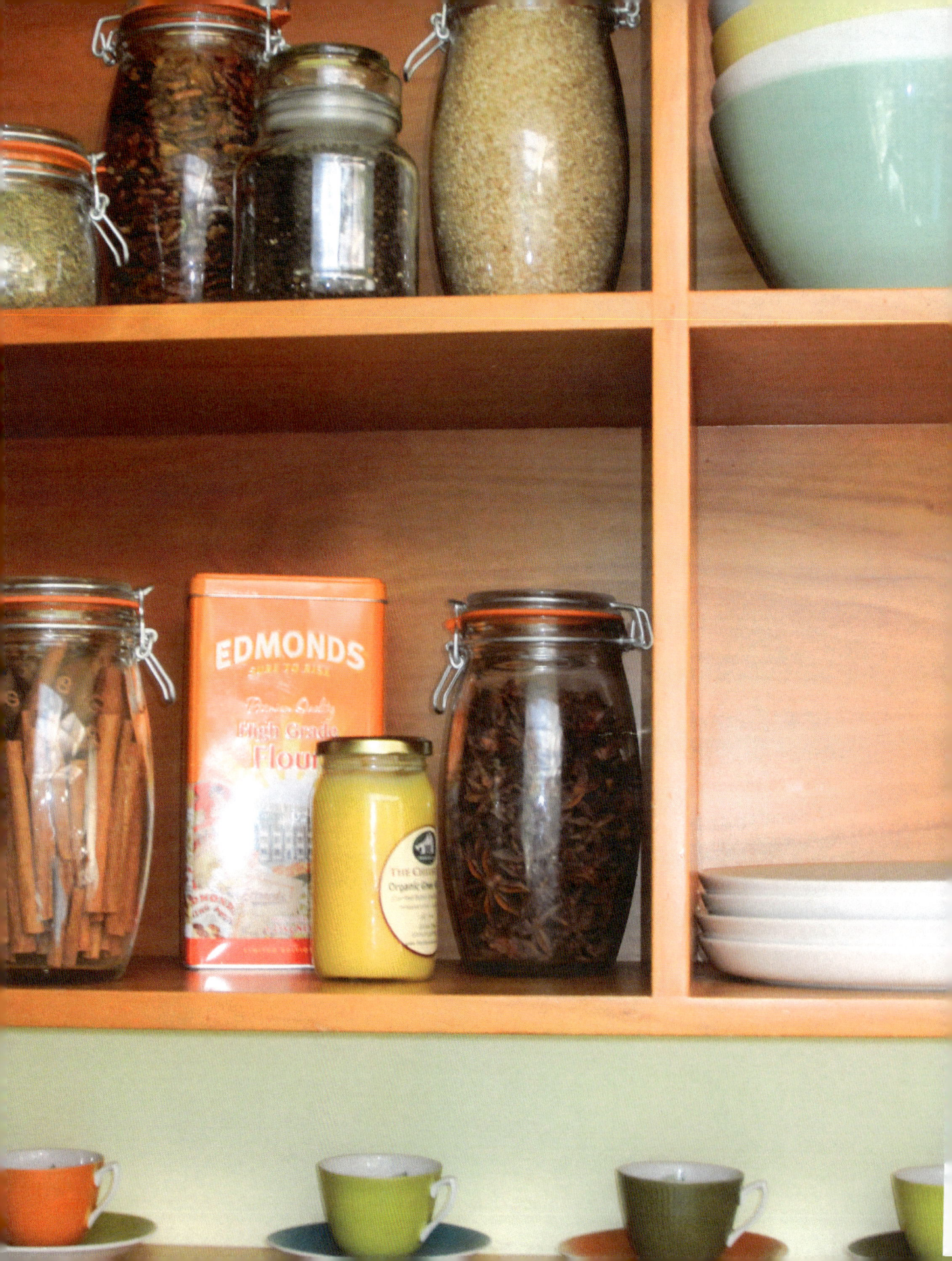

INTRODUCTION

Would you like to be healthier? Would you like to be able to better cope with the daily stresses of life? Would you like to have more happiness and balance in your life? The solution can be as simple as modifying your food choices to be in sync with your unique constitution.

Eat Well, Be Well is a wellness cookbook – a holistic approach to cooking that integrates the energetics of your body and your emotions to bring about a balanced state of health. I have taken the time-honored principles of ayurveda and interpreted them for use in a modern, western culture. My goal is to help you to understand and implement the theory so you can immediately experience the benefits.

Ancient dietary guidelines have been expanded into recipes designed for busy professionals, families and empty-nesters with discriminating taste and tight time schedules. The recommended ingredients are fresh, organic and whole foods. Many of the recipes can be prepared in a multitude of ways (dairy free, gluten-free, non-vegetarian and vegetarian) to accommodate various preferences. There are also suggestions for variations, so you can modify a "base" recipe to create fresh new dishes. Once you start, you will see the endless possibilities.

You don't have to be a great cook, but you have to be willing to cook. You don't have to have a lot of time, but you have to make a commitment of some time. By integrating a philosophy of wellness into your mindset, you can seamlessly transition to a healthy and happy body, mind and soul. Consider this book your personal wellness coach and let it guide you to a happier, healthier life.

To get started, it will be helpful to take a look at the big picture of the guiding philosophy of wellness called ayurveda.

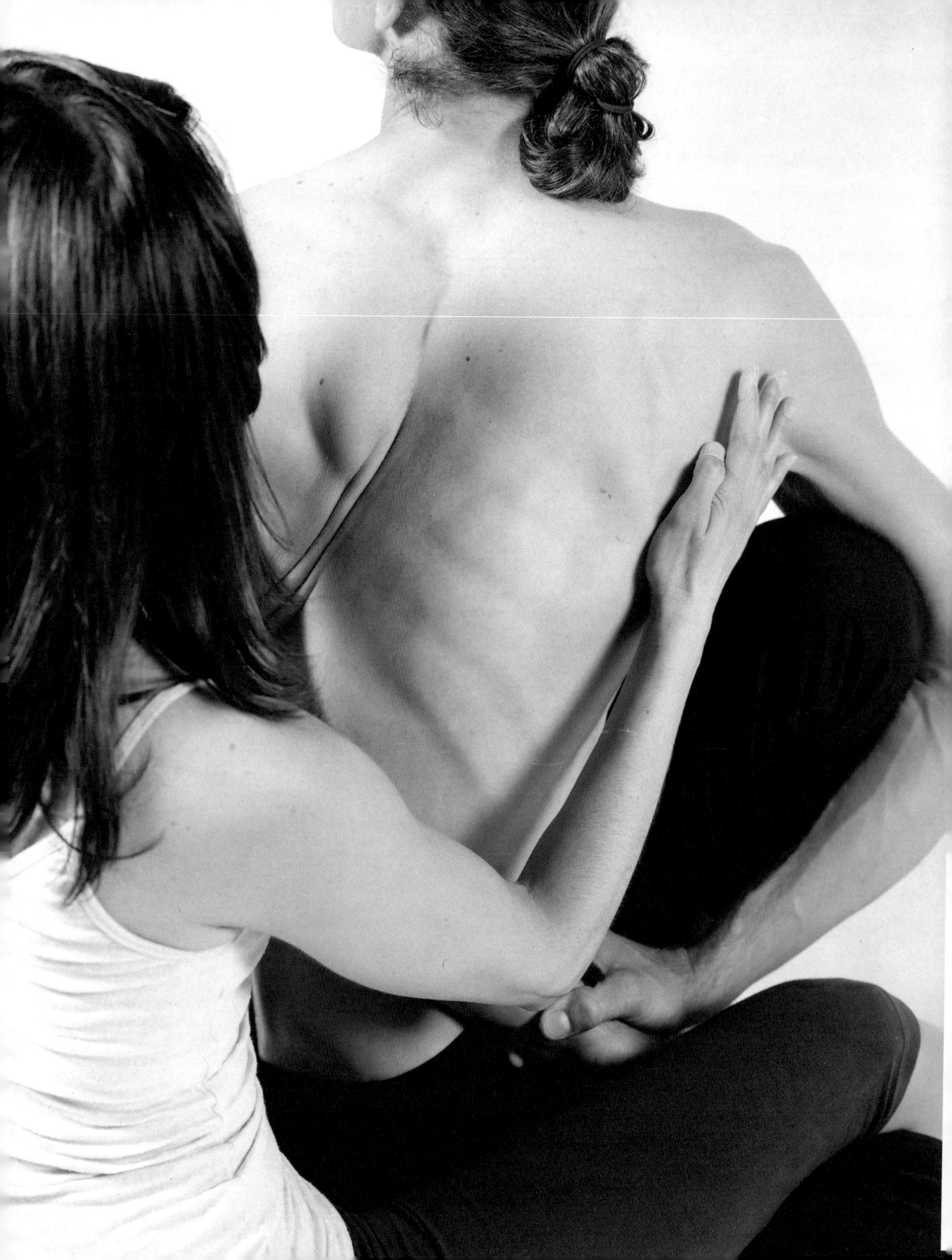

Chapter 1: About Ayurveda

Ayurveda is a Sanskrit term that can be translated as "science of life". It is an ancient system of natural healing that has been used successfully in India for thousands of years. Ayurveda is viewed as a universal truth - timeless in its application and effect.

Ayurveda is rooted in nature and came about during a time when man lived in sync with the natural rhythms of his body, the days and the seasons. There was great respect for the environment and preserving an ecological balance for the welfare of mankind.

During this time, the four aims of life were: virtue, wealth, gratification and spiritual fulfillment. A long, disease-free life was necessary to achieve these goals.[1] The ancients believed in an interconnectedness of the body, mind and soul – a whole body approach to well-being. To maintain a sustained state of well-being, ayurveda recommended diet and lifestyle advice designed to purify the physical and energetic channels of the body and promote longevity. These purifying measures were largely preventative in nature as they knew that an ounce of prevention was worth a pound of cure. Ayurveda was more than a healing science. It was a way of life.

Unlike most holistic healing systems, ayurveda is premised on the recognition that each person has a unique physical, spiritual and mental constitution. As such, diet and lifestyle recommendations were tailored to the individual – this was not a one size fits all approach.

Likewise, if a person fell ill, the physicians would custom design a remedy so as to achieve optimal results. The ayurvedic healer would look to find the root cause of an illness and advise the individual on how best to remedy the problem. The recommendations were tailored to the individual client and could consist of herbal formulations, cleansing therapies, rejuvenation therapies, dietary changes and lifestyle changes. The client was expected to actively participate in the healing process. Reversing the disease process took precious amounts of time, which is why there was so much emphasis on avoiding sickness in the first place.

The human body works the same today as it did in the past. Investing time and money to stay healthy makes sense, especially if you consider the alternative of getting sick. The costs of doctor visits, medicine, surgery and the time away from your life and work are enormous in comparison to the costs (time and money) to stay healthy with a preventative approach. Some insurance companies have done the math, and are now reimbursing for preventative programs for their policy holders. The time is ripe for a return to the time-honored practice of whole body wellness.

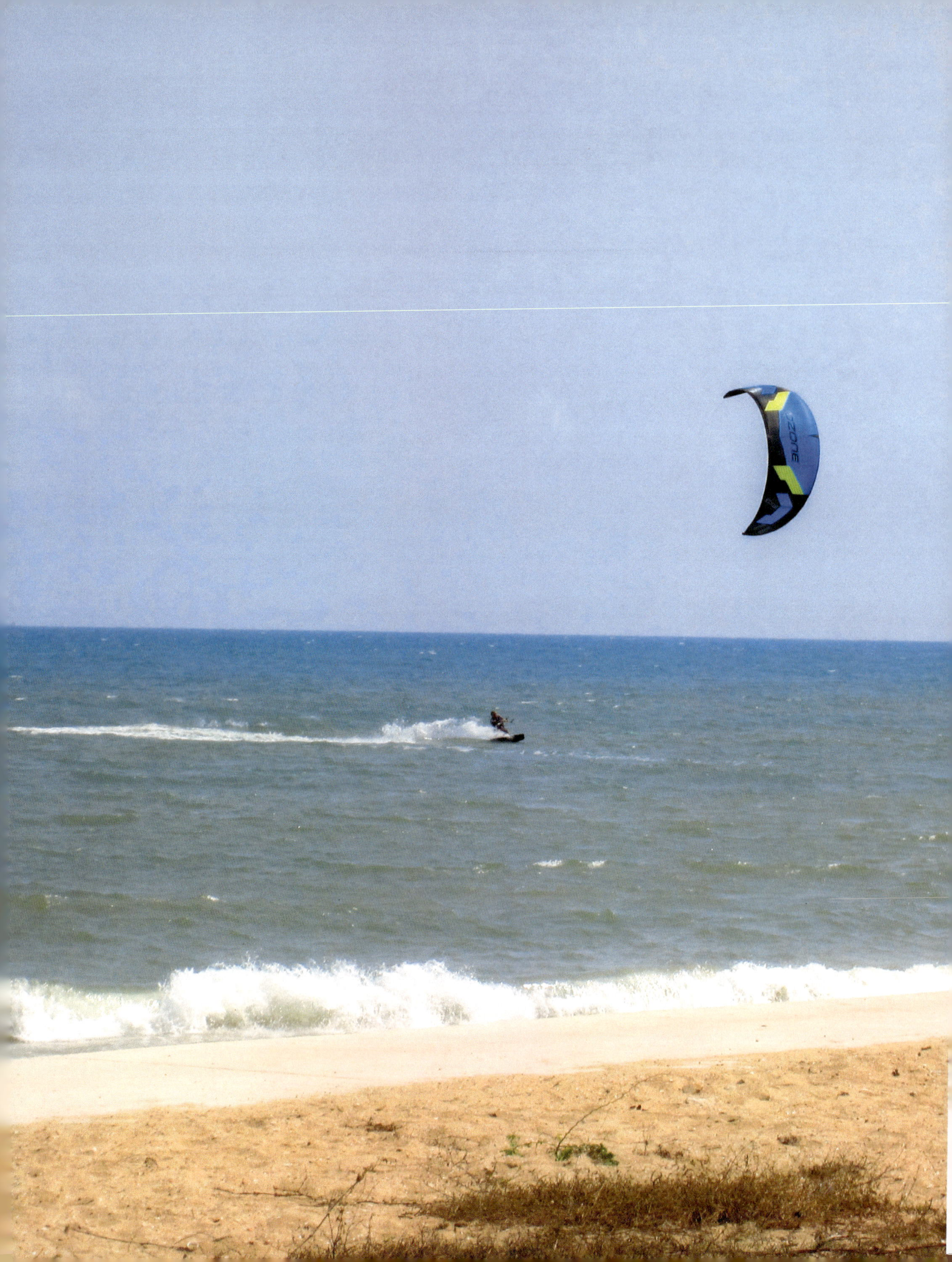

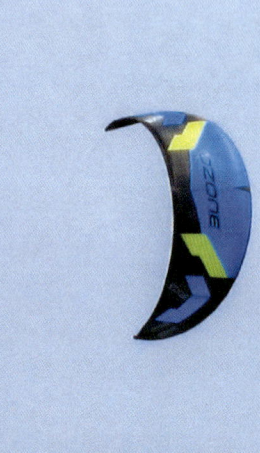

Chapter 2: The Five Elements:
The Key to Deciphering Your Unique Energetic Nature

The wisdom of ayurveda is based on the theory that everything in the universe is derived from various combinations of five elements, specifically: ether, air, fire, water and earth. Ayurveda does not define these elements in the literal sense that is used today. Rather, the elements can be thought of as metaphors which encompass physical qualities, energetic properties and biological functions. Ayurveda explains that the root cause of the manifestation of these elements is a form of energy; the elements come from energy then they further evolve into various types of energy (which are comprised of specific qualities). Listed below are the key qualities associate with each of the elements and examples of how they may manifest in an individual (physically and emotionally):

1. Ether (or space) has the qualities:

- clear
- light
- subtle
- expansive

In an individual, the etheric quality could be expressed as creativity, a vivid imagination or a tendency toward daydreaming. When the ether element is elevated, individuals easily pick up on subtleties; they can enter a room and without speaking to anyone can immediately sense the pulse of the situation (anger, fear, joy, sadness, etc.). When ether predominates, the default mood is joy and light-heartedness; the individual may also have a "willowy" frame. In the body, the ether element physically manifests as all the spaces (such as the spaces between organs). An excess of ether in the body can lead to insomnia, fear, memory loss, etc. Think about some people you may know who have these qualities. Maybe it was the person you met last night who was the "life of the party" or perhaps it was a child, joyfully playing in the park with his imaginary friend? Or it may be an office manager who proposes a grandiose vision of expanding into new territories (but leaves the task of completing the details for implementation and execution up to the staff)?

2. Air has the qualities:

- mobile
- dry
- light
- rough
- cold
- clear

Like a cool breeze, the air quality is expressed in an individual as movement (rapid speech, fast walking and quick thinking), coldness (in temperature) and perhaps an aloof attitude. The air element can create a tendency toward dryness (flaky skin, constipation) and roughness (cracked heels and elbows) or dry speech (choppy sentences). An "airy" person could also be very light in weight. In the body, this element manifests as all the movement but has an affinity to the nervous system.

An excess of air in the body can lead to stress, anxiety, bloating, gas, constipation, dehydration, etc. Examples of individuals with an abundance of the air quality include: the person in the office who is always cold, constantly requesting a higher temperature setting on the air conditioning; the non-stop talker who switches topics without taking a breath; the consummate multi-tasker; the person in the staff meeting that fidgets in their seat and taps (fingers, pens, toes) to release nervous energy.

3. FIRE HAS THE QUALITIES:
- hot
- sharp
- light
- dry
- subtle

Like a blazing fire, when this element dominates, the person is easy to spot; they often stand out (for great accomplishments or raging tempers). Hot headed, they may blow-off steam on a regular basis. Laser-sharp intelligence and focus, they can solve complex problems that require determined effort. They can make you cry with one of their sharp tongue lashings or have you laughing hysterically at their sarcastic wit. They can be intense, like the sun on a hot summer day without shade. While they can be light in weight, the light quality here is more precisely associated with the light of intelligence or luminosity. Their eyes and skin can be sensitive to the light of the sun. In the body, this element manifests as digestive enzymes, vision, the digestive fire and metabolism. An excess of fire in the body will lead to inflammation, ulcers, rashes, heartburn, indigestion, migraines, etc. Individuals with an abundance of the fire element may look red (red hair, flushed red face, sunburned skin). You are likely to find them giving a motivational speech to a captivated audience; or perhaps they're working on a spreadsheet of their 'life plan' plotting the necessary steps on how to achieve their lofty goals, then popping antacids because they have given themselves an ulcer trying to reach those goals; these are the overachievers! They are well-read and are so intelligent that their idea of conversation can often feel more like a debate as they expertly counter your every comment with a statistic or penetrating question seeking more details; they are expert at cross-examining a witness. Regardless of the season, these people are always warm; you can spot them wearing a t-shirt or sandals even after the weather has turned cool…and they will most likely be arguing with the "air" individual regarding the optimal thermostat setting in the office.

4. WATER HAS THE QUALITIES:
- cool
- liquid
- dull
- soft
- oily
- slimy

Like a glacier-fed lake, someone who has a lot of the water qualities will have a cool and calm personality. They will have a tendency to retain water and have a roundness to their shape. Their skin will generally be smooth, cool and clammy. Their default personality is to "go with the flow" and they have a loving disposition. In the body, this element manifests as all bodily fluids (plasma, urine, synovial fluids and mucus). An excess of the water element can lead to phlegm, mucus, swelling and profuse sweating. Examples of a person with a dominant water element include: the "chill" surfer dude …. or an enlightened monk who is not going to sweat the small stuff (or the big stuff) in life. This is the person you want in the exit row if your plane crashes as he will have the mindset to calmly assist passengers off the plane. When the water element is dominant, the person may always be wiping the sweat off his brow; or he is the first to break a sweat playing team sports. And at the end of a competition he is most likely to say with sincerity, "It's not whether you win or lose, but how you play". Can you think of someone in your office or family that has a relaxed, caring attitude and always remains calm even during a crisis?

5. EARTH HAS THE QUALITIES:

- gross
- hard
- dense
- static
- heavy
- dull

Like the earth that supports human life, the earth quality in the body serves as our foundation. In the body, it manifests primarily as our bones and cartilage. The earth element reminds me of a turtle – slow and steady with a hard protective shell. The earth quality manifests as someone who is very strong (physically and emotionally), stable (steady mind with unwavering thoughts) and heavy (large, heavy bones and weight; tendency for feeling heavy-hearted, gloomy or moody). They talk and walk slowly and are slow to take action, make decisions or grasp new concepts; they are immovable (in their faith, ideas and opinions) and can be stubborn. Because of the dense quality, subtleties are elusive; they are not going to perceive that you are upset with them; you will have to tell them quite directly. An excess of the earth element can lead to depression, obesity, lethargy, tumors, etc. Someone with an abundance of the earth quality would be a strong, supportive friend. If you have someone who you have been close friends with for many years (i.e., more than 10), that person likely has a lot of the earth element; if most of your friends are long-term close friends, then YOU are likely an earth person! Examples of individuals where the earth element predominates include: the college professor that puts the lecture hall to sleep with his slow, dull speech; the child that resists his mother's request to leave the playground by firmly rooting his bottom into the ground, defiantly folding his arms across his chest, pursing his lips shut and stubbornly refusing to move; the employee who "hunkers down" in his cubicle for the evening to meet a project deadline. [Note that the energy is slower and duller, as compared to a fire person, who would be blazing through the project with intensity.]

For our purposes, it is important that you understand the general metaphors as we will work with these throughout the book. As an exercise to help you become more familiar with the elements, you can practice observing how each element is expressed in your body and personality; then identify which elements dominate; you can expand the exercise to evaluating how the elements may be displaying in friends, family or co-workers.

Every individual is comprised of these five elements/energies in a unique combination. It is this unique combination of elements/energies that influences our constitutional make-up. While every individual is comprised of all five elements, typically one or two elements will express themselves more strongly. When the elements are in balance, energy is flowing smoothly, we are in harmony with our true nature and we are healthy and happy; our physical, mental and spiritual bodies are in sync. When the elements are out of balance, the energy stagnates and channels become blocked; we become prone to diseases of the body and mind which can bring physical and emotional distress.

Ayurveda teaches us that the five elements/energies are found in everything, including the food we eat. As with the elemental make-up of an individual, the elemental make-up of food also tends to have one or two dominating qualities (or energetics or elements). With an understanding of the energetics of the elemental make-up of food, you can balance the energetics in your body by eating "balancing" foods to target optimal health.

To understand the concept that food is comprised of the five elements (with the respective energetic properties), consider this simplistic example: chilies are related to the fire element. Recall that the qualities of the fire element include hot, sharp, light, dry and subtle. When you eat a chili, you can taste the hot sensation on your tongue. Then as the chili enters the digestive system, you may begin to feel warm; if the chili is really hot (or if you are ultra sensitive), you may feel a more intense, sharp, penetrating, burning sensation or perhaps even begin to perspire. Likewise, when you eat ice cream, you immediately feel the coolness or the water element spread to your core…you may even feel goose bumps on your skin.

We can also relate the elements to emotional states; our moods have an energetic make-up that can be linked back to the elements. As I mentioned, the feeling of joy is related to the ether element – the quality of lightness (think of light-heartedness). The opposite would be the feeling of sadness which is related to the earth element – a quality of heaviness (think of depressed or moody). The feeling of anger is related to the fire element (picture a cartoon character with a red face and smoke coming out of the ears to represent the inferno inside!). The opposite would be a feeling of calm which is related to the water element. Have you ever experienced a sense of calm when seated next to a water fountain or a lake?

If we understand the underlying elements that rule our constitution, we can shift to a diet and lifestyle that keeps those elements in balance. Let's look at an example of an individual with a fiery constitution. Fiery individuals would be predisposed to acid indigestion, heartburn or fits of anger. To cool down the flames, it is instinctive to add the water element (i.e., foods that are cooling on the physical level or practice meditation to cool at the emotional level) and avoid eating foods with the fire element (i.e., chilies!). If food affects our energetics, then perhaps this lends some credence to the expression "you are what you eat".

Now, imagine if that fiery-natured person was actually experiencing fiery symptoms (such as heartburn) and he proceeded to eat a bowl of chilies. He would be adding heat (chilies) to the fire (his fiery energetic). Can you see how that would be quite unbalancing?

This leads us to an intuitive formula for balancing the energetic qualities: opposites (energies or elements) balance; like (energies or elements) increase like (or create imbalance). Memorize this formula, because it is an important principle in ayurveda. If you feel like you need more practice understanding this concept, refer to Appendix A – Elements and the Twenty Qualities

On some level, most of us already know what will cause imbalance in our lives, but have we paid attention? If we have not learned to be present and honest with ourselves, how will we be able to make a committed effort to change? Ayurveda gives us a system that integrates body, mind and soul. It trains us to live and eat with awareness so we can make conscious choices for beneficial change; staying in balance becomes a conscious habit instead of a fleeting thought.

We are constantly being bombarded with elements that can create imbalance in our lives: a stressful, fast-paced job could be daily increasing the ether, air and fire qualities in your body; a diet rich in cheese, meat or beer accompanied by a lifestyle lacking vigorous exercise could be causing an excess of the earth element; living in a hot dessert and/or eating spicy, oily food could be creating an excess of the fire element. If we are not continually bringing in healthy opposites to balance our lives, our bodies eventually adapt to the new state of imbalance - our bodies acclimate to the new 'normal' imbalanced state. But this is not living in optimal health and eventually, the body will protest. First it will give you a warning sign (indigestion, insomnia, heartburn, diarrhea, constipation, bloating, lethargy, headaches, etc.). If you don't heed the warnings, the body will respond with an alarm bell (inflammation, ulcers, migraines, sciatic pain, low back pain, depression, etc.). And if you continue to ignore the distress signal, your body will put up a road block in the form of a serious disease requiring medical intervention to get you to contemplate the origin of your suffering (and hopefully discontinue its cause).

Ayurveda explains that disease can be avoided by simply understanding your "starting point" of balance and then modifying your diet and lifestyle to consistently be working toward maintaining that unique state of balance. The ayurvedic "starting point" is determined by using a logical classification system based on the elements. That classification system involves combining the elements into three main categories which are referred to as "three doshas".

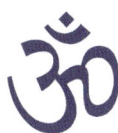

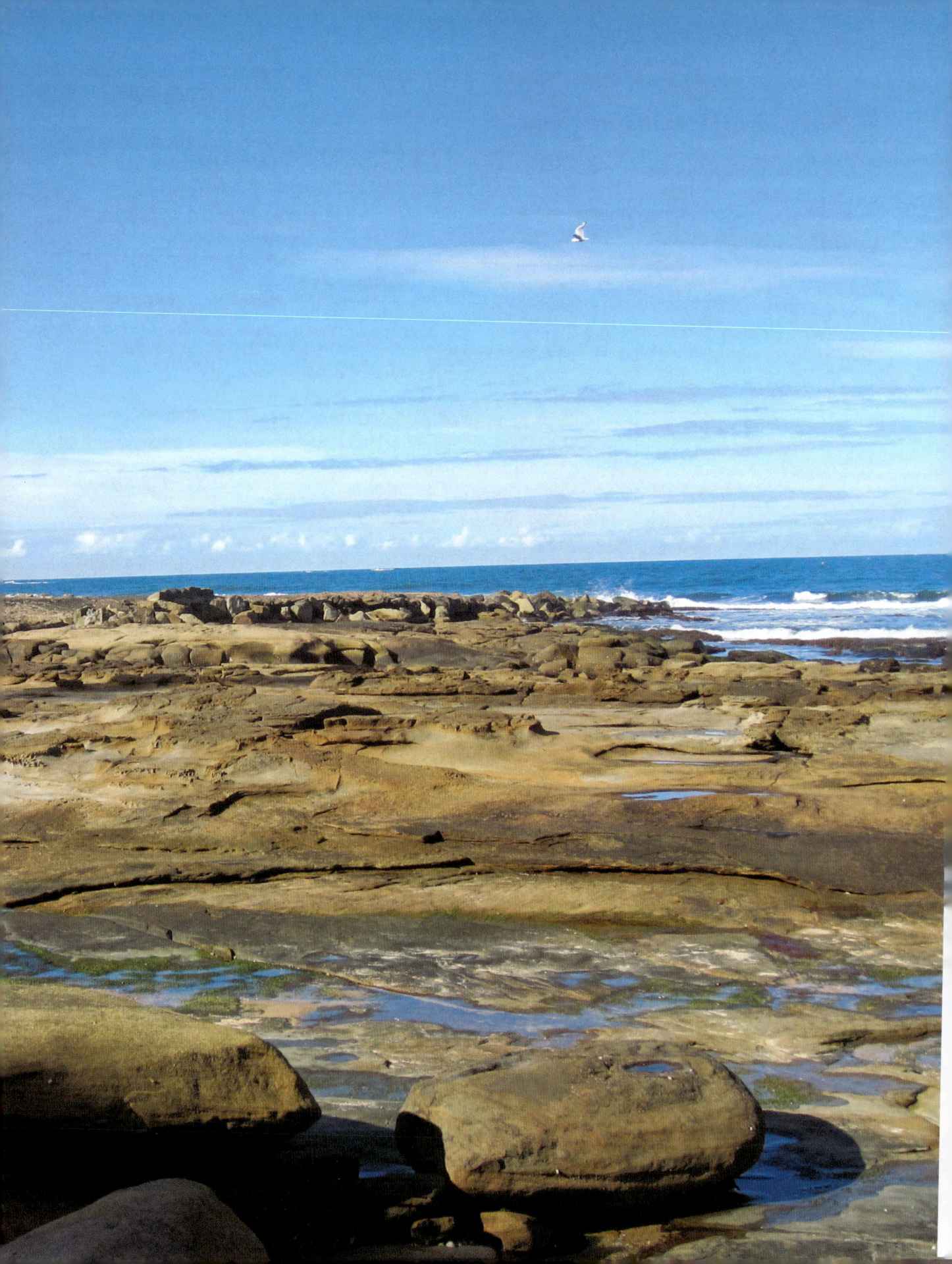

Chapter 3: The Three Doshas

The Sanskrit term "dosha" is used to broadly classify individuals into three unique combinations of body and mind elements or energetics: vata, pitta and kapha. These Sanskrit words have no direct translation in English, but are generally understood as follows: vata primarily represents the qualities of the ether and air elements; pitta primarily represents the qualities of the fire and water elements; kapha primarily represent the qualities of the water and earth elements. As you read through the following paragraphs elaborating how these qualities manifest in our bodies, relate them back to the metaphorical qualities of the elements that we described in Chapter 2.

Vata – Air

Vata is primarily influenced by elements of air and ether. For simplicity, it is referred to as the "air" dosha and it governs all movement in the body (i.e., respiration, circulation, nervous system, muscular skeletal system, digestion, absorption, assimilation and elimination). Nothing happens without vata. Vata is typically involved with degenerative functions in the body (such as in sickness or old age). The wind embodies the qualities of vata and we can understand this by visualizing a clear, crisp, autumn day in New England with leaves blowing off the trees; think of the drying effect that the cold air has on your exposed fingers (i.e., rough, chapped skin).

The colors associated with vata are blue, indigo and brown. The qualities of vata are: cold, light, dry, rough, mobile, subtle, clear and astringent. This translates into physical and physiological characteristics such as: a small frame, irregular features, a thin angular face, small eyes, wiry hair, cold dry skin, brittle nails, creativity, imagination, quick clipped speech, joyfulness, an erratic metabolism, an erratic appetite, a light sleeper, quick movements, an ability to perceive subtleties (clairvoyance or ESP), an eclectic fashion sense, a tendency to be a loner, non-committal in relationships, an ability to adapt and a flexibility to change. Vata out of balance can manifest as constipation, dehydration, excessive daydreaming, forgetfulness (i.e., "space cadet syndrome"), fear, loneliness, insecurity, nervousness, anxiety, flaking skin, rough cracking skin (especially at the heels or elbows), popping joints, difficulty with speech (i.e., stuttering), emaciation, black circles under the eyes, gas, bloating, vague abdominal pain and distention, neuromuscular disorders (tremors, spasms, numbness, tingling), inability to concentrate/racing thoughts, nightmares, sciatic pain, heart palpitations, breathlessness, hiccups, wheezing, asthma, fatigue and insomnia.

Pitta - Fire

Pitta is primarily influenced by the elements of fire and water. For simplicity, it is referred to as the "fire" dosha and it governs transformation. Cooking over a camp fire is a useful analogy when trying to understand the fire of pitta. Pitta cooks or digests our food; pitta cooks or helps us digest and understand our thoughts; pitta helps us to transform thoughts into feelings and feelings into emotions; ultimately, the thought is transformed into higher intelligence. Pitta regulates our body temperature; it is responsible for metabolic activities. To understand the qualities of pitta in the body, think of the interplay of fire with water. Water can put out a fire if water is in excess; but if the fire gets too hot, its heat can scorch everything in its path, drying all the water. When the fire is balanced, the water element can express its qualities and the individual will appear cool, calm and collected.The colors associated with pitta are red and yellow. The qualities of pitta are: oily, penetrating, hot, light, fleshy smell, spreading, liquid, pungent and sour. This translates into physical and physiological characteristics including: a medium frame, a heart-shaped face with a straight sharp nose and chin, almond-shaped eyes that are sensitive to bright light, shiny pink fingernails, oily and lustrous skin, shiny thin hair that is often red or with red highlights, a tendency for premature balding or gray hair, sensitive skin, a yellow undertone of the skin, a voracious appetite, skin that feels hot to the touch, an avid reader (especially accustomed to reading at night before sleep), highly intelligent, brave, passionate, a sharp (fashion-conscious) dresser, proud of possessions and family, predisposed to intellectual work (i.e., not manual labor in the hot sun), fleshy smelling perspiration, a desire to be in control and to be famous. Like vata, pitta has the ability to grasp subtleties in a situation; but pitta's understanding is based on laser sharp intelligence and logical analysis that combine to formulate an instantaneous conclusion. Whereas vata's understanding is based on intuition, subtle feelings and emotions. Out of balance, pitta can manifest as being angry, hateful, overly critical, judgmental, egotistical, mistrusting and fiercely competitive. Excessive pitta can lead to heart-burn, indigestion, inflammation, ulcers, rashes, jaundice, mononucleosis, depression, suicidal thoughts, dizziness, nausea, fever, diarrhea, migraines, sour taste in the mouth and bleeding disorders (i.e., bleeding rectum or gums and blood-shot eyes).

KAPHA - WATER

Kapha is primarily influenced by the elements of water and earth. It is generally referred to as the "water" dosha and its role is to support and nourish. Kapha provides oleation and lubrication to prevent wear and tear on the joints and their ligaments; it brings people together for compromise and understanding to create peace. Physically it manifests as serotonin and tryptophan that bring peaceful sleep. Kapha is the force that builds in the body and is especially active during the childhood and pre-adolescent years when the body is growing. The qualities of love and nurturing are analogous to the watery nature of kapha and can manifest as a desire to be liked by everyone, a need for connecting with people and a temperament that is compassionate and friendly. To comprehend the earth qualities of kapha you can think of the characteristics of a mighty oak tree. Oak trees are hardy, strong, unwavering and long-lived; they tend to retain water and can produce a lot of fruit (acorns). Likewise, kaphas are considered the heartiest of the three constitutions and likely to have long, healthy lives with the capacity to bear many offspring. In addition, they have a tendency to retain water and they can be unwavering in their views.

The color associated with kapha is white. The qualities of kapha are: heavy, slow, cool, oily, slimy, thick, soft, stable, liquid, sweet and salty. These translate into physical and physiological traits that include: a large frame, big strong bones, a soft curvaceous figure, a tendency to carry several extra pounds, a round face, large round eyes with thick eyelashes, a large spreading nose, cool clammy pale white skin, thick wavy hair, hairy bodies (especially backs and chests), large developed chests/breasts, slow talking, slow moving, slow to make decisions and a great memory (like an elephant, they never forget!). They are relaxed and content with the way things are and love to sleep. They tend to sweat…a lot. They often have a living/work space that is cluttered and untidy (think "pack rat"), a preference for loose-fitting casual attire, sleep soundly (can sleep anywhere through any amount of noise), thrive being in relationships, love working with a coach or partner to accomplish goals and have a sweet, loving temperament. Kapha babies often have very chubby cheeks, legs and arms. Out of balance kapha can manifest as stubbornness, selfishness, moodiness, depression, greed, miserliness, attachment (to possessions and relationships), and obesity (from emotional eating to replace lack of feeling loved). They are prone to congestion, phlegm, mucus, swelling/water retention, excess salivation, lethargy, diabetes, lipomas (benign tumors composed of fatty tissue), cysts, tumors and high cholesterol. They are also prone to constipation (like vata), but with kapha, the constipation is due to an excess of the "slow" quality (earth element) whereas with vata, the constipation is typically due to an excess of the "dry" quality (air element).

You may have read those three descriptions and identified with aspects of each dosha. Of course! That is because you are a combination of all the elements and all the underlying qualities. The key is to determine which doshas (combinations of elements) express most strongly in your constitution: it may be one; typically two; or perhaps you are a rare person in which all three are equally predominant.

My family provides a useful example of the dosha qualities in action. My older sister (kapha predominant) as a child was content to play in her crib; she was always happy and rarely cried; loving food and sleep, she ate and napped on schedule. As she grew up, she had to be mindful of her diet and benefited greatly from vigorous exercise. My mother (pitta predominant) would provide a "spark" to get kapha to move and make a decision, lest kapha mull things over too long and miss a deadline. Contrast me, the vata: needing more space and unable to sit still, I figured out how to escape from the confines of the crib – then instigated my older, content kapha sister to move beyond the borders of the crib. Vata had trouble digesting many foods and was a colicky baby with a tendency to become dehydrated; vata never wanted to nap.

My mother's head was spinning from the contrast of her first kapha child! In addition, I was a picky eater – hated broccoli, beans and salads (which perhaps was an intuitive reaction to my constitution's inability to handle these rough, cooling foods). In contrast, my kapha sister liked everything and would often help me with leftovers on my dinner plate so as not to waste food. I was a light sleeper and would have nightmares from watching anything with a scary plot line; gaining weight was a struggle for me. I assimilated the energy of my surroundings and at times felt unbalanced by the hubbub of my boisterous Italian family. On family road trips to grandma's house, vata was the instigator of many quarrels as I squirmed and poked my siblings in the crowded back seat of the car. "Am I going to have to separate you?" my parents would threaten from the front seat to try to settle down the commotion. As a young adult, I was a multi-tasker and would make quick decisions. My speech was very fast and clipped, often times finishing peoples sentences before they asked the question because I perceived what they were going to ask. I could quickly analyze a situation and make a decision, but I was reluctant to commit and would often change my mind. Discovering yoga helped to finally ground and balance my life.

My pitta mother was a fiery constitution and loved to keep things under control. When she set her intention, things would get done. She too would finish sentences of others, but in her case it was because she couldn't wait for them to get their information out. She had a stomach of steel and could easily digest beans and cabbage. She loved pungent and sour foods (pickles, tomatoes, garlic, scallions, etc.) and would eat them in spite of the acid reflux they often caused. These foods were increasing the "oily" quality of her pitta constitution and perhaps led to her gall stones. She was an avid reader and always had a book (or two, or three) going. Intelligent, she liked to analyze things and come to her own conclusion.

Take these family stories and relate them to your own families: who was the instigator and creative loner? Who was always content, loved to eat and made friends easily? And who was highly intelligent and liked to be in control?

I have given you a fine overview to help you understand the concept of dosha as it relates to your starting point of balance. In Sanskrit, the term "prakruti" is used to mean your "starting point" of balance; it is defined as your unique physical and psychological composition at birth. It is best to consult an ayurvedic practitioner to determine your individual prakruti. To make an approximation of it on your own, refer to Appendix B- Dosha Evaluation at the back of this book.

If we can understand the energetics of our prakruti, then we can follow dietary and lifestyle habits designed to keep those energetics (our doshas) in balance. More importantly, when we understand where our sense of balance should be (i.e., joy, proper weight, mental clarity, energy, sound sleep, etc.), then we immediately recognize when we are veering off track (sadness, weight gain, confusion, anger, jealously, greed, fear, indigestion, lethargy, insomnia, etc.) and can take action to get back to optimal health.

Some people have come to ayurveda looking to lose weight. That may happen. But it is more important that you gain an accurate concept of your optimal weight for your body type. It is futile to compare your body to someone else; you are a unique individual. Vata's are generally going to have smaller bones and be light in weight and angular in shape. Vata should not envy the beautifully curvaceous kapha bodies. Pitta will generally have moderate size bones and be average weight with a muscular shape; pitta should not try to emulate the willowy body structure of vata by constant dieting – that would lead to an emaciated look for pitta and would not be healthy. Kapha generally has the largest bones and, with a tendency to retain water, will generally weigh the most. Kaphas should love their curves and be grateful that there is 'more to love', but should not let this be an excuse to be sedentary or eat in excess. Ayurveda was intended to promote longevity and health. The ancient's description of health is: balanced energy, balanced tissues, and balanced digestion combined with proper elimination (of urine, feces and sweet) and an integrated concept of body, mind and soul. This whole body wellness approach is in stark contrast to the western concept of health - absence of disease. The western definition seems crude in comparison to the comprehensive, individualized approach of ayurveda. Understanding your energetic constitution will give you the tools to maintain overall wellness. Wellness that will radiate from your core.

DOSHA TIMES

Ayurveda also applies the concept of dosha to time by correlating the qualities of the "doshas" (vata, pitta, kapha) to the time of day, the season and the time of life. If you can imagine living during a time before the invention of electricity, you can perhaps understand how they were able to perceive a seamless relationship between man and nature via the underlying elements (and associated qualities).

Table 1[2]	Vata (Ether & Air)	Pitta (Fire & Water)	Kapha (Water & Earth)
Time of Day	2-6 am/pm	10-2 am/pm	6-10 am/pm
Season	fall	summer	winter & spring
Time of Life	old age	adult	child (birth to ~ age 16)

The vata (ether/air) time of day is dawn and dusk (2-6:00 am and pm). The vata season is fall; the time of life is old age. As we get old, we all will tend to "dry out" and have more vata tendencies like dry skin, popping joints, scattered thoughts, memory loss, etc. These are associated with the degenerative/vata forces in our body. During the vata time of life, one can benefit from vata-balancing foods (moist, oily, warm and grounding).

The pitta (fire/water) time of day is midday and midnight (10-2:00 am and pm). The pitta season is summer; the pitta time of life is young adult (this is the time period during which we have the "fire" to progress at school, advance in our careers and raise children). For women, menopause is the transition from pitta stage of life into the vata stage of life; women prone to vata imbalance in the years before menopause (i.e., dryness, memory loss, etc.) tend to experience an amplification of these imbalances during menopause. Likewise, women prone to pitta imbalance (i.e., heat, hot flashes, excessive irritability, etc.), tend toward an increase in these imbalances. During the pitta time of life, one can benefit from pitta-pacifying foods and drinks that are cooling in nature. It is really important to make time for adequate rest so you don't burn out (the flame of pitta).

The kapha (water/earth) time is midmorning and early evening (6-10:00 am and pm). Kapha season is spring and winter. Kapha age is birth to approximately age 16 (this is when we are in the developmental growth stage of our lives– remember, kapha is building). When we are young and growing, we need nutritious, energizing foods to help create a healthy body.

These "doshic times" are the origin from which the ancients derived diet and lifestyle recommendations. For instance, meditating before sunrise and at dusk was considered auspicious due to the vata/etheric qualities predominant at that hour; the subtle energies could easily be perceived. Midday, when the sun was strongest, correlated to peak pitta/digestive capacity and was thus recommended as the optimal time for the main meal of the day; manual labor or vigorous exercise was considered unbalancing during this fiery time of day. It was recommended being in bed before 10pm – during kapha, slow, sleepy time. At 10pm, pitta energy kicks in and provides a burst of energy that could keep you awake until 2am!

The correspondence of dosha classification to the seasons epitomizes how the ancients recognized a symbiotic way of living in harmony with nature. For instance, during fall, root vegetable crops are maturing and the cool, windy weather causes people to experience a little more vata than normal; eating the seasonal, grounding vegetables can help balance the effects of vata from the external environment on your body. Daily oil massage will greatly help to ground and balance out vata conditions. Likewise, in the heat of summer, emphasizing the cooling seasonal crops (fruits, bitter green leafy vegetables, etc.) will help to balance out the heat of the scorching sun/pitta flames. In the dead of winter, the kapha earth element is dominant and we need to eat warming foods and exercise regularly; avoiding stagnation will limit mucus build-up that can lead to illness. In the cool, damp season of spring, the water element of kapha tends to dominate leaving us vulnerable to spring colds and runny noses. During this season, we need to stay warm and dry, emphasizing foods that are balancing to kapha dosha such as mushrooms and barley. Avoiding mucus forming dairy products is also beneficial during the wet spring.

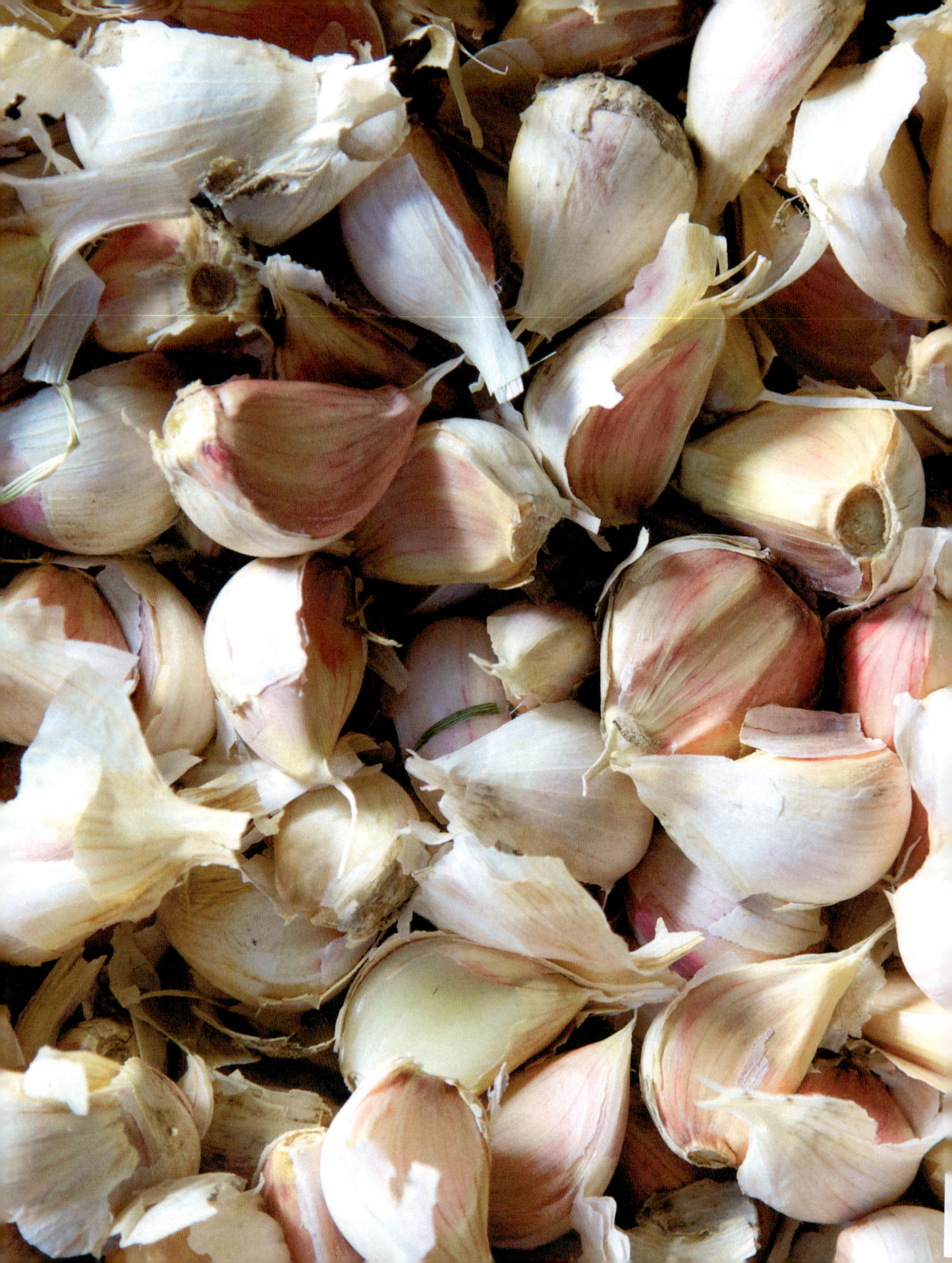

Chapter 4: The Six Tastes[3]

Now that we have an understanding of the qualities of the elements and the qualities of the doshas, we can look at the qualities of foods in more detail. As I mentioned earlier, food is comprised of the five elements. Ayurveda divides those elements among six "tastes" – sweet, sour, salty, pungent, bitter and astringent. All the elements (and all their qualities) are contained within each taste. However, there are typically two elements that dominate each taste. We can derive the energetic of the taste, based on the qualities of those dominating elements.[4]

Since the elements are merely forms of energy, the food we consume will correspondingly impact the energetics in our bodies, our state of balance. In general, vata (which has a light, dry, cool nature) will benefit from heavy, moist, oily, warming foods; pitta (which has a fiery nature) will do best with cooling foods; and kapha (which has a slow, dull, cool nature) will do best with heating, sharp (spicy) foods.

We can intuit the physical and emotional properties of food based on an understanding of the underlying elements. With practice, you will be able to understand the energetic affect of food by simply tasting and observing. For now, we can rely on ayurveda's perception of these underlying characteristics as outlined below[5]:

Sweet - earth & water
Sweet is comprised of the elements earth and water. The dominant energies of the sweet taste are cool, moist and heavy. The general effects on the dosha are to balance (or reduce) vata and pitta but increase kapha. The sweet taste is building in nature and is energizing. It is related to the emotions of love, joy and bliss. In excess, it can create a sluggish thyroid, thick blood (which leads to high cholesterol), diabetes, greed and attachment. Foods that have a sweet taste include: white basmati rice, barley, oats, amaranth (also astringent), asparagus, avocado, beets (cooked), cucumber, rabbit, milk, maple syrup, sugar, almonds (peeled and soaked), coconut, tarragon, coriander leaf (also astringent), fennel (also astringent) and vanilla (also astringent). Foods that have a sweet taste but a heating energetic include: molasses, honey, jaggary, corn, millet, carrot (cooked), buffalo, salmon, lamb/mutton and pork.

Sour - earth & fire
Sour is comprised of the elements earth and fire. The dominant energetic effect of the sour taste is hot, sharp and not too heavy. The general effects on the dosha are to balance (or reduce) vata but increase pitta and kapha. The sour taste can overpower all the other tastes and should be used in moderation. It creates moistness, reduces gas and stimulates the appetite and purgation. It makes the mind alert; something really sour will prompt the reflex action to close your eyes. In excess it can create: dampness and cold in the lungs; skin eruptions of acne and rashes; sensitive teeth; gastritis and diarrhea. Emotionally, an excess of the sour taste can influence your mind to be judgmental and overly critical. When these harsh thoughts are brought into a relationship, they can destroy the relationship leaving a "sour taste in your mouth". Foods that have a sour taste include: lemons, tomatoes (also sweet), tamarind, umeboshi plums (and salty), grapefruit, vinegar, fermented food, cheese, butter, sour cream, and yogurt (older than 3 days from manufacture date).

SALTY - FIRE & WATER

Salty is comprised of the elements fire and water. The energetic qualities of the salty taste are heating, heavy and oily. The general effects on the dosha are to balance (or reduce) vata but increase pitta and kapha. The salty taste is an appetizer, a digestive, anti-flatulent, anti-spasmodic and gives energy. Emotionally, the taste gives courage and enthusiasm. In excess, the salty taste will create water and sodium retention causing swelling. Salt is an addictive taste and attachment, greed and possessiveness are the emotions that are exacerbated when the salty taste is in excess. Excess salt can result in premature graying of the hair, hair loss and wrinkling. Excess salt can also induce vomiting. Common salty tastes include: sea salt, rock salt, seaweed and vegemite® (yeast extract).

PUNGENT - FIRE & AIR

The pungent taste is comprised of the elements fire and air. The dominant energetic effect of the pungent taste is heating but it is also sharp, light, drying and rough. The general effects on the dosha are to increase vata and pitta but to balance (or reduce) kapha. The pungent taste is anti-spasmodic and stimulates circulation, digestion, absorption and assimilation of nutrients. It thins the blood and removes clots, fat and worms. The pungent taste can cleanse sinuses by stimulating nasal secretions and dissolving kapha. The sharp, penetrating qualities generate the emotional states of enthusiasm and dynamism. In excess, it can cause dryness, kill sperm and ovum, cause irritation and ulceration. Emotionally, it can create anger, competitiveness and aggressiveness. Common foods with the pungent taste include: raw onion, raw beets, garlic, ginger, chilies, anise, black pepper, cayenne, mustard seeds, fenugreek (also bitter), star anise, cumin (also bitter), ajwain, basil (also sweet), cinnamon (also sweet) and paprika.

BITTER - ETHER & AIR

The bitter taste is comprised of the elements ether and air. The dominant energetic effect of the bitter taste is cooling but it is also light and drying. The general effects on the dosha are to increase vata but to balance (or reduce) pitta and kapha. The bitter taste is anti-inflammatory, anti-pyretic (reduces fever) and is a laxative. It is balancing to blood sugar levels and benefits the liver, pancreas and spleen. It is beneficial for introspection/withdrawing from the world. In excess, it can cause nausea and osteoporosis. It can deplete plasma, blood, muscle, bone marrow, fat, semen and sex drive. Neem juice is very bitter and it is the drink of choice for celibate sadhus as it eradicates their sex drive and helps them turn inward for meditation and away from the external world. Emotionally, an excess of bitter can create aversion, cynicism (the expression of a "bitter person" is an appropriate analogy), detachment, loneliness and depression. Foods that contain the bitter taste include most leafy greens, kale, aloe vera, collard greens, broccoli, chicory, arugula, radicchio, rhubarb, endive, dandelion greens, coffee, bitter gourd, neem juice (neem is also pungent and astringent) and turmeric.

Astringent - earth & air

The astringent taste is comprised of the earth and air elements. The energetic effect of the astringent taste is cooling but also drying. The general effects on the dosha are to increase vata but balance (or decrease) pitta and kapha. The astringent taste is anti-inflammatory, improves absorption, stops bleeding, binds stool, heals ulcers and scrapes excess fat. In excess it can create spasms, constipation, emaciation and a dry choking sensation in the mouth (so don't eat/drink an astringent taste before giving a speech!). Emotionally it is related to sensitivity or in excess, hypersensitivity. Foods that have the astringent taste include: Brussels sprouts, cabbage, cauliflower, celery, cranberries, green beans, lettuce, white potato, raw spinach, sprouts, zucchini, wheat pasta, rye (heating), quinoa (also sweet), amaranth (also sweet), rice cakes, legumes (adzuki, black-eyed peas, kidney beans, pinto beans and white beans), savi seeds, tofu (also sweet), venison, popcorn, cooked apple pulp, basil (also sweet), oregano (also sweet), parsley (also pungent), poppy seed (also sweet), rosemary (also sweet) and pomegranate. Spices that have an astringent taste but a heating energetic include: oregano, poppy seed, parsley, rosemary.

Exceptions to the Rules

You may have noticed that some of the foods have multiple, conflicting energetics (i.e., corn has a sweet taste but a heating energetic whereas the general rule is that sweet tastes have a cooling energetic). So how do you know whether eating corn will be balancing or unbalancing to the elements in your body? The dominant energetic of the food will be the one to express in your body. Eventually, you will be able to identify that dominant energetic by carefully observing how you feel (during and after eating).

For now, I have taken the guesswork out of knowing which energetic is dominant by compiling a book of tri-doshic (unless otherwise indicated) recipes. If recipes are not tri-doshic, then recommendations for condiments and spices are given to balance for specific doshas. If you want to move beyond the recipes in this book, you can reference Appendix C, D, E – Dosha Diet Aid for Vata, Pitta and Kapha respectively. These pages outline which foods and spices are balancing to specific doshas. They were derived from the "Qualities of Food Substances" table in Dr. Lad's book Ayurveda Cooking for Self-Healing.

But please consider these lists to be a general reference and not a mandate. The energetic impact of foods will vary depending on your unique energetic make-up, your present state of balance, the environment in which you are living, the environment in which the food was grown, etc. So use the "lists" as your compass to point you in the right direction. Over time, as you work with this system, your awareness will increase and your ability to discriminate what tastes and foods are most beneficial for your constitution will become clear.

Your goal should be to eat with awareness and feel how the food is affecting you personally (physically and emotionally) – that's what the ancient's did.

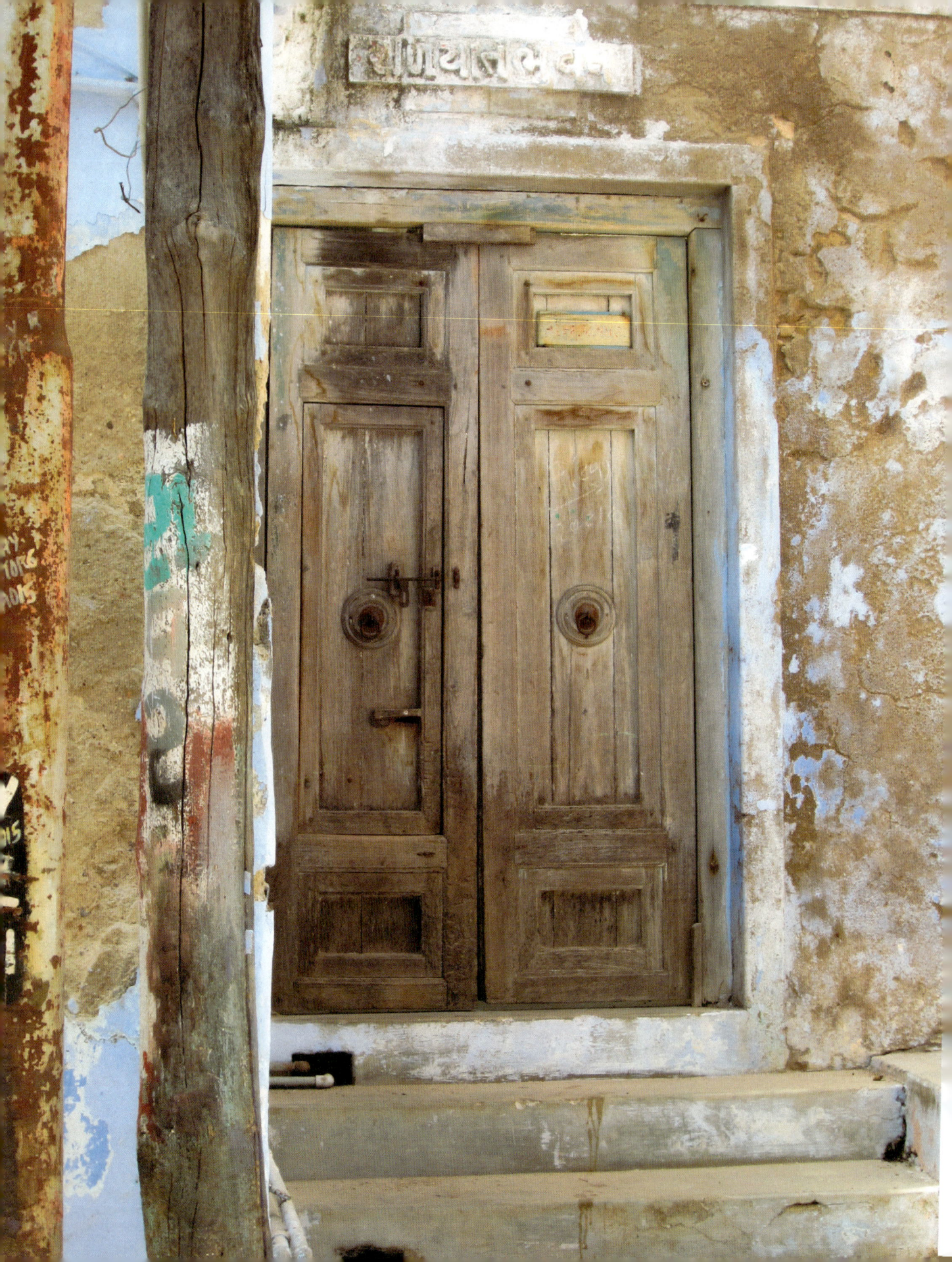

Chapter 5: Food Combining
Quality and Quantity

To further refine our dosha balancing skills, we should develop a general understanding of the interplay of energetics with the unique composition and capacity of our digestive systems – quality and quantity.

Using their understanding of the tastes and energetics of foods, the ancients established fundamental principles for efficient food combinations and optimal quantities. The intention was to optimize digestion, absorption, assimilation and elimination so as to promote health and longevity. The immediate effect of these lighter combinations is an alert mind and an energetic body.

Table 2 - Food Combining summarizes and expands on the basic principles. In general, for optimal digestion, absorption, assimilation and elimination:

- **Meats**, which are heavy, are best combined with light foods such as vegetables or salads. Most of the common serving methods in western society (i.e., steak and potato, chicken and bean burrito, spaghetti and meatballs, Philly cheesesteak sub, any meat sandwich, fried fish, etc.) are not considered optimal as they are excessively heavy and taxing on the system.
- **Fruits**, which are light and liquid, are best eaten alone. They combine well with other fruits. Raw fruits tend to be watery in nature and they move quickly through the digestive system; this movement gets delayed when the digestive system is full of other foods, resulting in fermentation, gas and bloating. An exception to the general rule is when the fruits are cooked or dried; this changes their basic characteristic and lends them suitable to be combined with other foods.
- **Cheese**, which is cold and heavy, is best eaten alone as it does not combine well with many modern serving methods (i.e., cheese and crackers; cheese and apples; macaroni and cheese, cheese with sandwiches, cheese pizza, etc. are all combinations that would be considered too "heavy").
- **Honey**, equal quantities by **weight** of ghee and honey are not good combinations, but mixing in a ratio of 2:1 (two parts ghee to 1 part honey) is fine[6]. Ayurveda believes that when honey is cooked, it will become toxic to the system.

The food combining principles essentially address the issue of the optimal capacity of our digestive systems in terms of quality and quantity of food inputs. Our digestive system was not designed to handle non-stop large, heavy, complex meals (as are commonly eaten in western society). The western eating habits place continual stress on the digestive system with inadequate "down-time" for the system to recuperate. Overworking the system in this manner can cause blockage downstream resulting in undigested food that putrefies and ferments, leading to gas, bloating and potential accumulation of "ama".

"Ama" is a Sanskrit word that describes a toxic end-product formed from improper metabolism of food and unprocessed emotions (refer to Appendix F - Ama for more details). It is caused by eating foods before the last meal has been digested. Ama clogs the channels of circulation in the body. It can prevent nutrients from flowing to the cells, organs and brain. Ama may also clog the channels that carry waste from the cells and tissues, resulting in a toxic build-up that may irreversibly harm cells over long periods of time.

Table 2 – Food Combining[7]

Uncooked Food	Combine well with:	Avoid eating with:
Fruits, fresh	other fruits except melons; eat as a snack or as breakfast	generally eat fruit alone; wait 1 hour before/after a meal to eat fruit.
Melons	other melons; eat as a snack	anything; wait 1 hour before/after meal to eat
Fruits, dried	salads, rice, grains, yogurt (in moderation due to high sugar)	meat, fish, eggs, milk, beans
Tomatoes	vegetables, rice (try corn chips & salsa)	fruit, cucumbers, dairy *
Lemons	vegetables, grains	fruit, cucumbers, milk, yogurt, tomatoes
Cheese	vegetables (except nightshades**), leafy green salads; eat as a snack	fruit, meat, wheat/bread, (i.e., cheese & crackers, pizza, pasta, grilled cheese, cheese tortilla, sandwiches, cheeseburger), nightshades**
Milk, raw	dates; best to boil and drink alone or with warming spices (cinnamon, cardamom, turmeric, cloves, nutmeg, etc.); boiling reduces mucus formation	anything with a sour energetic such as: bananas, sour fruits, yeasted breads, meat, fish, radish
Eggs	vegetables, grains	fruit, beans, dairy*, meat and fish
Meats	vegetables, rice	heavy foods, grains, nightshades, other meat (i.e., bacon cheese burgers), honey, milk, black lentils, radishes
Yogurt, fresh within 3 days of making	dried fruit, sweet berry smoothie, honey	bananas, sour fruits, dairy*, eggs, nightshades, hot drinks, meat and fish; avoid after sunset
Beans, lentils	vegetables, rice	fruit, dairy*(i.e., bean and cheese burritos), eggs, meat, fish
Wheat and pasta	pesto sauce (try variations with spinach, arugula, cilantro	fruit, tomato sauces, cheese, fish and meat
Honey, raw	yogurt, tea (allow water to cool until you can comfortably hold it in your mouth without burning your tongue)	equal quantities by **weight** of ghee and honey (i.e., 1 teaspoon honey with 3 teaspoons ghee); never combine with meat; NEVER COOK HONEY

*dairy- cheese, milk, yogurt; **night shades** – eggplant, tomatoes, white potatoes, peppers

We can relate the Food Combining Table to the modern scientific understanding of the biochemical digestion process, first introduced by Ivan Pavlov[8]. Digestion begins when we smell the aroma of food and the salivary glands initiate secretions. As food enters the mouth we begin to chew which serves three main functions: 1. It breaks down food into small particles that enzymes can further process downstream (ideally, chew until the food is liquefied); 2. It mixes the amylase enzymes in saliva with the food particles to start digesting starches; 3. It alerts the stomach to begin secreting digestive enzymes in anticipation of incoming food.

Different foods require different enzymes to break them into tiny molecules suitable for assimilation into the bloodstream. These enzymes require a specific pH environment for proper functioning and the enzymes will not be released until the pH has been regulated to the appropriate level. There must be the right amount of acid in the stomach, the right amount of alkali in the duodenum, and the right amount of time spent in each phase of digestion. The digestive process is a precisely designed mechanism comparable in its intricacy to a meticulously engineered German automobile. BMW® recommends premium fuel and regular maintenance for optimal performance. Similarly, ayurveda says optimal wellness can be achieved with high quality food, regular exercise (in accordance with your specific constitution) and adequate rest (in the amounts recommended for your constitution). While there have not been comprehensive modern studies encompassing the effects of food combinations on digestion, absorption and elimination, we do know the following[9]:

- Poor digestion of starches results in fermentation, causing gas and bloating.
- Poor digestion of fats results in high levels of fat in the stool, which can result in the loss of fat soluble vitamins (i.e., vitamins A, D, E and K).
- Poor digestion of proteins results in short chain polypeptides being absorbed into the bloodstream where they can mimic the action of hormones and cytokines (chemical messengers) thus interfering with normal biochemistry or potentially activating the immune system leading to food allergies and/or autoimmunity.
- Poor digestion can result in malabsorption (food being eliminated as waste without proper assimilation of nutrients), depriving the body of necessary nutrients resulting in anemia and other deficiencies.

Thus we may infer that efficient digestion of food is vital for long-term health and prevention of disease. Based on what we know about the digestion process today, the food combining rules that ayurveda prescribed thousands of years ago do not seem so far-fetched.

Many of us pass inefficient combinations of food routinely through our digestive systems with after-effects that we have learned to live with or perhaps are unaware of the cause. If you have a very strong digestive fire (as is common among young adults, those with pitta constitution or individuals who exercise regularly), then you will tend to be able to eat inefficient combinations with little or no symptoms. In most of us, inefficient combinations of food will create temporary discomforts (like gas, bloating, acid indigestion, acid reflux, drowsiness, constipation or diarrhea) that over time can cause longer-lasting changes (weight gain, food allergies, ulcers, irritable bowel, etc.). Ideally, after eating a meal, you should feel satiated, clear, alert and happy. To feel otherwise, is indicative of improper quantity or quality of ingested food. Your goal is to find a balance that does not place undue stress on your system.

If you are accustomed to large, heavy combinations, and would like to try the lighter ayurvedic approach, gradually introduce food combing over a period of several months. A gradual introduction will help coach your body to discriminate when your desire to eat is based on true hunger, versus a habit of eating because you like to always feel "full". Slowly eliminating inefficient combinations will help you to clearly recognize the impact that food is having on your body. To start, you can try eating one meal a day (breakfast, lunch or dinner) according to the food combining rules. Or maybe you want to focus on one rule for the day (i.e., always eating fruit alone). Slowly integrating the changes will be the key to lasting success.

Bread First, Salad Last

Ayurveda also recommended that the foods in a meal be eaten in sequential order according to their "tastes" and that all six tastes (sweet, sour, salty, pungent, bitter and astringent) be represented in the meal. This "eating order" corresponds to the digestive order, specifically: the "sweet" taste (i.e., bread, desserts, rice, wheat, barley, corn, etc.) should be eaten first; the "sour" taste (i.e., a pickle chutney, tamarind, lemon, tomato, etc.) should be eaten next; then salty; then pungent (i.e., chilies, onions, ginger, etc.); then bitter (i.e., green vegetables, broccoli, etc.); then astringent (i.e., dal, beans, lettuce, cauliflower, quinoa, etc.). This is easy to do when you are eating off a "thali" plate in India, where a plate (or banana leaf) is served with rice at the center, dessert and breads at one o'clock, followed in clockwise succession by small dishes containing each of the remaining tastes. But westerners don't generally prepare meals in this fashion. A simplistic way to adapt this to western style meals, is to eat your bread, rice and sweets first followed by a sour tasting appetizer, next the main meal and finish with the astringent taste – salad.

Don't Worry, Be Happy

Ayurveda was not intended to be a rigid approach, in spite of the myriad of "recommendations" that I have just outlined. In fact, the original teachings of ayurveda consisted of broad general guidance, like recommending people 'eat wholesome foods and avoid unwholesome foods'. To clarify "wholesome" versus "unwholesome", they provided definitions: wholesome foods were 'foods that maintain the balance of the tissues and the doshas, and unwholesome foods were 'those that imbalance the doshas and tissues'. There is a lot of flexibility in how this is interpreted and applied; flexibility that is necessary, to accommodate an individual's unique needs and present circumstances. Ayurveda is all about balance and happiness is essential to balance. The ancients also say that one should not suddenly avoid wholesome foods as it could lead to unhappiness. So don't suddenly remove beets from your diet because your predominant dosha is pitta (fire) and a "list" says that beets are warming and unbalancing to pitta. That would reduce happiness and being unhappy is definitely not in balance. Instead, observe how you feel after eating beets. If you experience symptoms of imbalance (heat, anger, rashes, diarrhea, heartburn, etc.), then consider adding cooling spices (such as coriander), removing the skin, cooking or reducing the quantity that you eat, gradually, over the course of several months. Eventually, you may even find a new favorite to replace them with – perhaps steamed kale?

Top 10 Essential Ayurvedic Tips for Wellness

At this point, you may be thinking that you will never be happy without eating pepperoni cheese pizza or apples with your brie or bacon double cheeseburgers. So I have compiled ten essential tips that help to minimize stress on your digestive system even if you are eating inefficient food combinations. This is not optimal as per ayurveda, but it is a good place to start while maintaining your sense of happiness; consider trying one tip a day and observing the impact on how you feel. Combine these rules with daily exercise and adequate sleep and you will be on your way to better health.

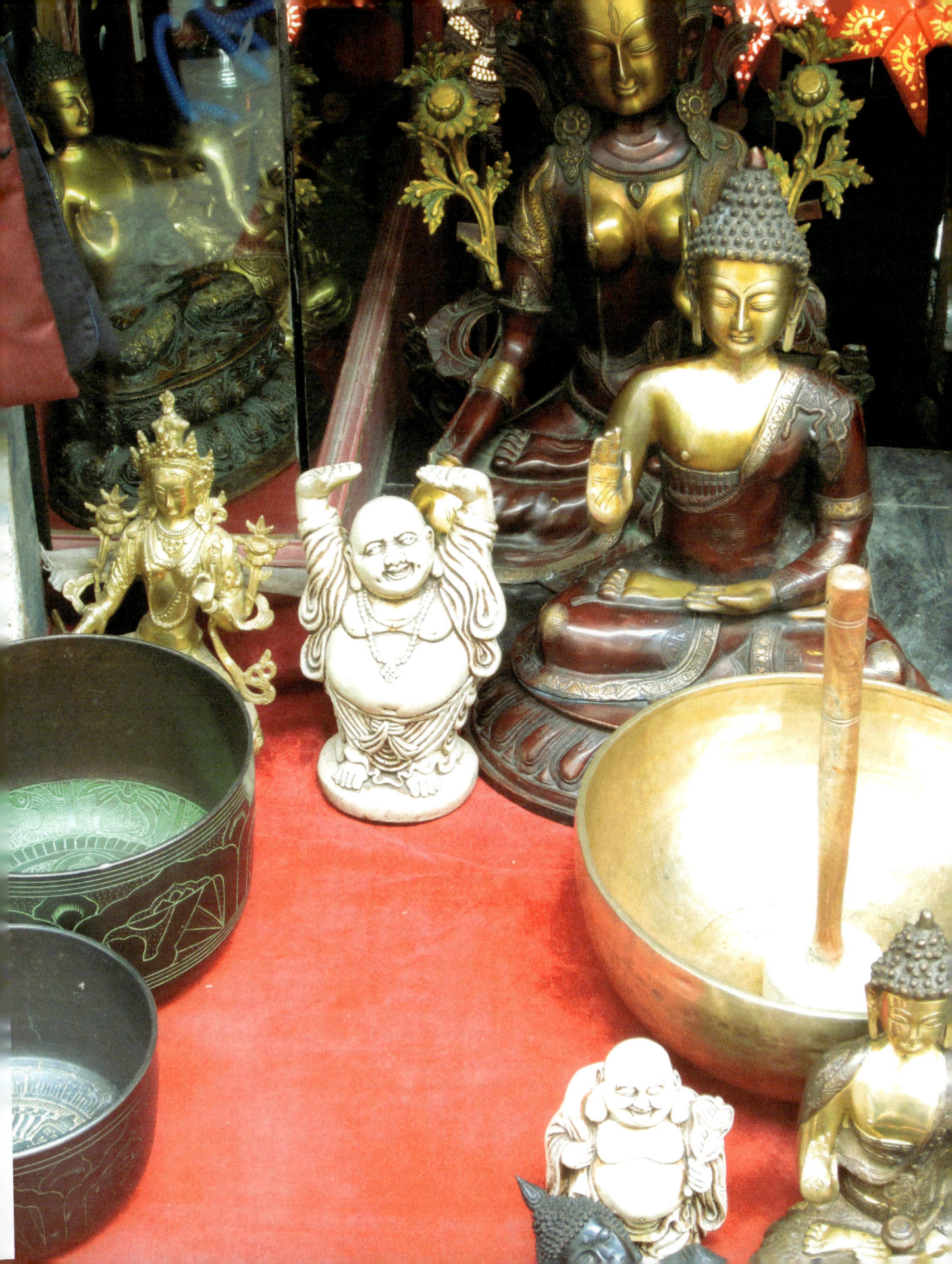

Table 3 – Top 10 Essential Ayurveda Tips for Wellness
1. Eat only when there is true hunger.
2. Wait six hours between meals.
3. Eat mindfully, in a harmonious environment and chew food thoroughly.
4. Drink warm water with your meals and upon rising.
5. Stop eating before you feel "full".
6. Eat your big meal at midday.
7. Cook your own food.
8. Emphasize organic, local foods in your diet.
9. Minimize leftovers.
10. Take a break with a mono-diet of kitchari.

1. **EAT ONLY WHEN THERE IS TRUE HUNGER.** Often times, our desire for food is not related to true hunger. To determine if your hunger is false, try sipping some warm water or herbal tea with honey. If that doesn't satiate your hunger and mealtime is a long time off, try eating fruit. [The natural sugars in fruit will provide energy and nutrients that the body can easily digest, absorb and assimilate; unlike a candy bar or other sweet made with refined sugars – natural is better.]

Ideally, establish a daily eating schedule to regulate your digestive system and minimize the potential for overloading your system. Identify the cause for your desire to constantly snack: is it emotional (are you eating because of loneliness, boredom or habit?) or are your meals too small or lacking proper nourishment? If you can identify the root cause, it is easier to find a solution that will bring lasting change. Conversely, if you have no hunger and it is a scheduled meal time, give yourself permission to skip a meal. Lack of hunger may be your body's way of telling you that it is still processing other food or there is some toxicity it is trying to purge. Try some ginger tea to assist the cleansing process. If you find yourself eating without hunger because you know when hunger arrives in a few hours, you will be in a meeting or otherwise unable to have a proper meal, then it is better to carry a "snack" with you for later than to eat without hunger now; as a modern practitioner of ayurveda, we need to be practical in our implementation.

2. **WAIT SIX HOURS BETWEEN MEALS.** It takes about six hours for an **average** western-sized meal to complete the digestion process (smaller meals or lighter/vegetarian meals will digest quicker). Waiting until the prior meal is digested will assist in proper absorption and assimilation by not overloading the system with more incoming foods. Constant snacking between meals means the digestive cycle is continually being asked to restart while the prior cycle is incomplete – you are asking your system to work overtime with no breaks.

3. **EAT MINDFULLY, IN A HARMONIOUS ENVIRONMENT AND CHEW FOOD THOROUGHLY.** The ancients had an implicit understanding of the mind-body connection. As it relates to the digestive system, they recommended eating in a harmonious environment with good company to aid digestion. Today we know that due to our physiological make-up, stress impacts every part of the digestive system through the release of hormones and nervous system responses. When our "flight or fight" response is activated, digestion is suppressed; blood flow, contractions of digestive muscles, and digestive secretions are all reduced. So when you sit down to eat, relax and take a moment to reflect and give thanks for the meal you are about to eat; embrace the nourishment as the food flows through your body.

Eating should not be too slow, as this encourages over eating (i.e., as is the case when we finish a large meal at a restaurant and feel full, but after 10 or 15 minutes we erroneously feel there is space enough to order dessert!). Nor should it be too fast. Rapid eating and inadequate chewing impedes optimal digestion. (Note: chewing gum creates the same response and "turns on" the digestive system by signaling incoming food and initiates the secretion of needless enzymes, taxing the digestive system. Gum chewing is like running your garbage disposal for a few hours without adding any food; it wastes energy and burns out the motor – avoid excessive gum chewing.).

4. **DRINK WARM WATER WITH YOUR MEALS AND UPON RISING.** The ancients believed that water was sacred and they had many methods of purification (boiling being one of the easiest to do in modern times); they believed water was purifying and once consumed it became auspicious and strengthening. Today we know that adequate water is vital for good health and a reactant in many of the digestive processes. It is the drink of choice with meals, in moderation. But if you drink too much water, it can dilute the digestive enzymes making your system work harder to process the food. Ayurveda recommends hot water because they believe that everything, even water, should be "pre-cooked" before entering the digestive system for optimal functioning. Don't want to drink hot water? Then at least avoid iced drinks with meals as it is believed that ice (cold) will be less than optimal for the digestive process. The use of soft-drinks, coffee, tea and alcohol taxes the system in general, and kidneys in particular; they can damage the vital energy in your body over time. Drink a cup of warm water upon rising; it will cleanse the GI tract and stimulate peristalsis.

5. **STOP EATING BEFORE YOU FEEL "FULL".** Ayurveda recommends eating the proper quantity of food broadly defined as 'that which gets digested in the proper time'. Food is more likely to get properly digested and absorbed if you don't over eat. A general guideline is to stop eating when you burp; this generally can indicate your stomach is filled to capacity. Ayurveda gives us the following practical guidance: your cupped hands approximate the size of your stomach, so this is the maximum amount of food you should consume at a meal. Although not optimal, smaller portions of incompatible foods will create less stress on your digestive system than larger portions. What if you don't like to "waste" food by leaving it on your plate, even though you know you are full? I can still hear my mother lamenting "there are children starving in Africa – finish what's on your plate." But maybe there was too much on my plate? Try placing smaller serving sizes on your plate (using your cupped hands as a measure); or save the leftovers for later. Over eating results in the food fermenting, putrefying and "wasting" in your stomach. As one of my teachers Jiwan Shakti used to say: "Once you're full you are going to waste the food whether you eat it or not. Do you want it to waste inside you, creating toxins, or waste outside where it could become beneficial compost?"

6. **EAT YOUR BIG MEAL AT MIDDAY.** The ancients lived in harmony with the rhythms of the day and seasons. They believed the digestion was strongest when the sun was strongest and identified midday (11am-2pm) as the optimal time for their main meal. Breakfast should be a lighter meal (i.e., fruit, porridge, crepes or a small veggie omelet). Dinner should be consumed before sunset; food intake at that time should be lighter and easy to digest (i.e., a warm lentil salad or soup, rather than a T-bone steak). Allow three hours after eating before going to bed. Allow one hour after eating before physical exercise (jogging or sex). Boiled, spiced milk before bed will aid sleep and can curb late night hunger.

7. **COOK YOUR OWN FOOD.** Commercially prepared foods are generally high in sugars, salts/sodium, fats and chemical preservatives. Cooking your own food gives you control over the quality and type of ingredients. Additionally, home-cooked meals are imparted with your energy which you will feel on subliminal levels thus reinforcing your objective of health and well-being. In general, lightly cooking foods is understood to prep the food for digestion (i.e., pre-digest it by starting to break it down) and aid the digestion process by promoting the elimination of flatulence and reducing mucus.

8. **EMPHASIZE ORGANIC, LOCAL FOODS IN YOUR DIET.** Emphasize local foods, in season that are fresh; vital energy and nutrients deteriorate quickly once the food has been harvested. Food that has been shipped across the country (or world) has lost much of its vitality. Emphasize organic or pesticide-free foods whenever possible to maximize taste and minimize potential long-term harmful effects of pesticide residue[10]. Washing produce does not eliminate all pesticide residues. Organic food or pesticide-free food is the best choice.

9. **MINIMIZE LEFTOVERS.** Ideally, eat food within a few hours of harvesting for optimal taste and nutritional content. Realistically, eating leftovers will save you some time and the alternative of eating commercially prepared food. So leftovers should be refrigerated in air-tight containers, reheated only once, and disposed of after two days. Frozen foods are likewise not ayurvedic, but a reality in a fast-paced modern society. If you must freeze food, use freezer-grade air-tight, single serving size containers; eat the frozen foods within a month; defrost only the portion that you are going to eat on that same day.

10. **TAKE A BREAK WITH A MONO-DIET OF KITCHARI.** Give your system a rest periodically (perhaps on a Sunday after an indulgent weekend? Or on the new moon to impart an attitude of new, healthy beginnings?) by eating a light, restorative mono-diet of kitchari for a day. This delicately-spiced stew of mung beans and basmati rice is easily digested, absorbed, assimilated and eliminated; it helps to neutralize the pH balance. It's a well deserved vacation for your digestive system.

FOODS FOR THE DOSHAS

With our knowledge of the five elements, the three doshas, the six tastes and food combining, we have a foundation to understand diet and lifestyles alternatives that can be balancing to specific doshas and those that can be unbalancing. Referring back to the ayurvedic formula - **opposites balance; like increases like** – we can recap with the following examples:

If you are trying to determine why you are feeling like a space cadet, full of anxiety and fear or are always constipated and have itchy hemorrhoids (symptoms indicating excess vata/air), analyze your food – have you been eating a preponderance of pungent, bitter or astringent tastes? Are you consuming a lot of cold (raw), light, mobile, dry, rough foods such as potato chips, crackers, beans, caffeinated drinks or raw salads? Or has your lifestyle included a lot of mobile activity – travel, running, non-stop talking at meetings with no down time? When vata (cold, light, dry, rough, mobile, subtle, clear) is in excess, then we need to bring in the opposite qualities to decrease vata. The opposite qualities of vata (i.e., warm, heavy, moist, smooth, stable, dense, thick) can be introduced easily through diet by emphasizing the sweet, sour and salty tastes with warming foods; drinking a cup of herbal tea, warm spiced milk, a hearty root vegetable stew or beef broth, bananas or sweet oranges. Lifestyle recommendations include meditation, grounding yoga asana postures and daily oil massage (self massage: leave oil on for 15-20 minutes, follow with a warm shower). The general advice for vata is to slow down, keep to a routine, stay hydrated and get plenty of rest.

If you are feeling angry, irritable, judgmental and your skin is breaking out in hives, pimples and rashes or your stomach is burning with acid (indicating an excess of pitta/fire), analyze your food – does it have a preponderance of pungent, salty and sour tastes? Have you been eating a lot of spicy Mexican food, pickles, lemons, tomato sauce or fried foods? Have you been working long hours? Have you been in a hot climate or under pressure at work or in your relationships? When pitta (oily, penetrating, hot, light and liquid) is in excess, then we need to bring in the opposite qualities to balance it out (such as dry, slow/dull, cold, heavy and dense). We can reduce pitta with sweet, bitter and astringent tasting cool foods and drinks; salads, bitter green leafy vegetables, organic ice cream (or coconut ice cream), apples, avocado, cilantro, organic milk, coconut water, *pitta cooling coriander milk drink*, relaxing near a calm, cool lake, avoiding sitting in the hot sun, avoiding chilies and avoiding eating oily, fried foods. The general advice for pitta is to stop burning the midnight oil, meditate and "chill out".

If you are feeling lethargic, sad, clingy, full of excess mucus and you can't fit into your skinny jeans (indicating an excess of kapha/water), analyze your food – does it have a preponderance of sweet, sour and salty tastes? Have you been eating a lot of cheese, meat, dairy, wheat, fried foods, Philly cheesesteak subs, ice cream, bananas and chocolate? When kapha is in excess (heavy, slow, dull, cool, salty, static, etc.) we can bring in opposite qualities to balance it out (such as light, mobile, sharp, warm, etc.). We can reduce kapha by: emphasizing pungent, bitter and astringent tastes; eating cooked leafy green vegetables; liberal use of garlic, onion, ginger and spicy foods; eating drying foods such as beans and barley and corn. The general advice for kapha is to get moving which can be done by eating lively, spicy food, varying their routine, participating in new adventures and group activities, but most expeditiously through vigorous exercise.

ॐ

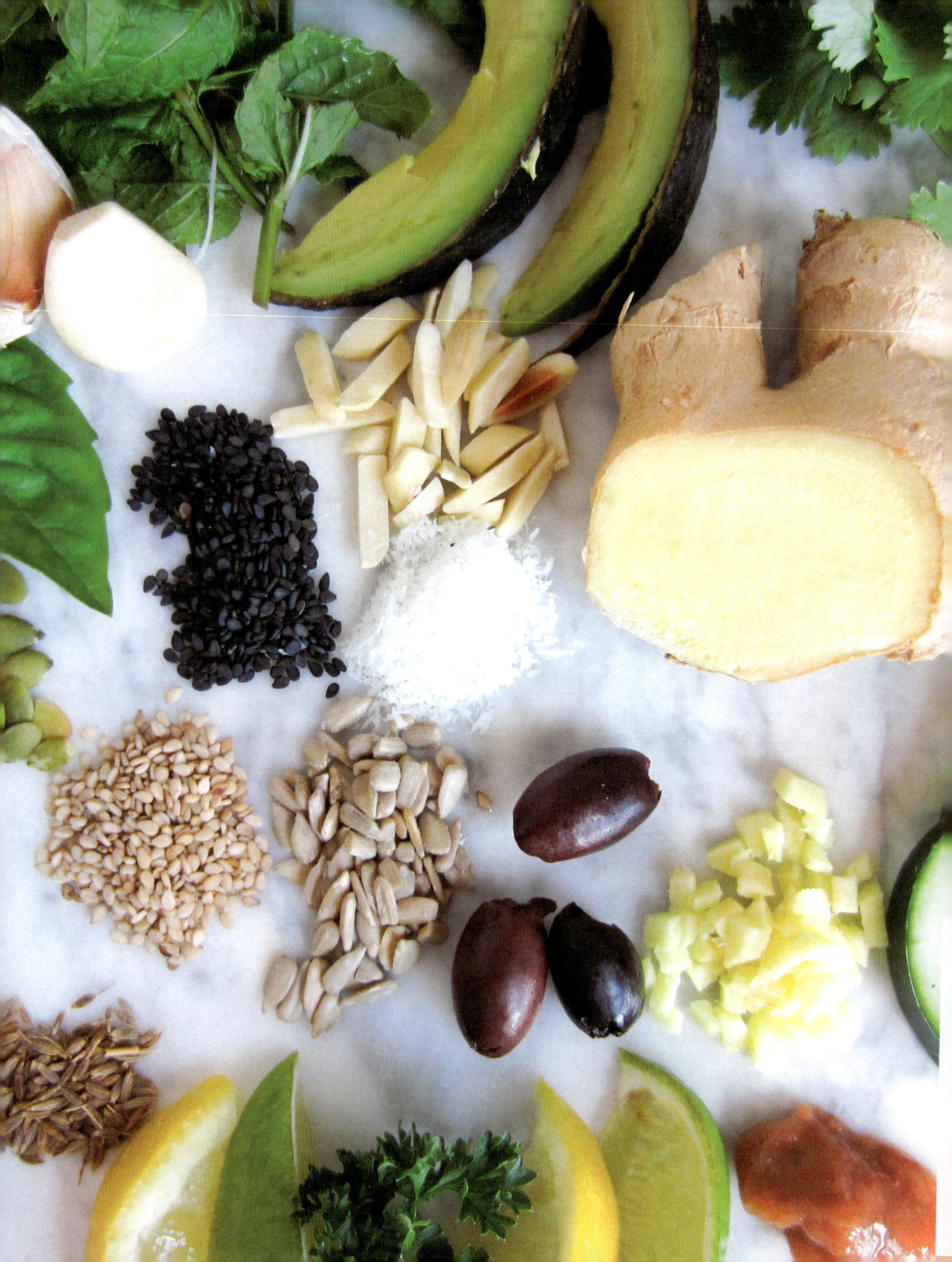

Chapter 6: Ayurevda for the Family

I trust you are now getting a general feel for how to incorporate the knowledge of the energetics of foods and the doshas. When cooking for more than one person, recipes can be cooked so as to be tri-doshic (balancing to all doshas) by way of their combinations of ingredients and spices or they can be adapted at the table via addition of suitable *"churnas"* (spice combinations designed to balance specific doshas) or condiments (sauces, chutneys, seasonings, etc.). The recipes in this book are generally tri-doshic and many provide variations to target specific doshas.

You can apply the general rules to adapt your meals to be tri-doshic for the family. For instance, let's say it is a sweltering summer day and you want to prepare a cool salad for the family. Prepare a base salad, using tri-doshic ingredients (see *"build your own salad"* recipes), and top with dosha-specific dressings for added balancing. Ayurveda does not recommend raw foods (especially for vata). But in the appropriate time, season and quantity, with dosha-balancing condiments, a salad could provide some happiness (ease of preparation) without a major disruption to your balance.

Let's say you are serving that salad with brown rice and steamed vegetables. To make it more balancing for vata, serve it with tahini sauce or tamari to provide additional grounding and warmth; for pitta add some fresh coriander or shredded coconut to provide additional sweet and cool qualities; kapha could add some chili sauce, scallions or sprouts to add heat or lightness to the meal.

In general, vata needs moisture (sauces, soups and dressings); pitta needs cooling (coridander and coconut); kapha needs movement and dryness (spices, garlic, raw onions and no sauces).

Cooking within the ayurvedic framework for a family is not complicated, it simply requires a bit of forethought. Many of the condiments can be prepared in advance (or purchased) and stored in the refrigerator so that will create some ease in your life. Refer to Table 4 "Dosha Condiment Table" for more ideas.

The dosha condiment table is your go-to reference for finding a condiment, sauce, chutney, salad dressing, drink or juice that will help to balance your dosha. Here's how it works: Let's say vata wants a salad, but understands that the energetic of lettuce is cold, dry and light (unbalancing). The solution is to select some condiments and salad dressings from the "vata" column to help warm and ground the salad. Feel like going to the juice bar with your friends? Check out the balancing blends for your dosha before you go! Items highlighted in the table are names of recipes that you will find in the recipe section of this book; they can be referenced at the beginning of each recipe chapter.

> To further assist you in implementation of the ayurvedic wisdom into your life, I have summarized diet and lifestyle tips for each of the doshas in **Appendix C, D & E - Dosha Diet Aid for Vata, Pitta and Kapha**, respectively. Use these as guidelines to help you get started on your ayurvedic journey. Remember, the ultimate determination of what foods are balancing is how you feel after eating. Relax, enjoy your food and bring awareness to the effects the food has on your body -- physically and emotionally.

Table 4 - Dosha Condiment Table

	Vata	Pitta	Kapha
Condiments	avocado	avocado	basil pesto
	basil pesto	cilantro (fresh)	chilis
	chives	coconut, dried shredded	chives
	creamy yogurt	*creamy yogurt*	flax seeds
	cucumber	cucumber	ginger
	dulse	dill	mushrooms
	lemons/limes	jicama	mustard and mustard seeds
	olives (black)	lime	onions, raw
	nuts and seeds	mint	radish
	salt		sprouts
	umeboshi paste/plums		wasabi
Sauces & Chutneys	*vata plum compote*	*cool coconut chutney*	*hot pepper sauce*
	vata lemon cashew cream sauce	tamari	*kapha hot onion chutney*
	tamari	*pitta cooling date chutney*	*kapha spicy pear chutney*
	vata sweet onion chutney		
Salad Dressings	tahini dulse dressing	fresh squeezed lime juice	*pitta kapha pomegranate dressing*
	vata tamarind honey dressing	*pitta kapha pomegranate dressing*	*kaphi wasabi dressing*
Drinks	*vata pitta ginger tea*	*vata pitta ginger tea*	*kapha ginger tea*
	masala tea	*pitta soothing mint-rosewater*	*mint tea*
	mint tea	*pitta cooling coriander milk*	
Juices*	carrot-ginger-beet	apple-cranberry	apple-lemon
	orange-lime	apple-lime	kale-carrot-parsley
		coconut-water	pomegranate-lime-ginger-apple
		kale-carrot	
		watermelon	
*no added sweetners			

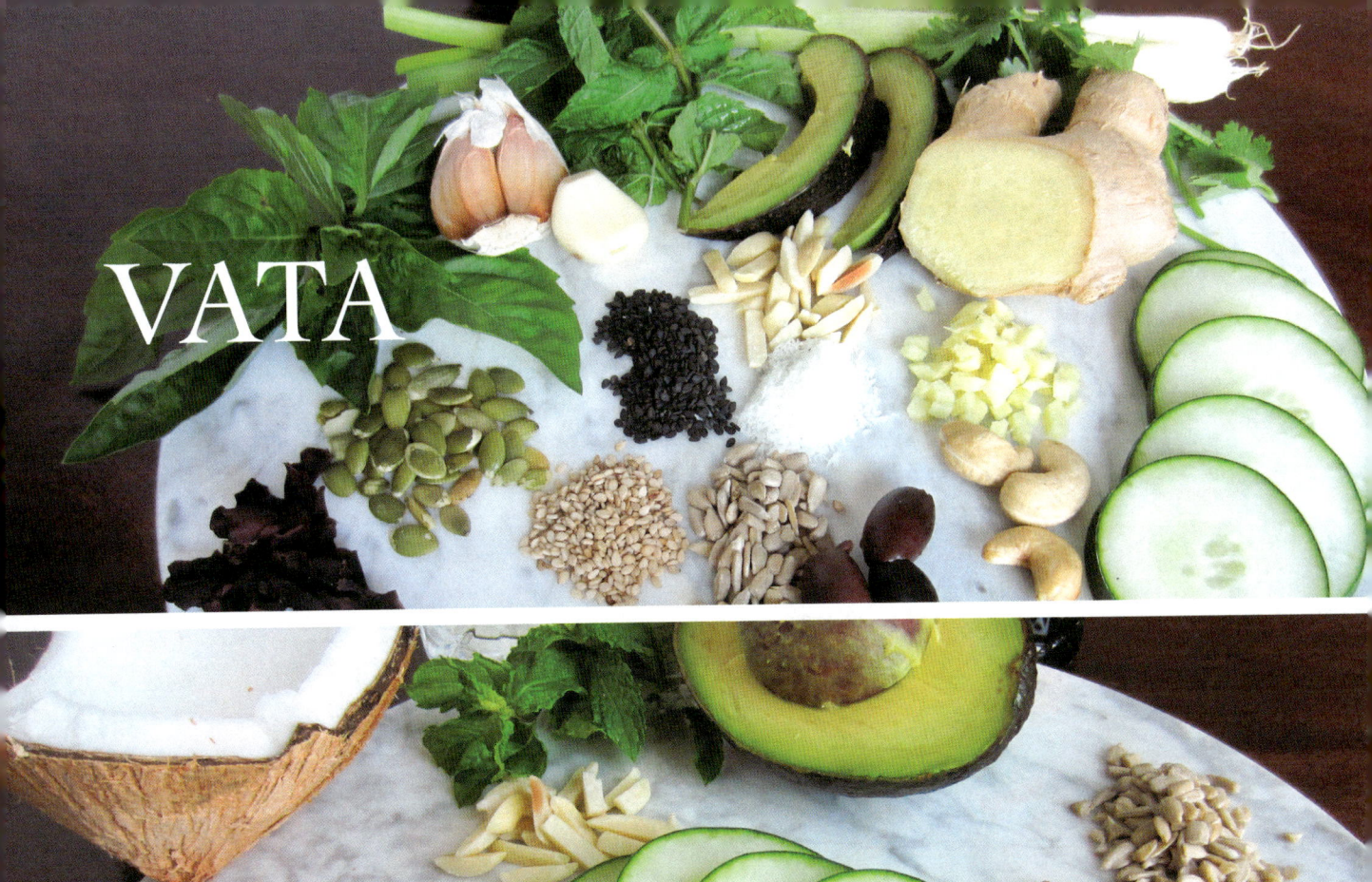

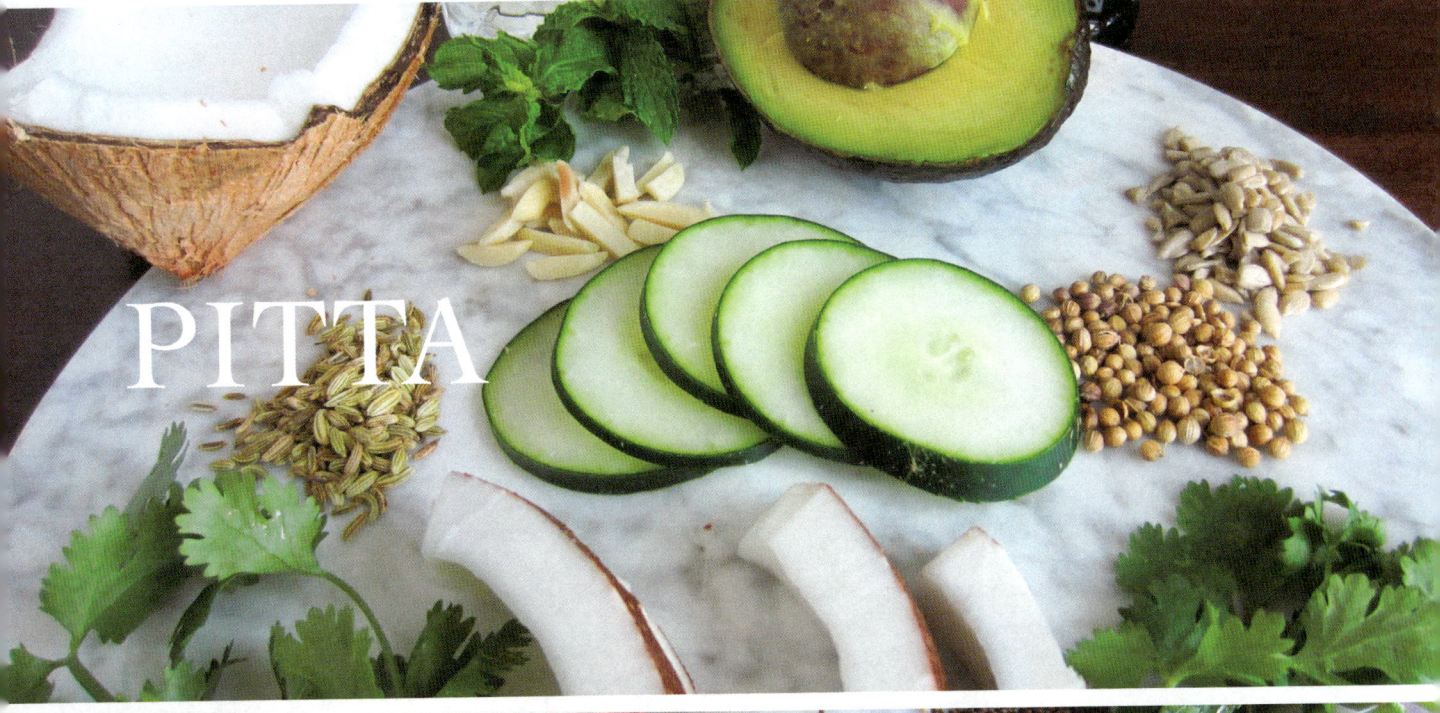

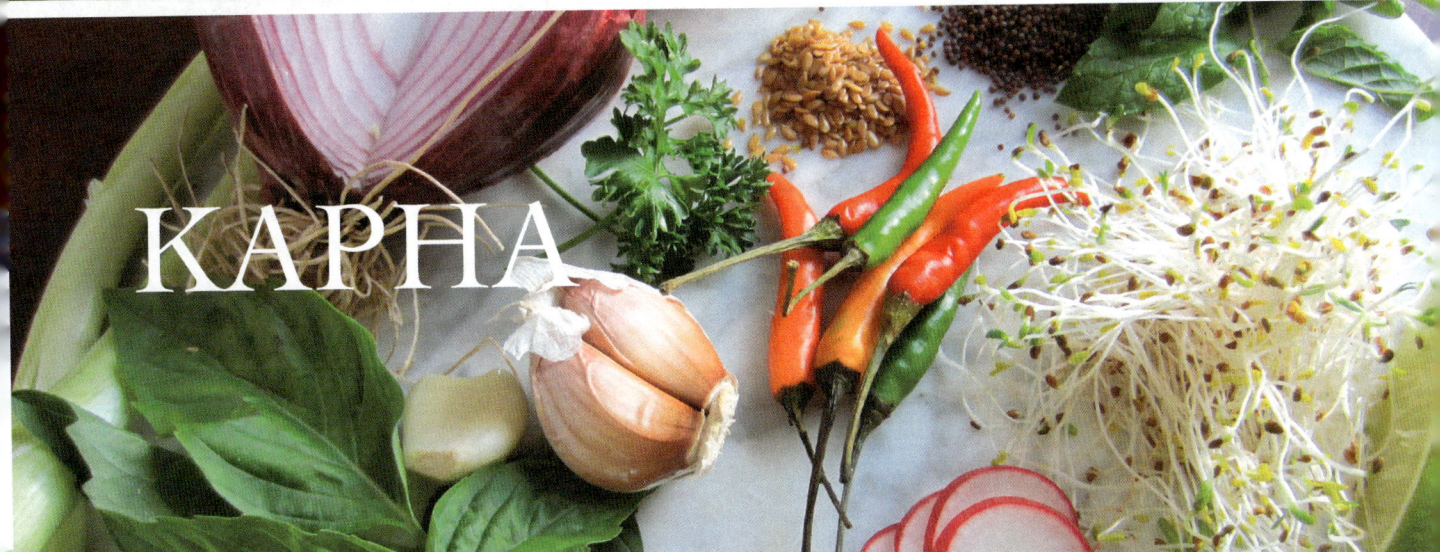

VATA

PITTA

KAPHA

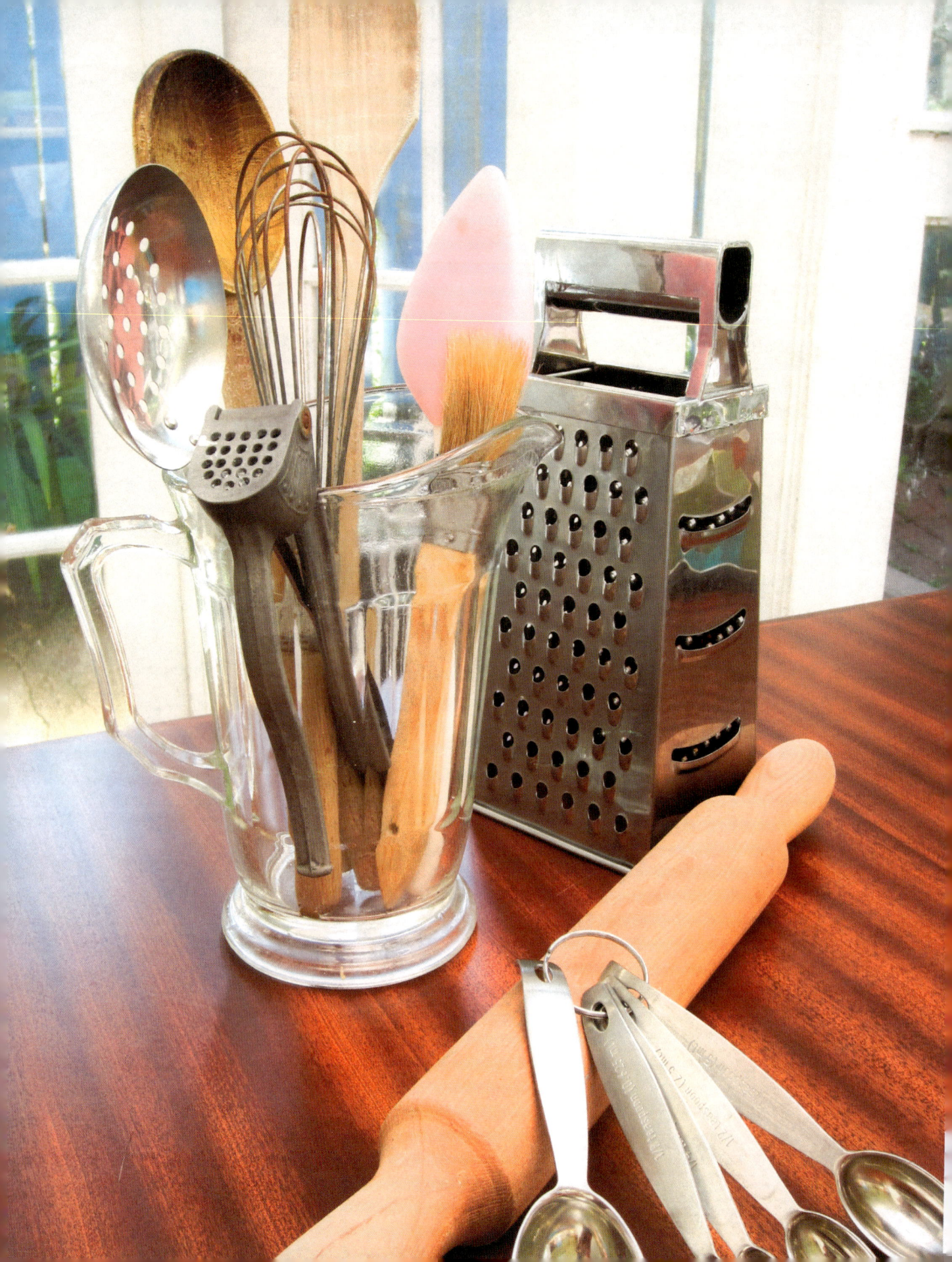

Chapter 7: Kitchen Essentials

A well-stocked kitchen with proper tools and core ingredients will greatly ease your transition to the ayurveda approach to wellness. The items included in the tables in this chapter will help ensure that you always are prepared to whip something up for yourself, family or friends.

Many of the items you likely already have on hand, so peruse the tables in this chapter to help fill any gaps. The last section of the chapter includes tips that came to mind as I was writing. I hope you will benefit from them.

Table 5 Pans, Utensils, Gadgets*

Pans & Miscellaneous	Utensils	Gadgets
fry pan 8"	chef's spatula 4"x2" silcone	blender, handheld immersion (Cuisinart® 3 in 1/200 watts
fry pan 10"	garlic press	can opener
sauce pan, 5 quart		chef's candles, Prices®
sauce pan 1 quart	knife, bread	citrus juicer
sauce pan, 2 or 3 quart	knife, chef 8"	coffee grinder
saute´ pan, 3 quart	knife, pairing 4 "	cutting boards (wooden + jelly board®)
vegetable steamer		food processor, Cuisinart® 9-cup
	measuring spoons & cups	french coffee press
rice cooker (3 or 5 cup)		grater citrus
	ladle, stainless steel, 4 ounce	grater, ginger
baking pan, 13"x9"x2"	pastry brush, 1½ "	grater, 4-sided box grater
cooling rack, metal 10"x15"	stirring spoon, wooden 14"	
baking sheet, 14"x17"		knife sharpener (Wűsthof® 2-stage)
loaf pan, 8"	strainer, 5" fine metal mesh	vegetable peeler
pie pan,glass, 9"	strainer, 10" fine metal mesh	mortar & pestle
springform pan, 8"		
square baking pan, 8"	turner, slotted, non-stick 13"	rolling pin
	flexible scraping spatula	sauce wisk, 8" (silicon & metal)
mixing bowls (3) 1-4 quart		thermometer, oven
ramekins (4)		thermometer, baking
air tight containers (glad® freezer safe) (6) (2-cup)	Zojirushi® lunch box	

*Brand names listed are products which I have found to be of superior performance, long lasting and backed by strong warranties; I do not receive compensation from the manufacturers of these products.

Table 6 - The Pantry

Grains	Sweeteners	Seeds
amaranth	coconut sugar	sunflower seeds
couscous (Israeli)	honey (raw)	flax seeds
whole grain barley	maple syrup	pumpkin seeds
polenta, Food Merchants® pre-cooked organic	pomegranate syrup (or pomegranate molasses)	sesame seeds
quick cooking oats		
quinoa (red and white)	**Condiments**	**Asian**
rice, basmati	artichoke hearts (canned)	chilies*
rice, brown	rosewater	coconut milk (canned)
rice, purple (forbidden rice)	tamari	coconut, fresh shredded*
rice, wild	tamarind concentrate, seedless (Neera's®)	curry leaves*
	vinegar (apple cider)	kombu (dried kelp)
Beans	vinegar (white balsamic)	kuzu root starch (or arrowroot)
adzuki beans		lemongrass stalks*
black beans	**Oils**	lime (kaffir) leaves*
cannellini (white) beans	coconut oil	fine rice vermicelli noodles
garbanzo beans / chickpeas	olive oil	nori sheets
	sesame oil	shitake mushrooms (dried)
Lentils	sunflower oil	soba noodles
mung dal (split, hulled)	ghee	tofu
puy lentils (or French)		umeboshi paste
red lentils	**Dried Fruit**	wakame (seaweed)
tur (toor) dal	apricots	rice vinegar
urad (urid) dal	cherries	wasabi powder
	cranberries	
	raisins	

Most beans (and lentils) can be purchased from bulk containers at the local natural food store, food co-operative or Whole Foods Market®. This allows you to purchase small quantities to meet your immediate needs; beans and lentils will begin to dry out after about six months and will become tough, so only purchase what you need to ensure freshness. Beans may also be purchased in cans where they are pre-cooked, packaged in water and sometimes kombu (dried kelp that aids digestion). Read the labels and select brands that do not contain added salt, sodium and preservatives. I prefer beans packaged in BPA-free cans.

Grains should be stored in an air-tight container in a cool, dry, and dark location. A sealed container is very important for maintaining freshness and reducing the possibility of infestations.
*Fresh frozen shredded coconut, curry leaves, lemongrass, lime (kaffir) leaves and chilies are available at Indian, Asian and ethnic markets. Sometimes they are difficult to find, so buy in bulk and

then freeze extras in a Ziploc® freezer bag for up to 3 months. To use, remove amount that you need and return the rest to the freezer, being sure to seal tightly; the coconut will take 15-20 minutes to thaw, but the other items will thaw in 5 minutes at room temperature.

SPICES

Dried spices should be purchased in small quantities and used within six months of purchase to ensure optimal flavor, quality and freshness. Many stores now sell organic spices in bulk bins so you can purchase a quantity to meet your specific needs, often at a lower per unit cost.

If you have the resources (time, space and suitable climate), consider starting an organic spice garden for year-round fresh quality spices. Mint, tarragon, thyme, chives, oregano, basil and rosemary are relatively easy to grow and can liven up salads and most meals.

To help you set up your spice cabinet, I have included a spice table with all the spices that are used in the recipes in Eat Well, Be Well. In some instances, I have included the same spice in seed and in powder form (i.e., coriander, cardamom, etc.). This is because I use the spices in various forms depending on the recipe. In curries, soups and stews I like to use coarsely ground or whole spices; in sauces, desserts and vegetable seasonings, I like to use a finely ground powder. Freshly ground seeds are the most flavorful and give you the flexibility of grinding to your desired consistency (coarse or fine). But grinding adds a few extra minutes (grinding time and cleaning) to meal prep. So I like to have both options available. Set up your kitchen to suit your needs. I have recommended Frontier® chili powder; I like their blend as it is not heavily salted and well-balanced.

Table 7 - Dried Spices & Fresh Herbs

Dried Spices	Dried Spices (Continued)	Fresh Herbs
anise (star)	dill	basil
ajwain	ginger powder	chives
allspice	nutmeg, ground	cilantro
basil	oregano	garlic
bay leaf	parsley	ginger
cardamom, ground and seeds	roesmary	lemons/limes
cayenne	saffron	mint
chili powder (Frontier*)	salt, rock (Himalayan salt)	oregano
cinnamon, ground and sticks	savory	parsley
cloves, ground and whole	tarragon	rosemary
coriander, ground and seeds	thyme	scallions
cumin, ground and seeds	tumeric	

TIP – When substituting fresh herbs for dry herbs, the general rule is 1 part dried herbs is equivalent to 3 parts fresh herb. (i.e., 1 teaspoon of dried oregano is equivalent to 3 teaspoons or 1 tablespoon of fresh oregano). Dried herbs have a smaller water content and a higher concentration of essential oils resulting in a stronger flavor than the fresh herbs.

Table 8 - Stocking the Refrigerator

Vegetables	Nuts	Flour
beets	almonds (slivered, blanched, peeled)	arrowroot flour
carrots	cashews	almond flour
ginger, fresh	coconut (unsweetened, shredded)	amaranth flour
greens (kale, bok choy, swiss chard, broccoli)	pecans	corn flour
onions	walnuts	brown rice flour
potatoes, red or Yukon		wheat flour
potatoes, sweet	**Nut Butters & Dairy**	
squash or pumpkin	butter, almond	
	butter, cashew	**Fruits**
	butter, unsalted	seasonal/dosha-specific
	milk (cow, rice, soy or almond)	
	yogurt, unsweetened, plain	

The essential items that you should have stocked in your refrigerator for cooking recipes in this book include: onions, root vegetables, leafy greens, nuts, seeds, butters and flour. Nuts have a high oil content and can go rancid quickly. So I recommend storing nuts in the refrigerator. I also store flours in the refrigerator or freezer in an airtight container or Ziploc® freezer bag to preserve freshness. I typically make my own nut (and seed) butters; see *basic nut butter* recipe in the book.

The essential fruits that you will need are lemons and limes. In addition, you can stock seasonal and dosha-specific fruits as indicated in the *dosha-diet aids* in the appendix. If you don't know your dosha, then sweet berries are generally tri-doshic.

ORGANIZE YOUR SHOPPING

You may have seen some items on these lists that are not at your supermarket (i.e., certain lentils or Asian ingredients). They are typically found at an Asian or Indian market. To find the nearest international market, you can ask a local Indian or Asian neighbor or co-worker or search on the internet or ask your Facebook friends! When I have lived in small towns, I have been able to find an international store that has everything I need within an hour's drive. Most of the items can be kept for 2 months or more (either frozen, in the refrigerator or in the pantry) so if you plan in advance, you can minimize driving. Pick up an inexpensive Chinese cleaver while you're there – they are perfect for cutting squashes, pumpkins and other hard-skinned items. You may consider asking your local grocer to carry some of the items (like the split mung dal, chilies, lemongrass or frozen coconut). If all else fails, you can purchase online and have the items delivered; I have referenced some websites in this book to help you. Peruse the recipes and make a list of ingredients you do not have; then head to the market! I often get recipe ideas from shopping in international markets; I'll pick up something that looks interesting and bring it home and experiment. I hope you will enjoy the shopping adventure as much as I do.

Tips – The Healthy Kitchen & Specialty/International Foods

- **Cutting Boards** – Choose a wooden board that meets your needs by considering: weight, dimensions, groove for juices and ability to fit in your kitchen sink. Sanitize your cutting board after use as follows: rinse the board under hot running water, using a dough scraper or putty knife to remove any meat or particles stuck to the board; wash with mild detergent and hot water, rinse, then dry with a clean towel. Spray the board with distilled vinegar (5% acetic acid/full strength white vinegar is a good disinfectant, effective against E. coli, Salmonella, and Staphylococcus which can cause food poisoning); let dry. To deodorize, pour baking soda over the surface and spray undiluted white vinegar on top; let it foam and bubble for five to ten minutes, then wipe down with a damp cloth. To remove beet stains from a wooden board, scrub with lemon juice then sprinkle baking soda; let set for 5 minutes then rinse with water. Note that hard cutting surfaces (such as glass, marble, granite, bamboo and plastic) will tend to dull your knife blade. Some people find it easier to designate a separate, dishwasher-safe board for chopping meat, fish and poultry. Epicurean® and Dexas Jelli® Boards will suit this purpose; they are thin and lightweight, so you may need to anchor them by placing a thin damp dish towel underneath.
- **Prices® Chef Candles** – are made with oils of basil, patchouli and geranium. They are an excellent way to remove smells from the kitchen (especially when using turmeric or cooking curries). Burn the candles during cooking and the kitchen will be free of odor when the meal is served.
- **Chef Knives, blades** – Selecting a knife blade is a trade-off between cutting precision and toughness. The chart below ranks blade type from highest performance/sharpest edge to lowest performance. High carbon stainless steel chef knives are durable, versatile knives that can perform tasks ranging from hard cutting (i.e., cantelopes) to fine slicing (i.e., tomatoes). They hold their edge longer than stainless steel knives and do not require as much maintenance as carbon steel blades; these knives are not recommended for cutting tough skins (like pumpkins and squash). Instead, use an inexpensive cleaver ($15 at an Asian market) for chopping these items. The back edge of the clever can be used to open a coconut: hit firmly along the mid-line of the coconut, multiple times (turning the coconut to hit all sides) until it cracks open.

Table 9 - Knives				
Blade Type	Cost	Performance	Corrodes and/or reacts to acidic foods	Maintenance*
Carbon Steel Blade	$$$$	Extremely Sharp	Yes (can blemish knife with stains and corrode edge)	Highest, wash and dry promptly
High Carbon Stainless Steel	$$$	Very sharp/holds edge	No	Moderate
Super Stainless Steel	$$	Difficult to sharpen due to hardness	No	Moderate
Stainless Steel	$	Does not hold edge	No	Moderate

*For lasting performance, wash and dry your knife promptly after use, regardless of the blade type.

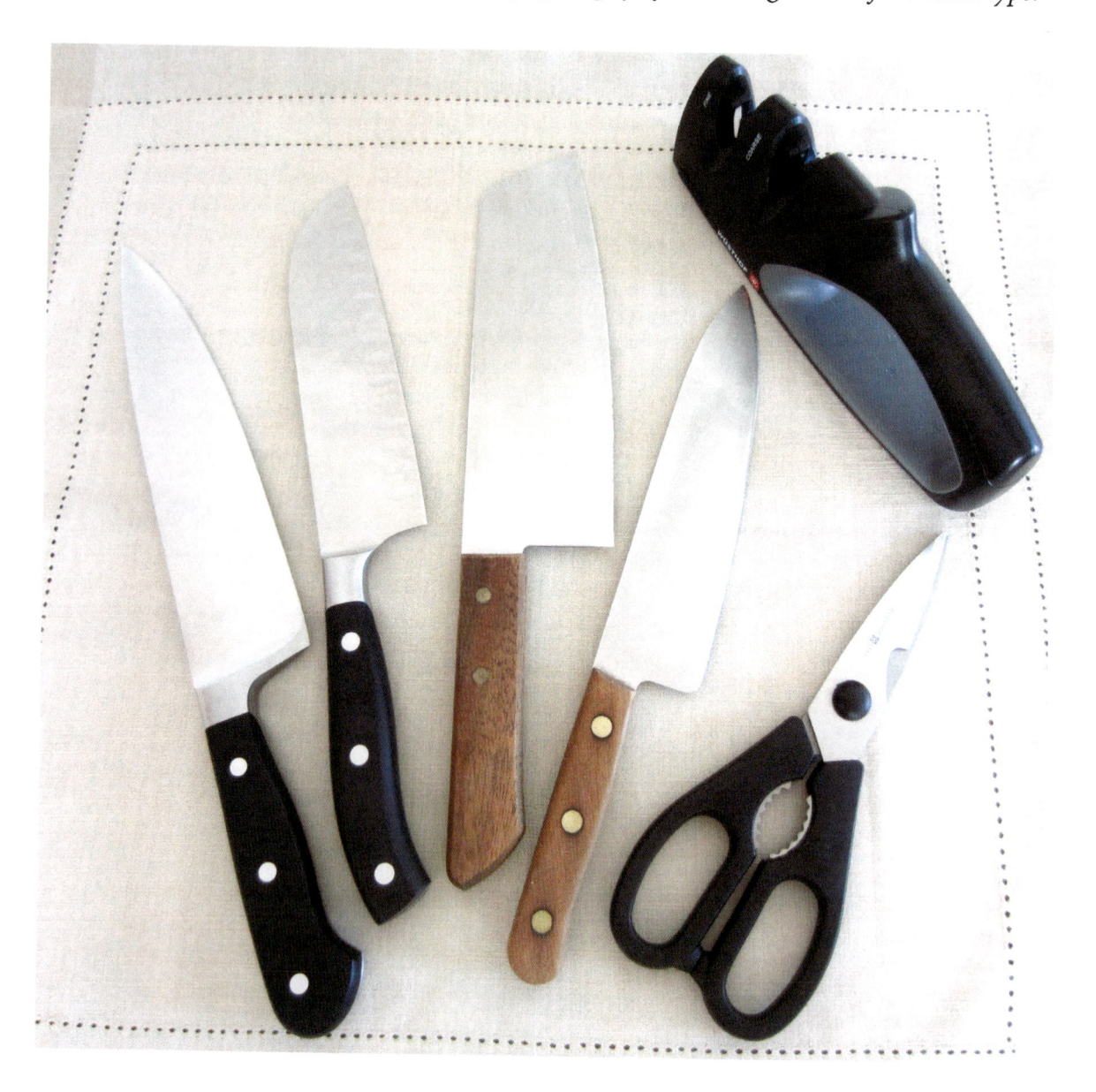

- **Healthy Cookware** – When choosing pots and pans, select cookware that will not react with your food (or only minimally react with your food). Reactivity is based on: the composition of your cookware, cooking temperature (i.e., a higher temperature will increase the rate of reactivity), food composition (i.e., acidic and fatty foods will be more reactive) and time (cooking and storage time in the cookware container)[9]. When using plastic containers for storage, look for containers labeled BPA-Free with the numbers 1, 2, 4 or 5 on the bottom; The Mount Sinai School of Medicine recommends **avoiding microwaving food in ANY plastic containers and avoiding putting ANY plastic containers in the dishwasher**[13]. Research has linked some plastics to causing endocrine disruption which could be a causal factor in cancer. If using a microwave, glass containers have so far proven to be the safest.

Table 10 - Healthy Cookware		
Healthiest - Non-reactive	**Moderately Healthy - Moderately reative**	**Reactive - NOT recommended**
enamel coated cast iron (LeCruset® & Chantel®)	stainless steel (18:10 density)	aluminum
glass (Pyrex®)	cast iron	non-stick, Teflon®, T-Fal®, Silverstone® (toxic fumes are emitted at temperatures over 570°F; chemical coating is susceptible to scratches that can flake into food)
anodized aluminum (All-Clad®, Caphalon®)		copper (excess exposure is considered toxic to the brain and liver)
earthenware & ceramics (test for lead in antique pieces)		
	Utensils	
wooden paddles	stainless steel	plastic
bamboo steamers		aluminum
wooden and stainless steel spatulas and spoons		
	Cold Storage (NOT FOR HEATING)	
glass (Pyrex®)	stainless steel	aluminum foil
paper, wax or butcher (in lieu of plastic bags)		plastics containing BPA (#3, #6, #7)
plastic, BPA free (#2, #4, #5 – (Glad BPA Free, Ziploc® Freezer-safe, double zip) cling wrap (low-density polyethylene/LDPE or PVC-free)		cling wrap containing polyvinyl Chloride (PVC) or Bisphenol A (BPA)

- **Lunch box/Zojirushi ®** - This is a well-made insulated lunchbox from Japan that is fitted with multiple stacked containers inside; it is ideal for soups, rice, vegetables and stews. It will keep your foods hot/warm for hours if you follow the instructions included in the packaging (i.e., pre-warm the outer insulated container with boiling water; the bottom container insert should be filled with soup or other steaming hot dish; the next container should have your vegetable and the top dish should contain your rice or grain. The steam from the bottom container rises and keeps the upper containers warm). The containers are NOT spill proof, so you must be careful to keep the thermos top side up especially when commuting to/from work or school (i.e., don't place it in the trunk of your car or on the car floor where it can roll over on its side).
- **Asian Noodles (Soba versus Udon)** - Soba noodles are traditionally made with buckwheat flour which is gluten-free, but always check the labels to make sure wheat flour was not added. The noodles are thin, dark in color and have a nutty, firm texture. They are often served cold as salads. Udon noodles are thicker, white noodles and made from wheat flour. They are often served in a warm, soy-based broth with scallions and mushrooms.
- **Bread crumbs, gluten free** – You can make your own gluten free bread crumbs by toasting a few slices of gluten-free bread (such as rice-millet blend) and then chopping them in your food processor until they become a coarse crumb; store in a Ziploc® bag or airtight container in the freezer to avoid mold growth.
- **Coconut milk** – Coconut milk can be purchased in most grocery stores in the international food aisle. It comes in 13.5 ounce cans and has a long shelf-life. Once opened, you should transfer unused contents to an airtight container and store in the refrigerator for up to one week. Coconut milk is a good alternative to cow milk, cream or yogurt (with the addition of some lemon juice) in most recipes due to its smooth creamy texture; when used in small amounts, the coconut taste is not noticeable. It is a great addition to quick baked goods, puréed vegetables, porridge and Asian soups.
- **Honey** - Ayurveda believes that raw honey has many benefits including scraping fat and cholesterol from the body's tissues making it the "go to" sweetener for kapha or anyone trying to reduce kapha in their body. However, eating a jar of honey is not going to create weight loss -- ayurveda is about balance so let moderation be your guide. Ayurveda cautions that heating honey above 108°F will render it toxic at the cellular level which could cause blockage of subtle energetic channels. Today we know that when honey is heated its molecular structure changes; it coagulates and becomes sticky. This sticky glue-like substance can clog mucous membranes and arteries leading to cellular toxicity. Heating honey denatures the active enzymes and alters the molecular structure of the chemicals inside[13]… so perhaps the ancients may have been on to something with honey.
- **Manuka Honey** – Manuka honey comes from bees who feed on the flowers of the Manuka bush, (or the "Tea Tree") in New Zealand. It has long been used by the native Maori people for its medicinal properties and its unique, delicious earthy taste. The honey has grown in popularity and there are several systems being used to market and "rate" the bio active potency levels. It is said that a rating over "10" will have therapeutic value and anything less will not; the price increases significantly with the bio active rating. While the marketers quibble over ratings and potency, I'm going to enjoy manuka that fits my budget.

- **Kuzu Root Starch** (Pueraria lobata) – Kuzu root is also called Japanese arrowroot and is sold in small white powdery chunks; use a mortar and pestle to crush the chunks into a powder before measuring. It is a gluten-free thickening agent that will create smooth, glossy, thick sauces for soups, desserts and gravies; it balances the acidity of sweets and can be used in icings, pie fillings, puddings and gelatins. You can substitute in recipes calling for arrowroot powder, corn starch or potato starch. In Traditional Chinese Medicine it is known as ge-gen and was historically used to treat minor indigestion, the common cold, fever and alcoholism.
- **Miso** – Miso is a traditional Japanese seasoning produced by fermenting soybeans with salt and the fungus kōjikin (rice and barley may also be used). During fermentation the protein of the soybeans and grain are disassembled into amino acids, including all nine essential ones. Miso should not be boiled in order to retain the health benefits. When adding to a dish, dissolve the required amount in a little water and add after cooking is complete. White miso is fermented for a lower amount of time and is milder in flavor and less salty than the other darker (yellow and red) varieties. It can be used in soups, sauces and dressings.
- **Mizuna** – Mizuna is a Japanese green with a mild peppery taste (i.e., less peppery than arugula). Its energetic is mildly warming, but generally suitable for all three doshas. It can be used raw in a salad, steamed with some noodles and an Asian dressing, or added to soup. Sometimes I find this at Whole Foods Market®, farmers markets or local food co-operatives; more consistently I find it at Asian specialty stores.
- **Mushrooms, rehydrating** – Try using a French press to rehydrate dried mushrooms; the plunger can be pressed down to keep the mushrooms submerged under the water.
- **Nuts, chopping** – For chopping small quantities of nuts, try using a coffee grinder or spice grinder; for larger quantities, use a food processor.
- **Nut storage/preparation/as a dairy substitute** – It is difficult to judge the quality of nuts in the shell, and some nuts are difficult to shell, so we tend to purchase shelled nuts for convenience and practicality. Nuts purchased from a health food store are typically stored in the refrigerator section and meet their standards of natural processing – inquire at your local health food store for specific details. If you purchase commercially-packaged nuts from a general supermarket, be aware that they may have been processed using ethylene gas, methyl bromide fumigation, hot lye or glycerin/sodium carbonate solution for loosening their skins, and citric acid for rinsing.

The ancients favored almonds (soaked overnight and peeled to eliminate pitta-aggravating qualities in the skin) for their reputed value of building vitality and being easy to digest. These insights are supported today as we know almonds are nutrient dense and are moderately alkaline forming. (Consuming alkaline-forming foods helps to keep your pH balanced). Most other nuts available in the U.S. are primarily of benefit to vata, as they are oily and heavy. Pitta is best with coconuts (and almonds in moderation); kapha should avoid nuts as they will directly increase kapha.

Consider using nuts as an alternative to dairy products (i.e., cheese, milk, butter, etc.). Nuts can be ground to a paste or butter with the addition of a little oil and can be used in place of regular butter in many recipes. Cashews (and almonds) have a mild flavor and are a good place to start when you don't want to alter the taste of your recipe. Nut flours are also becoming more popular as a gluten-free alternative, but they don't rise, so they generally need to be mixed with other flours for baking.

- **Pomegranate Syrup or Pomegranate Molasses** – Pomegranate syrup is a sauce with a sweet and astringent taste. It is made from pomegranate juice concentrate that has been boiled with a sweetener (typically cane sugar) until reduced to a thick syrup. It is used frequently in Mediterranean cuisine and can be purchased at international grocery stores or in the international aisle of major grocery stores.
- **Salt** – There are a wide variety of salts available today to suit every taste and budget. The coarser texture salts are ideal for soups and stews, but a fine texture salt is preferable when seasoning delicate dishes and dips. Rock salt (i.e., Himalayan pink salt) is tri-doshic and an excellent choice. In comparison, table salt is less natural as it is heavily processed (which eliminates minerals) then supplemented with iodine and a chemical additive to resist clumping. The U.S. recommended daily allowance of salt is 2,300 milligrams (1 teaspoon) per day or 1,500 milligrams (~ ½ teaspoon) per day if you are over 51 (or are black, have high blood pressure, have diabetes or have chronic kidney disease).
- **Sesame Seeds** – Sesame seeds appear in Hindu legend symbolizing immortality. Unhulled (brown or black) sesame seeds are high in calcium and a good dairy-free solution to supplementing your calcium intake. When the raw, unhulled seed is crushed, as in tahini or sesame butter, its nutrients are more easily digested. When left whole, the seeds do not break down as well during digestion. Ayurveda recommends chewing a small handful of sesame seeds on an empty stomach each day to support your bones. Today we know that calcium inhibits the absorption of iron, so eating the sesame seeds separately in the morning is sound advice to ensure it does not interfere with absorption of iron[14].
- **Tamari versus Soy Sauce** – Soy Sauce contains wheat while Tamari is "wheat-free" (however, always read labels to make sure the manufacturer did not add wheat and to make certain "traditional brewing" methods were used as this ensures the highest quality). Since they contain fermented alcohol, they should be stored in the refrigerator after opening. Tamari is brewed from whole soybeans, sea salt, water, and koji (Aspergillus hacho). Since it is not diluted with the sweet tasting wheat, it has a stronger flavor than soy sauce; it is traditionally used to season longer cooking food such as soups, stews, and baked dishes. Tamari can be used for marinades, salad dressings and as a condiment or dipping sauce. Tamari is not as heating as salt, so pitta can use it in substitution of salt in many dishes. Kapha should avoid; vata can benefit from tamari.
- **Tamarind paste** – Tamarind paste is made from the fruit of the tamarind tree which was indigenous to Africa, but now grows widely in Asia and Mexico. The fruit is contained in large brown pods that resemble bulbous snap peas. The fruit is extracted from the pods and boiled into a thick, sticky paste, then strained to remove the seeds. The remaining seedless paste is sticky and sour and heating. It is ideal for vata as the sourness aids digestion. Pitta and kapha can use in moderation. Many Thai and Indian dishes use tamarind. You can find seedless tamarind paste in most Asian markets, but they typi-

cally contain some other ingredients (written in an Asian language so I'm not sure what they are!) and have a funny taste. I recommend Neera's® tamarind paste because it's not watered down and has no chemical preservatives or additives; a little goes a long way. Whole Foods Market® and larger supermarket chains carry her brand, or you can order easily online at: cinnabarfoods.com

- **Tomatoes** – Tomatoes are highly acidic so it is best to avoid cooking/storing tomatoes in an aluminum pan/container because aluminum is a reactive metal. The metal reacts with the acid in the tomatoes imparting a bitter flavor to your food along with health concerns related to the aluminum leaching into the food.

I always peel and seed tomatoes. This habit was ingrained by my Italian grandmother who said that the seeds and skin would make the 'gravy' (spaghetti sauce) bitter; she never added sugar to her gravy and it was delicious. It's very easy to do using plum tomatoes; simply chop off ¼ inch from each end of the tomato, then use a sharp vegetable peeler to remove the skins. Slice the tomato in quarters and scrape out the seeds using the sharp point of a knife. If you are using round-shaped tomatoes, you will need to carve out the area where the tomato was attached to the stem, and then peel with a sharp vegetable peeler.

- **Chewing food** – It is important to chew food adequately. Chewing is the first stage of digestion and it preps the food for further processing downstream in the digestive tract. But how much is enough? IDEALLY, you should chew your food until it becomes liquid. This could be anywhere from 20-50 bites, depending on: the quantity of food you put in your mouth and the type of food you put in your mouth (i.e., think of an apple versus steak versus mashed potatoes). This seems like a lot of chewing, especially if you are trying to have a conversation during your meal. I encourage you to try it at least once and observe the effects. This will give you a base line measurement of where you should be. Perhaps a more manageable alternative for time-pressed westerners is to take smaller bites and wait until you have swallowed before taking another mouthful of food; this will slow down your rate of eating and as an added benefit may help you from mindlessly eating beyond the capacity of your stomach.

- **"Dirty Dozen"** – Refers to a yearly study generated by The Environmental Working Group (www.ewg.org) that ranks the pesticide content on a variety of produce. The produce is washed and peeled then analyzed and ranked for pesticide residue. Refer to their website for the most up to date results as this list changes yearly in accordance with varying pesticide use. Generally apples, grapes, berries, celery and leafy greens consistently make the list for their high pesticide residue content. If organic foods are not readily available and/or you feel the cost of organic produce is prohibitive, this list provides an option to limit your exposure to pesticide, by avoiding the foods on the list, or purchasing them from organic producers.

- **GMO/GM Foods** - Genetically Modified Organisms or genetically modified foods refers to foods that used genetically modified seeds. GM refers to a laboratory technique that re-programs a plant with new and/or enhanced properties by inserting gene units into its DNA. These gene units are created by joining fragments of DNA, usually derived from multiple organisms (i.e., the GM gene in herbicide resistant soy beans grown since 1996 is pieced together from a plant virus, a soil bacterium and a petunia plant[15]). Independent, peer-reviewed studies designed to assess longer-term and subtle health effects have not been conducted. The U.S. currently has no labeling requirements for GM foods; however, some companies are voluntarily adding "GMO-free" labels onto their packaging. In addition, foods in the U.S. labeled "100% organic" cannot contain GMO's.

- **Organic** – Foods labeled "organic" in the U.S. meet USDA standards that minimize harm to the environment by emphasizing renewable (or sustainable) resources and the conservation of soil and water, thus protecting the environment for future generations. Synthetic fertilizers, sewage sludge, irradiation, and genetic engineering may not be used. Meat, poultry, eggs and dairy products labeled "organic" must come from animals that are given no antibiotics and no growth hormones (i.e., rBGH or rBST). Meat and dairy products labeled organic in the US cannot have come from animals that have been fed GM food (i.e., GM corn, hay, feed, etc.).
- **Read labels** – Salts and sugars will increase your desire to eat, potentially leading to over eating and the consequential ill health effects. Read labels and look for no-salt/no-sodium alternatives. Opt for low-glycemic index sweeteners such as coconut sugar, brown rice syrup and fruit-juice sweeteners when cooking or when purchasing commercially prepared foods (i.e., jams, dried fruits, baked goods, etc.).

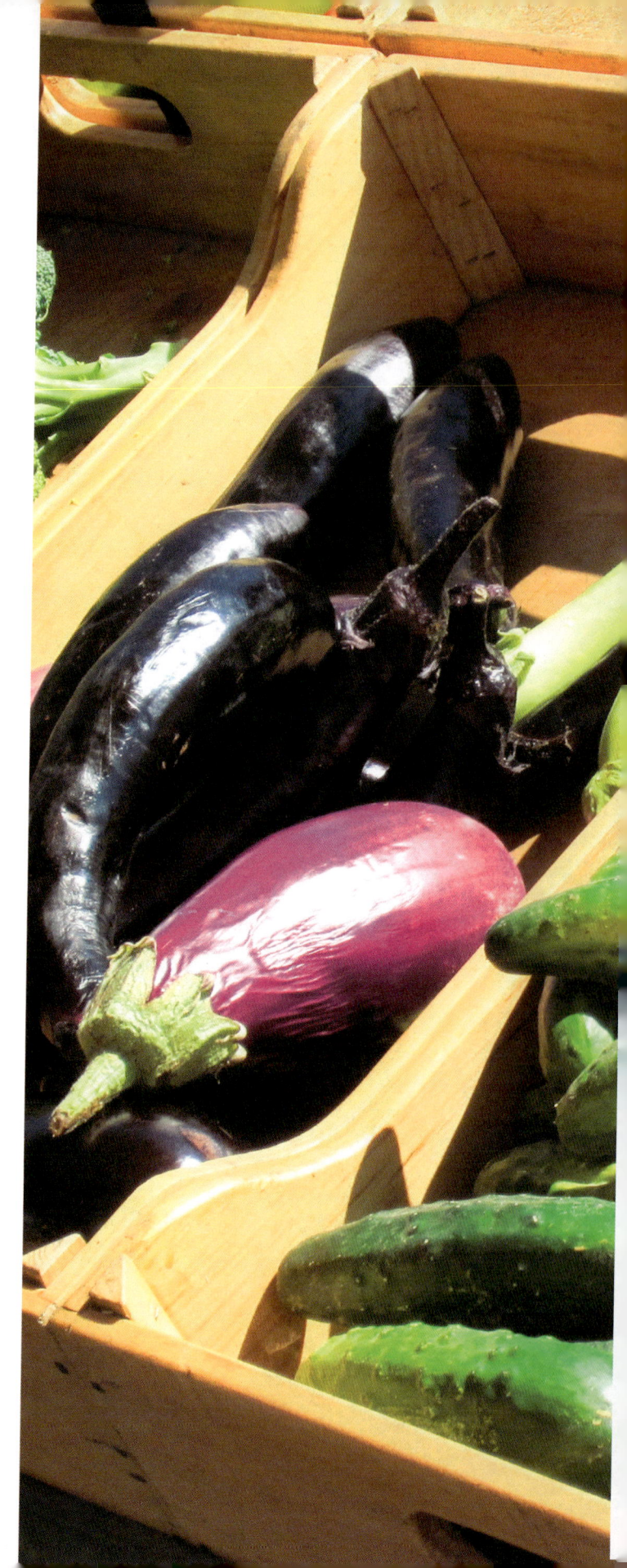

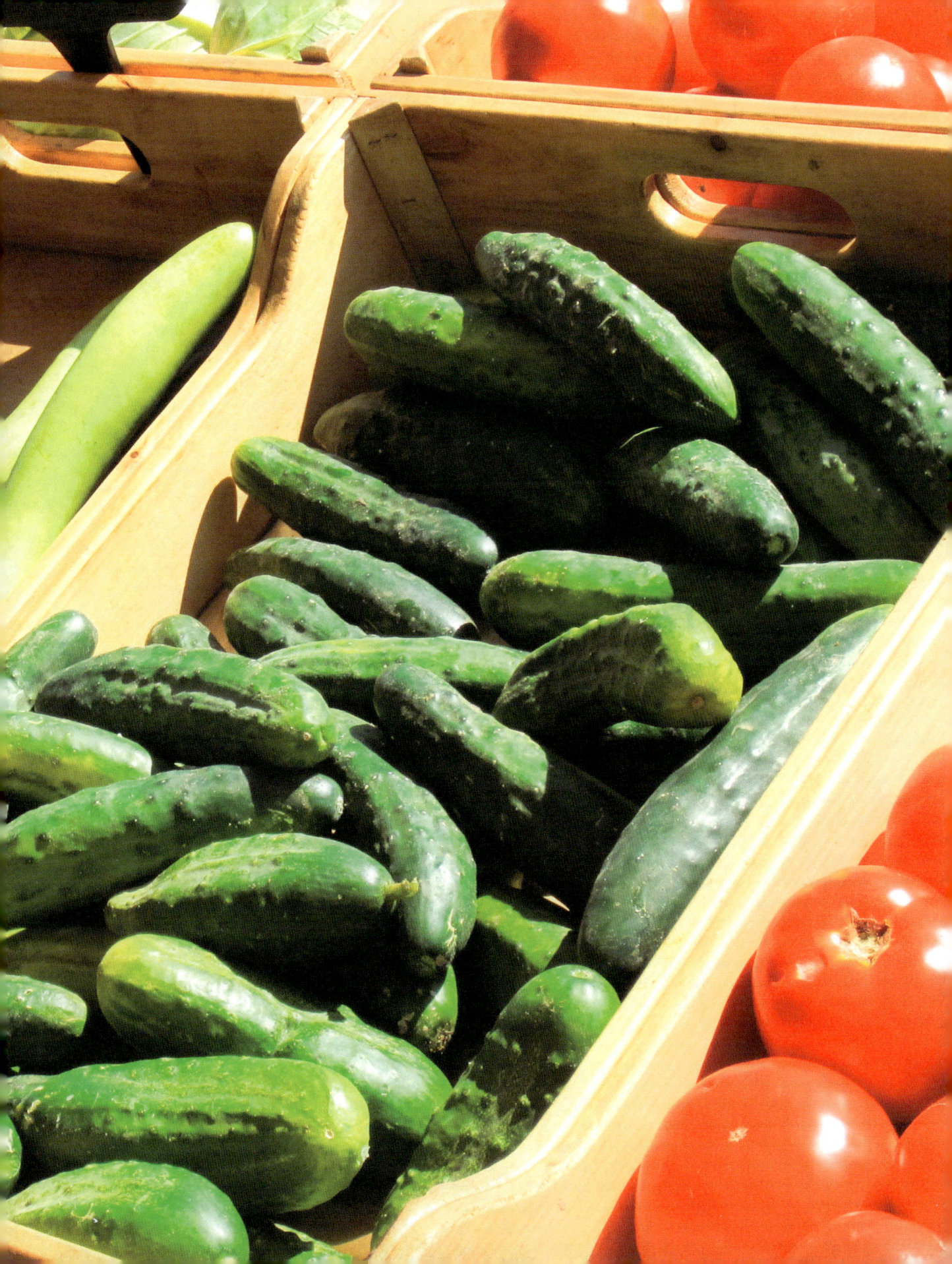

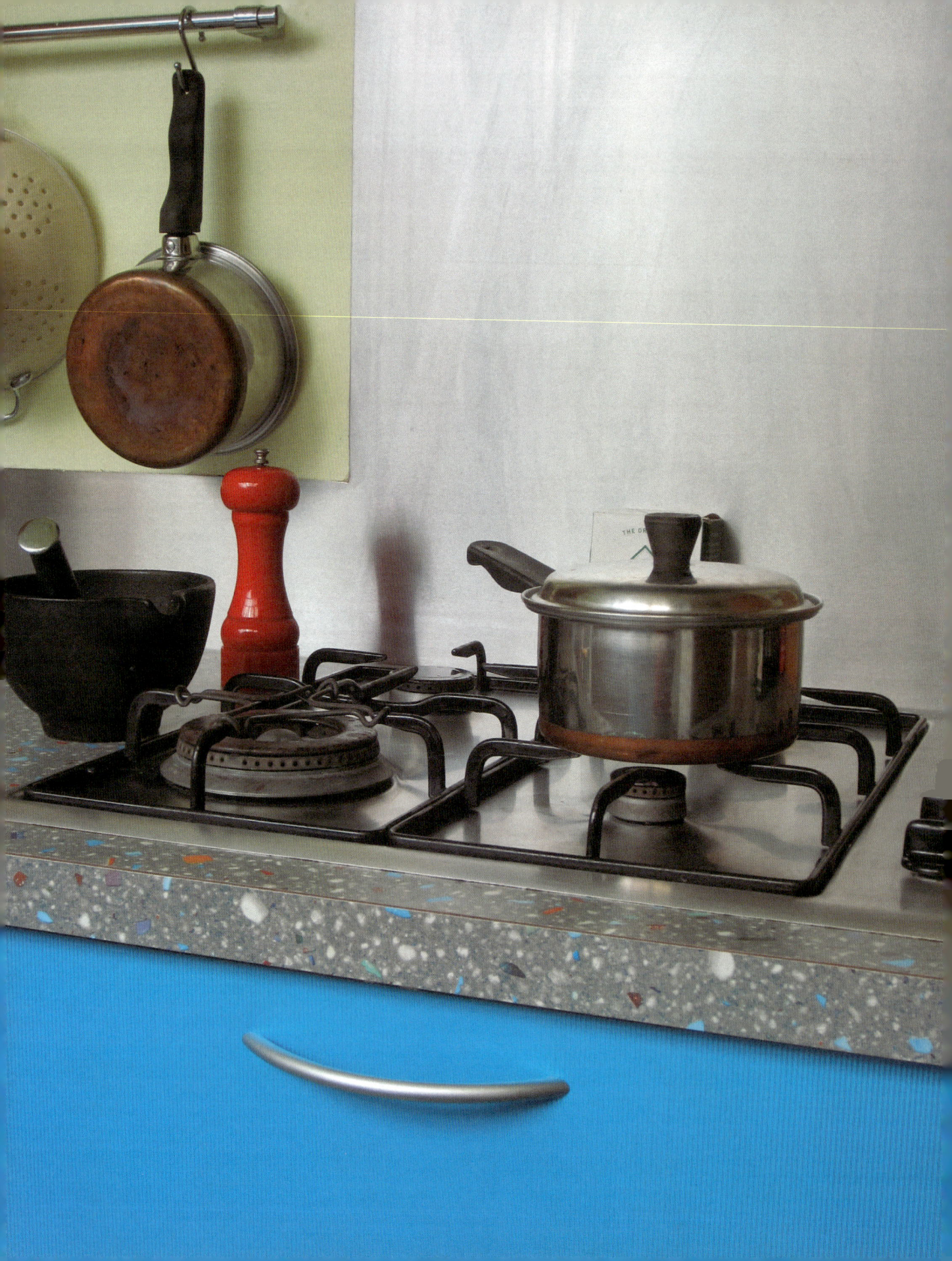

Chapter 8: Let's Cook

Preparing a meal can be a meditation on giving love and healing energy to yourself and those who are eating your food. As you chop, stir and arrange ingredients, affirm your intentions for creating a meal that provides sustenance, health and happiness. I often will chant a mantra during cooking with the express intention of imparting the food with that energy; that energy can then connect with the subtle energy channels of the body. I consider food to be a gift that nourishes life and I always like to offer my gratitude prior to eating the food.

The following recipes were created to be balancing to all doshas or tri-doshic, unless otherwise indicated. In the heading of each recipe is a quick-read code to indicate if the recipe is dairy-free (DF), gluten-free (GF), soy-free (SF), or vegetarian (V). I categorize eggs under "dairy" so please note that a dish labeled "vegetarian" may contain eggs. Also, if a recipe has dairy, but I provide non-dairy alternative in parentheses, then I classify the recipe as "dairy free" because it can be made without the use of dairy. The recipes include the following:

SERVING SUGGESTIONS – I have provided suggested combinations of food to serve with certain recipes to maintain a tri-doshic meal. The serving suggestions will round out the energetics of the dish, especially if that dish is skewed toward one dosha.

VPK – I have indicated condiments, spices and recipe modifications that could be used to target a specific doshas (i.e., I may suggest "add more coconut milk to cool the dish for pitta", etc.).

VARIATIONS – In some of the recipes I will offer substitutions to accommodate gluten-free, dairy-free and meat based diets.

If you read through the entire recipe first, you will get a feel for the flow of the recipe. Some of the recipes have long lists of ingredients/spices, but they generally whip up pretty quickly once all the ingredients have been measured and prepped. I understand that your time is precious so I've indicated when things can be made ahead or frozen for later use; and how to utilize leftovers. If you gradually incorporate the recipes into your life, I trust you will get into the flow of ayurveda in no time.

In testing these recipes, I used a gas stove and All-Clad® pans. Your cooking times and temperatures may need to be adjusted if you use a different heat source and/or pans of differing quality.

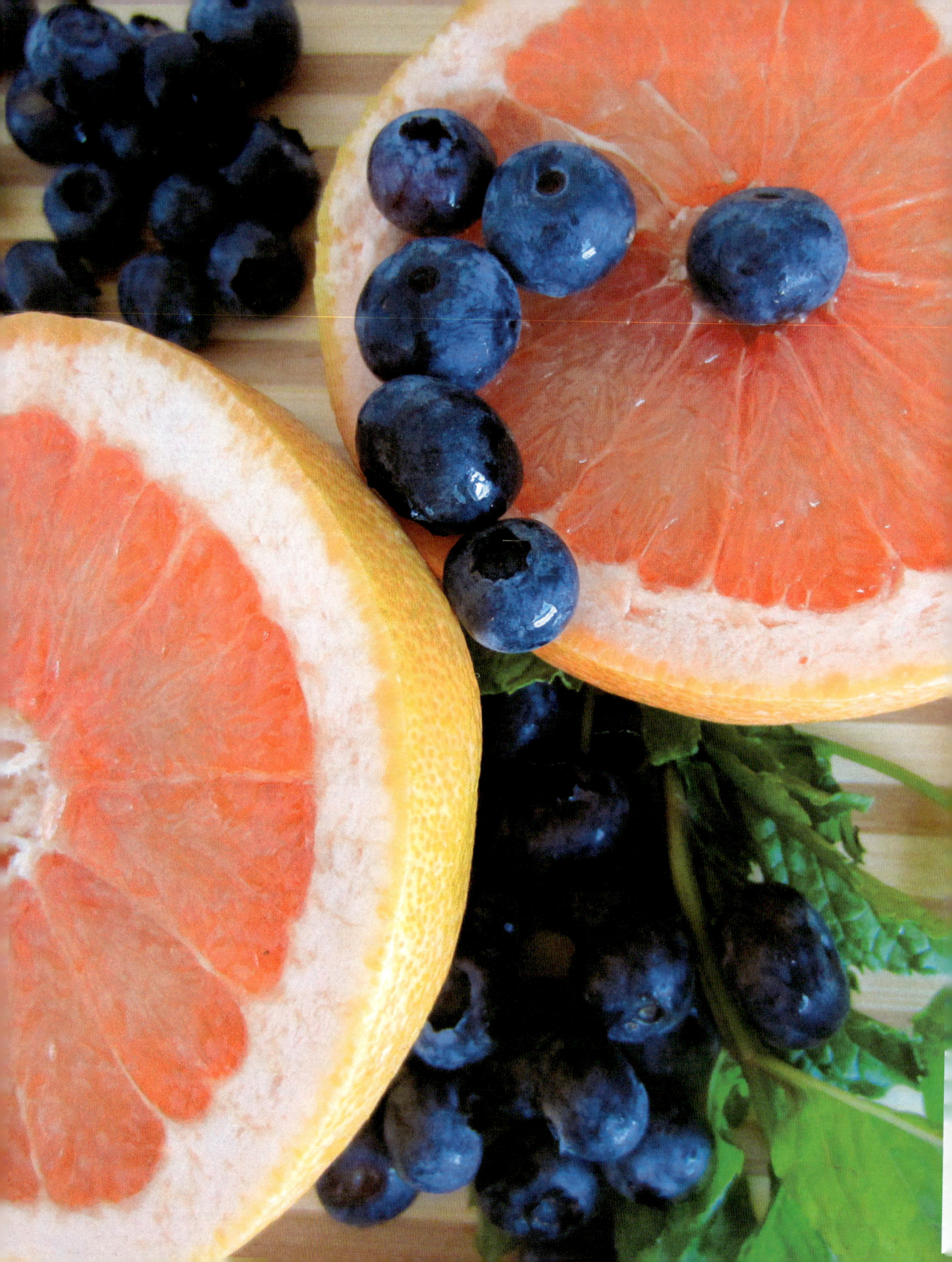

Chapter 9: Morning Meals

If you are working with an ayurvedic practitioner, they will typically prescribe for you some additions to your morning routine to aid with balancing your energy. A simple routine may involve tongue scraping, oil pulling, teeth brushing, yoga, meditation or prayer, self-massage and bathing. This sequential routine helps to set the tone for your day. It's like when you hear your favorite song on the radio and you instantly feel happy; the residue of the song stays with you for hours. The morning routine is important time for you. The length of the routine is less important than the regular commitment; it should be manageable, not stressful. Record it on your calendar as a recurring appointment that has no end date.

After you have completed your morning routine, your body is ready for food. In ayurveda, the morning meal is typically a light meal designed to kindle the digestive fire for the day. Eat according to your appetite and the seasons. In the hot summer months, our digestive fire is generally low so you may feel satiated with a simple bowl of minted fruit (grapefruit, blueberries, apricots, strawberries, etc.) or some home-made yogurt topped with raw honey and granola. Amaranth crepes with pomegranate syrup are suitable for the summer and they are gluten-free. In the cooler fall and winter months you may opt for a warming porridge made from amaranth, quinoa, oats or barley. Or you may want the grounding qualities of eating some protein in the form of poached or scrambled eggs. Lighter, drier variations of porridge (i.e., no added milk, yogurt or sweeteners) are suitable for the wet spring climate when our bodies will be trying to remove excess water/mucus build-up from the winter. The millet breakfast patties are great in the spring as they are dry and light; but they are versatile to be used year round by pairing them with condiments or topping with poached eggs, avocado or sprouts to compliment the seasonal digestive needs.

ॐ Recipes - Morning Meals

- AMARANTH CREPES WITH POMEGRANATE SYRUP
- AMARANTH PORRIDGE WITH PEAR JUICE, CURRANTS & ALMONDS
- YOGURT PARFAIT
- NUTTY QUICK OATS
- SCRAMBLED EGG WHITES
- POACHED EGGS FOR VATA
- MILLET BREAKFAST PATTY
- VATA BREAKFAST BANANA
- ZUCCHINI TRAIL BREAD
- MAPLE ORANGE SCONE
- COCONUT CRANBERRY QUINOA PORRIDGE
- CREAMY YOGURT
- YOGURT LASSI

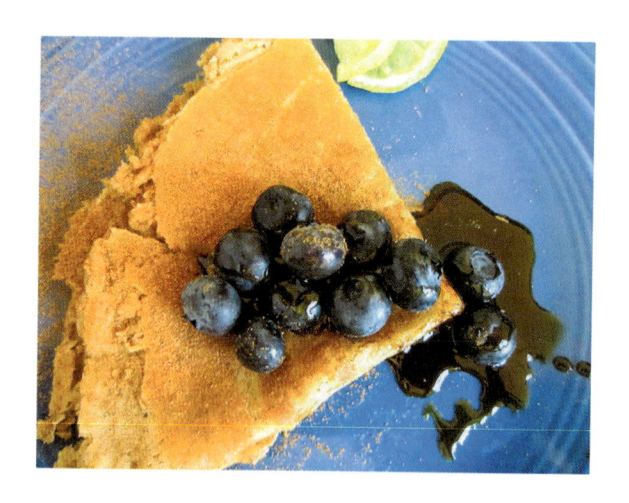

❀ Amaranth Crepes with Pomegranate Syrup
GF/SF/V
Yield: two 10-inch crepes

1 whole egg
1 egg yolk
2 teaspoons pomegranate syrup
4 ounces of coconut milk
(cow, almond or soy milk can be substituted)
2 teaspoons grated lemon rind
⅛ cup amaranth flour, sifted
⅛ cup brown rice flour, sifted
½ teaspoon cardamom powder
(do not substitute)
1 teaspoon cinnamon powder (do not substitute)
⅛ teaspoon Himalayan salt
2 teaspoons butter, melted

Place eggs in a 2½-quart bowl and whisk until frothy. Add the pomegranate syrup, coconut milk and lemon rind, whisking until combined. Add the amaranth flour, rice flour, cardamom, cinnamon, salt and butter, then whisk again until the batter is thin and smooth. **Cover and let the batter set for 10 minutes in the refrigerator.** Remove from refrigerator and whisk briefly.

Pre-heat a 10" non-stick skillet over medium heat. When a drop of batter placed on the pan sizzles, you are ready to cook. Lift the pan off the burner and pour a thin layer of batter into the pan (approximately ¼ cup). Note that it is difficult to have wafer-thin crepes using gluten-free flour; set your expectations accordingly. Gently tilt the skillet in a circular motion to spread the batter evenly across the bottom of the pan. Rest the pan on the heat source and patiently wait.

When the bottom is done, you will see a change in color and the crepe will easily lift from the pan. Test it by running a spatula around the edges. When the spatula can easily slide under the center of the crepe, it will be time to flip (about 2 – 3 minutes). Flip the crepe and cook for 30 seconds on the second side. Remove from pan and place on a warming dish in an oven at 200°F, while preparing the other crepes. Leftover batter can be stored in the refrigerator for up to 3 days, but the amaranth flavor starts to overwhelm the spices with each day.

SERVING SUGGESTIONS: Top with pomegranate syrup, *vata plum compote*, seasonal berries, yogurt, whipped cream or raw honey; garnish with mint leaves, pomegranate seeds, sifted cinnamon powder or lemon wedges.

VPK: The astringency of the amaranth flour and pomegranate syrup is balanced by the sweet rice flour, coconut milk and butter.

VARIATIONS: Try adding ½ teaspoon of almond, orange or vanilla extract.

About: The lemon peel and cinnamon mellow the strong flavor of the amaranth flour. Using butter or ghee will give the crepe a caramel taste and help with browning; this will be lost if you substitute with oil. Making smaller crepes will be easier to flip, but they will be more difficult to fold due to the inflexibility of the gluten-free batter. Have fun making these. The first crepe may be a disaster – but don't fret; it doesn't count; use it to contemplate how to modify your techniques so as to create the causes and conditions for future crepes of higher quality.

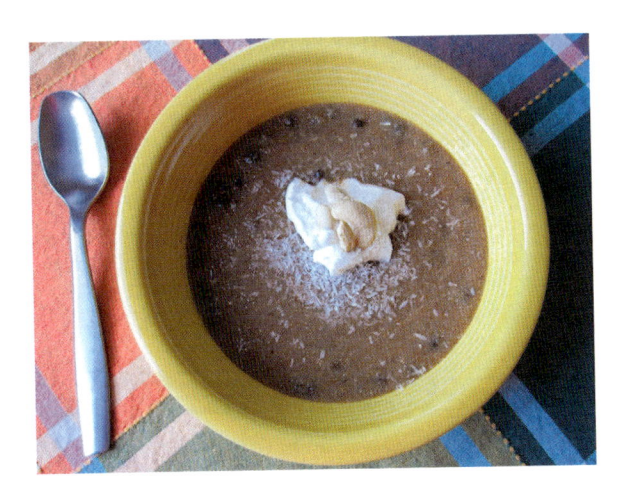

Amaranth Porridge with Pear Juice, Currants & Almonds
DF/GF/SF/V
Servings: 2

½ cup amaranth, rinsed well
½ cup pear juice
½ cup water
¼ cup dried currants (or raisins or apricots)
1 teaspoon cardamom powder
1 tablespoon almonds, blanched and peeled and slivered

Combine the amaranth, water, pear juice, currants and cardamom in a 2-quart pan. Bring to a boil over medium heat stirring constantly. Reduce heat to low, and simmer for 10-15 minutes, stirring occasionally.

SERVING SUGGESTIONS: Top with fresh cream, yogurt, coconut milk, or almond milk.

VPK: Vata can make this more "soupy" by adding more water; kapha may prefer a drier porridge. Vata and kapha can substitute cardamom powder for cinnamon, ginger or allspice. Pitta and vata can substitute toasted almonds for unsweetened coconut flakes.

VARIATIONS: Replace pear juice with water, apple juice, pomegranate juice, orange juice, etc.; substitute currants for dried apricots or dried cranberries.

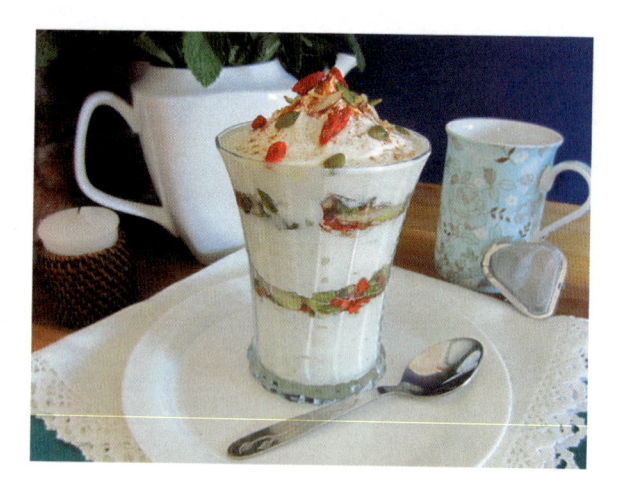

Yogurt Parfait
GF/SF/V
Servings: 1

1 cup home-made unsweetened, plain yogurt
Trail Mix:
>   2 tablespoons pumpkin seeds
>   2 tablespoons toasted almonds
>   2 tablespoons goji berries
>   2 tablespoons sunflower seeds

1 teaspoon honey
¼ teaspoon cardamom
¼ teaspoon cinnamon

Combine the trail mix ingredients in a small bowl and set aside. Spoon 4 ounces of yogurt into an 8-ounce cup. Sprinkle 4 tablespoons of the trail mix over the yogurt, making an even layer. Spoon 2 ounces of yogurt on top of the trail mix; add another layer of trail mix and then yogurt; drizzle the honey on top of the yogurt; sprinkle cardamom and cinnamon on top. Serve.

SERVING SUGGESTIONS: Eat for breakfast or as a mid-morning snack. It is best to avoid eating yogurt after sunset.

VPK: This is grounding for vata and cooling for pitta; pitta could substitute maple syrup for the honey. Kapha can eat on occasion and should add ¼ teaspoon ginger powder to balance out some of the heaviness of the yogurt.

VARIATIONS: Vata and pitta could add shredded, unsweetened coconut; vata and kapha can add dried apricots.

Bulk Nutty Quick Oats
Yield: 10 servings

10 cups quick oats, unsalted
10 tablespoon raisins, unsweetened
10 tablespoon dried fruit-sweetened cranberries, chopped
10 tablespoon coconut, shredded, unsweetened
1¼ cup slivered almonds, toasted
5 teaspoons cinnamon
2½ teaspoons cardamom

Combine all ingredients in Ziploc® bag. Scoop out desired amount as needed and add boiling water to bring to desired consistency. Store in refrigerator for up to three months.

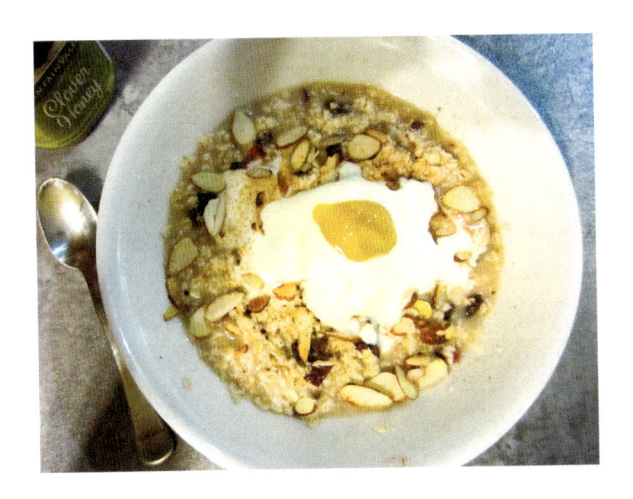

🌸 Nutty Quick Oats
DF/GF/SF/V
Servings: 1

1 cup quick oats, unsalted
1 tablespoon raisins, unsweetened
1 tablespoon dried fruit-sweetened cranberries, chopped
1 tablespoon coconut, shredded, unsweetened
2 tablespoons slivered almonds, toasted
½ teaspoon cinnamon
¼ teaspoon cardamom
1½ cups of water, boiled
1 teaspoon raw honey
3 tablespoons plain yogurt, unsweetened (optional)

In a serving bowl combine the oats, raisins, cranberries, coconut, almonds, cinnamon and cardamom. Add the boiling water to desired consistency and stir; let sit for 1 minute. The oats will absorb the water and become a thick porridge consistency. Adjust the water until you achieve the consistency you desire.

SERVING SUGGESTIONS: Top with the yogurt and honey.

VPK: If you are trying to reduce pitta, you could use coconut sugar or maple syrup in place of the honey; kapha may want to spice it up with the addition of ⅛ teaspoon of powdered cloves.

VARIATIONS: Try adding sunflower seeds, pumpkin seeds or sesame seeds; vata can experiment with different nuts – walnuts, hazelnuts, pecans; variations of the dried fruit are endless – dried apricots, dried blueberries, goji berries, etc. Dried fruit has a different energetic than raw fruit, so while the "rule" is to eat fruit alone, the exception is when the fruit is dried. Dried fruits work well with oatmeal and porridge; bananas and juicy fruits do not.

ABOUT: This can be made ahead in bulk quantity and stored in a Ziploc® baggie for an instant healthy breakfast. Great for travelling when you want a quick breakfast in your hotel room without refined sugar, salt and cholesterol.

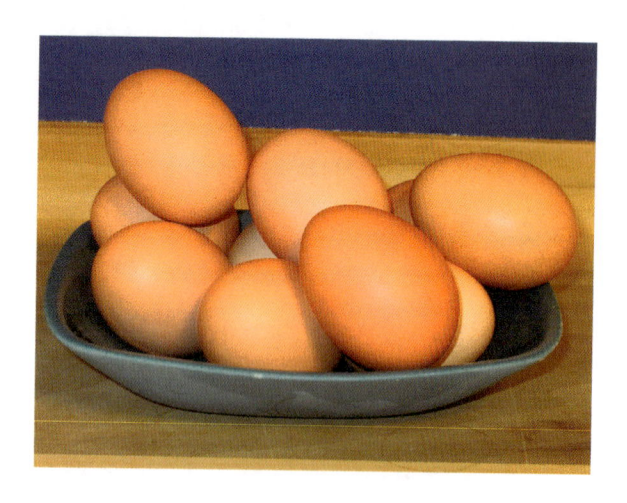

🌸 Scrambled Egg Whites
GF/SF/V
Servings: 1

2 egg whites
2 tablespoons water
1 teaspoon cilantro, chopped

Whisk the egg whites, water and cilantro in a 1-quart bowl. Heat an 8 inch non-stick skillet over medium heat. Pour the batter into the pan and immediately reduce the heat to medium-low. Using a wooden spoon, begin to scrape around the edges of the pan, moving soft, cooked eggs toward the center of the pan. Continue this action of scraping the bottom of the pan and redistributing the cooked eggs toward the center of the pan until all the liquid has been absorbed.

SERVING SUGGESTIONS: Serve with *millet breakfast patty*.

VPK: This is a tri-doshic recipe for breakfast eggs. If cooking for vata solely, then they can use the whole egg as the yolk is warming; due to the cholesterol in the yolk, kapha is generally better with the egg whites only. The cilantro is balancing to all the doshas. Kapha could also add a little Tabasco® Sauce or a side of *kapha hot onion chutney* with their portion.

VARIATIONS: Try adding ¼ cup chopped arugula in place of the cilantro.

🌸 Poached Eggs for Vata
GF/SF/V
Servings: 2

2 eggs
1½ quarts of water

Pour the water into a 2-quart saucepan and heat on medium high to just below boiling. Bubbles should form on the bottom of the pan, but don't let them risen to break the surface. Adjust the heat if necessary.

If your eggs are old, add a teaspoon of white vinegar to the water to help the white coagulate faster, and help the poached egg keep its shape; otherwise, skip the vinegar.

Crack the egg into a small bowl. Transfer the egg into the pan, by slowly sliding the egg down the side of the pan into the water. This helps keep the egg intact. Allow to cook for 3-4 minutes to desired consistency (3 minutes will be soft, longer will be a firmer yolk). Remove the egg with a slotted spoon and transfer to a paper towel-lined plate to drain before serving.

SERVING SUGGESTIONS: Serve on top of *millet breakfast patty*. Top with pumpkin seeds.

VPK: This is best for vata; pitta can eat on occasion and top with cooling cilantro or sprouts; kapha should likewise only have on occasion and should top with sprouts.

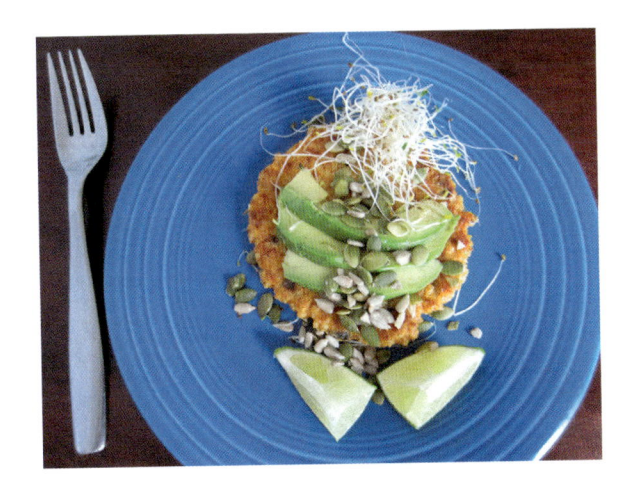

🌸 Millet Breakfast Patty
DF / GF / SF / V
Yield: 4 patties

1 cup leftover *fluffy cinnamon currant millet* (or plain cooked millet or quinoa)
½ cup sweet potato, peeled, boiled and mashed
1 egg, lightly beaten
3 tablespoons arrowroot flour
⅛ teaspoon Himalayan salt
1 tablespoon grapeseed oil (or olive oil)

In a 2-quart mixing bowl, combine the millet, sweet potato, egg, flour and salt. Scoop out ⅓ cup of the batter and form into a patty. Warm the oil in an 8-inch skillet over medium heat. Add a patty to the skillet and cook until the first side is browned. Then flip the patty and finish cooking the second side (about 3 minutes each side).

SERVING SUGGESTIONS: Serve with avocado slices or a *poached egg* or *scrambled egg whites;* top with sunflower or pumpkin seeds or sprouts; garnish with a lime.

VPK: Millet is dry and light so vata will benefit with additional liquid and grounding such as: a squirt of lime juice and slice of avocado or a poached egg; pitta will benefit from the hearty protein of an avocado garnish. Kapha can garnish with sprouts to keep things light and moving – and a squirt of lime for more zest.

VARIATIONS: If you use plain cooked millet or plain quinoa, you should add some seasonings to the patty – 1 teaspoon in total of one or a combination of spices (i.e., cardamom, cinnamon, allspice, etc.).

🌸 Vata Breakfast Banana
GF / SF / V
Servings: 1

1 ripe banana, peeled, cut into ¼ inch slices
2 teaspoons ghee
½ teaspoon coconut sugar
⅛ - ¼ teaspoon each: cinnamon, cardamom, ginger powder

In an 8-inch non-stick skillet, melt the ghee over low heat. Add the sugar, cinnamon, cardamom, ginger and cocoa powder, stirring to combine. Place the banana slices in a single layer on top of the ghee / spice mixture. Cook for one minute. Flip to coat the other side. Cook for one minute. Remove from heat and transfer to a serving dish.

SERVING SUGGESTIONS: This is best eaten alone as a small breakfast, mid-morning snack or afternoon snack.

VPK: Ripe bananas are sweet, but they have a sour energetic effect which makes them heating and mucous forming. They are smooth and heavy so they are ideal for vata. Pitta and kapha should avoid. If pitta or kapha want to eat bananas, they could opt for unripe (green) bananas which are soft, light, astringent, and cooling.

VARIATIONS: Substitute 1-2 tablespoons of molasses to supplement your iron intake.

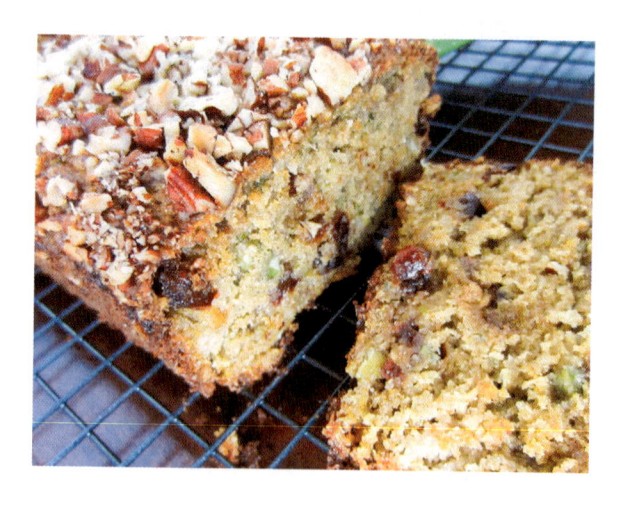

Zucchini Trail Bread
GF/SF/V
Yield: one 8-inch loaf

1 egg
½ cup avocado oil
½ cup coconut sugar (do not reduce)
1 tablespoon grated ginger
3 tablespoons cashew butter
½ teaspoon almond extract
1 cup zucchini, shredded (about 1 small zucchini)
¼ cup amaranth flour
¼ cup arrowroot flour
¾ cup almond meal (or almond flour)
½ teaspoon Himalayan salt
½ teaspoon baking soda
½ teaspoon baking powder
¼ teaspoon cardamom
⅛ teaspoon nutmeg
⅛ cup pumpkin seeds, coarsely chopped
⅛ cup sunflower seeds, coarsely chopped
¼ cup dried cherries, fruit-juice sweetened, chopped
¼ cup almonds, sliced

Preheat oven to 350°F. Lightly grease an 8" non-stick loaf pan.

In a 3½-quart bowl, beat together the egg and oil. Stir in the sugar, grated ginger, cashew butter and almond extract. Add the zucchini. In a 2-quart bowl, sift together the amaranth flour, arrowroot flour, almond flour, salt, baking soda and baking powder. Stir in the cardamom, nutmeg, pumpkin seeds, sunflower seeds and cherries. Pour the flour mixture into the bowl with the zucchini mixture; stir briefly until just combined. Transfer to the loaf pan and sprinkle the almonds on top in a thick layer. Bake about 60 minutes or until toothpick inserted in center comes out clean. Remove from oven and set on a wire rack to cool for 10 minutes. Invert to remove from the pan; cool completely before cutting. Store the bread in an airtight container for up to 3 days.

SERVING SUGGESTIONS: Serve warm with butter. This is a good snack for travel, at the office or any other time you may be missing meals.

VPK: It's heavy, so eat in moderation.

VARIATIONS: Substitute toasted pecans for the almond; substitute chocolate chips for the cherries.

❁ Maple Orange Scone
SF/V
Yield: 5 scones

1½ cups whole wheat pastry flour
2 teaspoons baking powder
¼ cup wheat germ
1 tablespoon flaxseeds
½ teaspoon Himalayan salt
½ cup quick cooking oats
⅜ cup ghee
2 tablespoons maple syrup
2 tablespoons orange zest
2 tablespoons plain whole milk yogurt
½ cup pecans, toasted, coarsely chopped
1 egg, beaten (for glaze)

Preheat the oven to 400°F. Grease a cookie sheet with butter.

Sift together the flour, baking powder, wheat germ and salt. Add the flax seeds and oats, stirring to combine. Add the ghee and combine with a fork until the mixture is crumbly but starting to cling together. In another bowl, combine the maple syrup, orange zest and yogurt. Add the wet mixture to the flour mixture and combine using a fork. Add the pecans, then use your hands to finish working the dough until it becomes soft and firm. The dough should not be sticky; add more flour if necessary. Transfer the dough onto a lightly floured surface and pat down to 1¼ inch thickness. Shape into desired form (triangles, circles, etc.) and place on cookie sheet. Brush top and sides of each scone with the beaten egg. Bake 18-22 minutes until tops are lightly golden and scones feel slightly firm when pressed with finger.

SERVING SUGGESTIONS: This is good for breakfast on the run or with afternoon tea.

VPK: Eat in moderation by all three doshas.

❁ Coconut Cranberry Quinoa Porridge
DF/GF/SF/V
Servings: 2

½ cup quinoa, rinsed
1½ cups water
1 tablespoon coconut, shredded, unsweetened
½ teaspoon cinnamon (or cardamom)
1 tablespoon dried cranberries (or currants, raisins, dried cherries, dried apricots), chopped
½ teaspoon lemon juice
1 teaspoon honey

In a 1½-quart sauce pan, combine the quinoa, water, coconut and cinnamon and bring to a boil. Reduce heat to simmer; cover and cook for 20 minutes, stirring occasionally, until the grains are soft. For a thinner consistency, add more water. Remove from heat and top with cranberries and honey. Leftovers can be refrigerated overnight and reheated the next day.

SERVING SUGGESTIONS: Stir in plain yogurt for a creamy porridge. Add almond, rice or soy milk for a dairy-free creamy porridge. Garnish with fresh mint.

VPK: Quinoa is considered tri-doshic but I find it to be drying. I feel the addition of the yogurt or milk adds some balance for vata.

VARIATIONS: Add sliced, blanched almonds, pumpkin seeds or sunflower seeds for a heartier breakfast. Other dried fruits and nuts can be added as per the **dosha diet aids** in the appendix. Bananas and fresh fruit would not be an optimal combination here. You can vary the recipe substituting quinoa for amaranth or using half amaranth and half quinoa.

❀ Creamy Yogurt
GF/SF/V
Yield: about 28 ounces

1 quart (32 ounces) whole milk, raw or regular pasteurized
¼ cup (2 ounces) plain organic yogurt (I prefer Siggis®)

1 candy thermometer
32 ounce glass jar with lid, sterile and dry

Pour 3 cups of water into the bottom of a double boiler pan; pour the milk into the top of the double boiler and heat to just below boiling (about 185-190°F). Stir the milk slowly for 20 minutes (to make thinner yogurt, cook for 10 minutes). Turn off heat and let the milk cool until it is tepid warm/115-120°F (about 15 minutes); if a skin forms on the top of the milk as it cools, remove and discard the skin. Whisk in the yogurt.

Incubate in a warm place for 4-7 hours (refer to the table "Incubation Methods" in *about making yogurt*). Place in a refrigerator to cool for **about two hours** before using. Yogurt can be stored for up to 1 week in the refrigerator.

SERVING SUGGESTIONS: Fresh yogurt is sweet and can be served with sweet blueberries, dried fruits and toasted nuts. The yogurt can be spiced with cinnamon, cardamom or ginger to reduce mucus formation. Honey is a good sweetener, especially for kapha. Use in a *yogurt lassi* or as a cooling condiment for pitta with dal dishes.

VPK: Great for vata and pitta; kapha should use in moderation and add warming spices.

❀ Yogurt Lassi
Servings: 1

½ cup of home-made yogurt
½ cup of water

Savory Lassi/vata
¼ teaspoon cumin powder
1 teaspoon cilantro
pinch salt

Sweet rose lassi/pitta
2 drops rosewater
½ teaspoon maple syrup

Spicy lassi/kapha
½ teaspoon ginger powder
⅛ teaspoon cinnamon
⅛ teaspoon cardamom

Combine the yogurt, water and seasonings (savory, sweet or spicy) and mix well. You can use an immersion blender, a whisk or shake in a jar with a covered lid.

🍴 About Making Yogurt

Yogurt is fermented whole milk that has been cultured with live bacteria. The following steps are involved in making yogurt[16]:

1. Heat the milk to just below boiling (about 185-190°F) to change the structure of the protein molecules.
2. Allow to cool to a temperature that will be friendly to the live cultures – about 115-120°F.
3. Add the live cultures. You can either use store-purchased yogurt or a starter culture.
4. Incubate the cultures at 115°F (see incubator options below). The cultures will feed on the sugar in the milk (lactose) creating lactic acid. The lactic acid causes the milk to coagulate slowly. If the coagulation is too fast, it will curdle the milk. The optimal temperature for the bacteria to grow is 115°F. Incubate for 4-7 hours at approximately this temperature.
5. Place in refrigerator to cool for **about two hours** before using. The Lactobacillus will continue converting lactose to lactic acid until the temperature reaches 41°F; at that time Lactobacillus will become dormant.

The cultures remains active between 98°F and 120° F. The ideal temperature is 115°F.

	Incubation Methods	
Heating Pad Incubator	**Wide-mouth thermos Incubator**	**Yogurt Maker**
2-quart glass, wide-mouth jar with lid	2 quart thermos	
Thin cotton towel		
Electric heating pad		
Pour fermenting milk into the jar and close tightly; wrap the towel around the jar and the heating pad around the towel; secure towel/heating pad in place with thick rubber bands; turn to the low setting on the heating pad. Remove wrappings when finished.	Pour fermenting milk in the thermos and close the lid tightly. After six hours, remove the lid and put the jars in the refrigerator to complete the process.	Follow instructions per manufacturer.

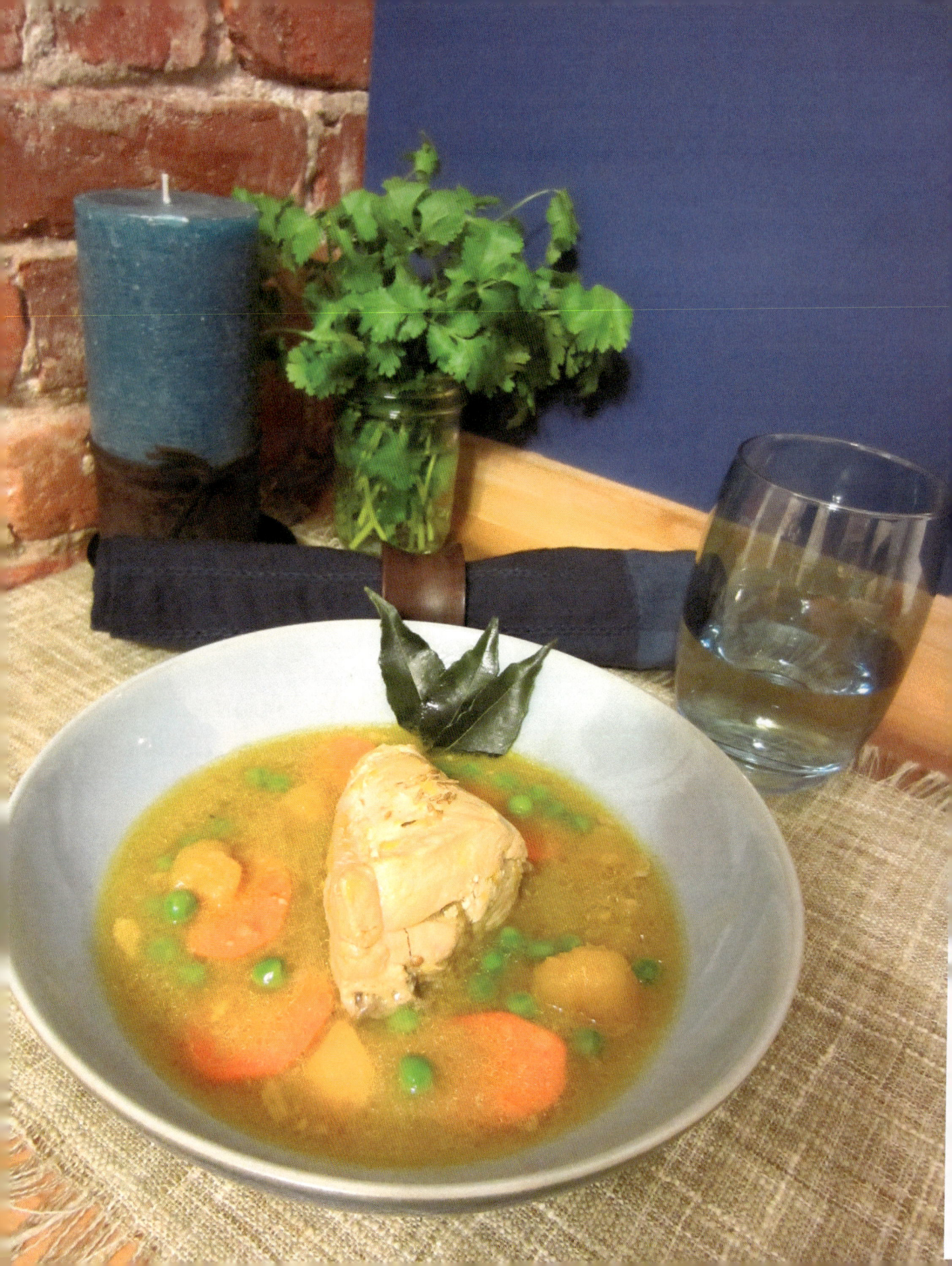

Chapter 10: Midday Main Meals

The main meal should be eaten around noon (11:30am – 1:30pm). This is when the digestive fire is strongest so plan accordingly. If you are eating animal protein, which tends to be heavy and requires several hours for proper digestion, this is the optimal time for consuming. Likewise, if you are new to eating lentils and beans, you may want to introduce them into your diet midday when the digestive fire is strongest.

Tips for the Aspiring Vegetarian

I was not raised in a vegetarian household, so it took me many years to be able to digest lentils and I am still unable to digest beans on a regular basis without experiencing some digestive discomfort. Lentils and beans tend to be dry, light, rough and cold, which you may recall is identical to the vata constitution. So vata needs to add moisture (i.e., water, broth), warmth (i.e., spices) and oil (ghee, coconut oil, sunflower oil, etc.) when preparing beans or lentils to improve digestibility. Vata especially should not skimp on the ghee/oil when cooking lentils and beans; their dryness can be balanced out by liberal amounts of the opposite quality (oily). If you are new to lentils and beans, I would recommend the following guidelines (especially if you are vata constitution or have a challenged digestion system):

1. **Soak lentils and beans overnight in water**. When you ingest lentils/beans, they travel through your digestive system absorbing water. This can create dryness and lead to constipation, gas and bloating. As the beans soak, they absorb the soaking water, so use clean, filtered water; if there is any soaking water left, you should discard the water and use fresh water for cooking.
2. **Experiment with lentils in soup and combine with meat**. Lentils are easier to digest than beans. Cooking them in a soup or stew provides added moisture that will help your body acclimate to the dryness of the beans. Combine them with a small amount of meat to add warmth and grounding.
3. **GO SLOW**. Start by incorporating a lentil dish into your diet one day a week for the first month. If you have no problems with this (i.e., no constipation, gas, belching, bloating, malabsorption, etc.), then you can introduce another day of lentil/beans the next month and continue until you are eating lentils/beans as many days a week as you desire. If you have problems, try different recipes and smaller quantities of beans. Consult your ayurvedic practitioner for assistance.
4. **Drink a lot of water throughout the day**. Lentils are drying and it may take some time for your body to adjust.

Due to your cultural habituation, it may be extremely difficult to convert to a 100% vegetarian diet without experiencing (major) imbalances to your system. I've been trying for years and always seem to become quite depleted if I abstain from meat for more than a week. I have yet to find the protein shake or supplements that will not upset my digestion/elimination. I feel like I've tried everything. At one point, I even consulted with my astrologer in desperation. Perhaps out of a sense of compassion, he informed me that my planetary positions predisposed me to eating meat, saying I would have much difficulty with a vegetarian diet. I told him about a classmate who teased me that I would return as a butcher in my next life because of my meat eating now. So he told me a story about a butcher who became a saint…conceivably there is some hope for me yet!

Chakrapani explained that if a person is raised vegetarian, then they have no problem abstaining from meat in their diet. But if one is not raised vegetarian, then SOME people may have difficulty in adjusting to a diet that is 100% vegetarian. Chakrapani, like my ayurvedic doctor and teacher, is a strict vegetarian (no meat, fish or eggs) but he suggested eggs as a good starting point for people trying to reduce meat who feel a need for extra protein. Consuming lighter meat such as fish and chicken, would also aid in the transition from animal protein.

I hope these tips help you to find a balance that will work for your body. I continue my quest for supplements that my body will tolerate and will be happy to make a switch someday.

Legumes: Lentils, Dal & Beans

Lentils

Lentils are an edible pulse/bean and part of the legume family. They are dried and are available throughout the year. They are sold prepackaged (in boxes or bags) or in bulk form. Prepackaged lentils should be in undamaged packaging with no signs of moisture damage. When buying in bulk, be sure that the lentil bins are covered. Lentils should be fairly uniform in size and color, and they should be free of insect damage (i.e., no small pinholes in the lentils, cracked or broken pieces). Lentils should be stored in an air-tight container out of the sunlight in a cool, dry place for no more than six months (assuming that most lentils have potentially already been in storage at the store or in a warehouse for up to six months). After one year, the color of lentils will fade and they will dry out, taking longer to cook. Do not mix newly purchased lentils with older lentils in your cupboard because the old lentils will be dryer than the ones you just purchased, resulting in uneven cooking times.

Lentils have good nutritional value, containing dietary fiber, B-vitamins, protein and are low in calories. To prepare lentils, sort and remove any debris or stones and rinse under cold water. Place in a pan of boiling water and cook (uncovered) until tender. (See **Table 11 – Lentils, Dals, Beans** for cooking times using the boiling method.)

The lentils used in this cookbook can be found in most grocery stores, health food stores, international grocery stores and specialty stores. Lentils cook much faster than dried beans and they do not require pre-soaking. However, if your digestion is sensitive or if you are new to lentils, you may want to pre-soak every bean and lentil (except red lentils which would turn to mush during pre-soaking) to aid digestion.

The lentil recipes in this cookbook primarily use: Puy lentils/French lentils and red lentils. I find these the easiest to digest, with a nicely balanced flavor and super easy to cook. They cook in 10-20 minutes, making them perfect for when your time is tight and you need a quick meal. Start with the lentil recipes in this cookbook and I trust you will be a lentil lover in no time.

Puy lentils are grown in a region in France called "Le Puy" that has mineral-rich volcanic soil. The lentils are nutrient dense and have a mild, peppery smell. They are pricey, so a great alternative for the budget conscious are "French" green lentils which are a tad less earthy. I use Puy and French lentils interchangeably in this cookbook; the difference in taste is comparable to substituting a California sparkling wine for French champagne. Note that "French lentils" are not the same as "green" lentils (or dried green peas), even though French lentils have some green in their coloring; when purchasing, look specifically for a label that says "French lentils" or "Puy lentils". In terms of energetics, they are a little dry, a little heavy and slightly heating. Vata loves these in soups; pitta and kapha will find a salad of French lentils to be most balancing. *French lentil salad with lemon vinaigrette* is a nicely balanced dish suitable for all the doshas (vata can apply liberal amounts of the vinaigrette). They retain their shape after cooking and are ideal in soups, stews, casseroles and cold salads.

Red lentils do not need any pre-soaking (in fact, they must not be pre-soaked); they will cook in 10 minutes. They are delicate and do not hold their shape when cooked and instead turn to mush. That's how you know they are done; so don't be upset that your red lentils didn't stay round. They are best added to soups to lend texture or add protein. In spite of their mildly peppery flavor, they are sweet, cooling and light making them ideal for pitta. Vata needs to add warming spices and ideally eat them in stews or soups; kapha likewise needs to add spice to warm them up. Check out the *Moroccan veggie burger recipe* made with red lentils; gluten-free, dairy-free and soy-free – it will please everyone!

DALS

Beans or lentils that have been split and had their outer shells removed are called "dal". This refining of the bean improves the digestibility and taste, but it decreases the nutritional benefits (especially the fiber content). Dal generally cooks quicker than beans, but not as quickly as lentils. Dals

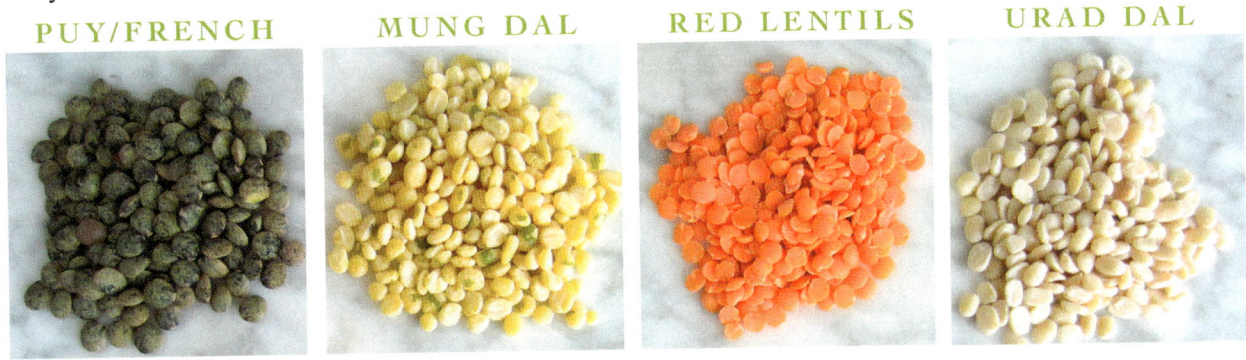

PUY/FRENCH   MUNG DAL   RED LENTILS   URAD DAL

tend to lose their shape and become creamy after cooking. They are typically used in soups, stews, salads and desserts. In this cookbook, I have included recipes for mung dal, urad dal and tur dal which I find to be the most flavorful and easiest to digest for the aspiring vegetarians or those with sensitive digestion. Mung dal is available at most supermarkets in the international or bulk foods aisle. Urad dal and tur dal is generally only found at Indian or Asian supermarkets.

To prepare dal, sort and remove any debris or stones. Rinse the dal several times until the water runs clear. Place one cup of dal in a four cup bowl and cover the dal with fresh, filtered water; soak for two hours or overnight. The dal will absorb the water and expand. Drain the dal. At this point, you can cover and place in the refrigerator for later use (for up to a week). So every Sunday night I soak some dal; on Monday morning, I drain it and place in a covered container in the refrigerator. At some point during the week, I am happy to find some pre-soaked dal in the refrigerator that I can whip up into a tasty meal. To cook the dal, place it in a heavy-bottom stainless steel pan with 3 cups of water. To aid digestibility you may want to add any of the following to the cooking water: turmeric (⅛ teaspoon), 1 bay leaf, a pinch of hing powder or a 1-inch piece of kombu (edible kelp). The bay leaf or kelp should be removed prior to serving. You may add a teaspoon of oil to the water to keep the water from boiling over during cooking. Bring the water to a boil, then reduce heat to medium and simmer uncovered until the dal is tender.

Alternatively, you may cook dal using a pressure cooker, which will reduce cooking times, or use a slow-cooker and cook the lentils overnight. (See Table 11 – Lentils, Dals, Beans for cooking times using the boiling method.)

Mung Dal (or moong dal or yellow dal or split hulled green gram) is commonly used in ayurveda cooking. It is used to kindle a weak digestive fire or to give the digestive system a rest. Mung dal is sweet, cooling, light and nutritious. Mung dal soup is often given after an acute illness to aid recovery. Kitchari is a traditional mung bean/rice dish that is delicately spiced according to dosha and eaten during restorative and cleansing therapies to heal the digestive system. Mung dal cooks relatively quickly with minimal soaking. However, if you are new to lentils or have a fragile digestive system, you may want to soak overnight.

Note: Whole mung beans are green and readily available in most U.S. supermarkets, whereas the split, hulled yellow mung dal may require a visit to an international market, food co-operative or health food store. You can purchase fresh, organic split mung dal online at http://www.banyan-botanicals.com/. If you decide to substitute mung beans in a recipe calling for mung dal, the mung beans will require overnight soaking and a longer cooking time. The mung beans are heavier than the mung dal and will be more difficult for vata (or someone new to eating beans) to digest. Recipes in this book use the split mung dal because that variety is considered balancing for all constitutions.

Tur dal (or toor dal or split pigeon pea) is heavy, heating and astringent. It is yellow in color and sometimes it is packaged with an oil coating (which is used as a preservative). Tur dal is excellent for vata and kapha; pitta can eat in moderation with cooling spices and light side-dishes. Tur dal takes about one hour to cook using the boiling method. I have adapted a traditional *tur dal Bangalore sambhar* recipe to be tri-doshic and spiced to a western palate.

Urad dal (or white dal or Urid dal or split hulled black matpe bean) is heavy, sweet and heating. When cooked, it becomes creamy, heavy and grounding containing lots of protein and iron; ideal for vata, pitta can eat in moderation, kapha needs to add lightness. They can be heavy to digest, so should be prepared with heating spices (i.e., garlic, ginger cayenne and tamarind).

They have a distinct earthy taste and are rich in vitamins. In India, urad dal is used in curries, soups, idlis (steamed breakfast cakes) and dosa (a fermented, stuffed lentil pancake). I first experimented with urad dal when I was feeling exhausted on one of my vegetarian stints. My supportive friend from India recommended I eat urad dal which he described as the food of the mythical figure Lord Hanuman – a vegetarian monkey-God with otherworldly strength! He shared with me his favorite recipe of *urad dal with tamarind* which I've adapted and included here. I'm still not vegetarian, but I do love my urad dal! Urad dal is most suitable for vata. Pitta can eat in moderation (with a cooling chutney). Kapha on occasion (with lots of heating spices to lighten the dal). Urad dal takes 60-90 minutes to cook using the boiling method.

BEANS

Beans tend to be hard, heavy, rough, dry and cooling, well-suited for balancing pitta and kapha, but potential digestive torment for vata and those new to beans. The best way for vata to eat beans is in a soup, where the added moisture and warmth of the broth will balance the dry, cold qualities of the beans. The beans used in this cookbook (aduki, black, garbanzo and white beans) are readily available in cans where they have been rinsed, pre-soaked and cooked. Read the labels to find the brands packaged with the least amount of salt/sodium and no preservatives. I also look for cans that were manufactured without the use of BPA. Canned beans will often be cooked with kombu (kelp) which is a natural digestive aid that doesn't impart any flavoring on the beans; I prefer this to the cans that have added sodium. The pre-cooked canned beans are a huge time-saver. If you opt to purchase dry beans, then you must pre-soak overnight and cook for a minimum of one hour if using the boiling method, so understand that additional planning is involved. (See "*Table 11 – Lentils, Dal, Beans*" for recommended cooking times.) If you are new to beans or have a sensitive constitution, try the soup recipes such as *puréed lemon garbanzo soup*.

Aduki (or adzuki or red beans) – Aduki beans are astringent and cooling with a pungent post-digestive affect. They are often sweetened and used in Asian desserts or added to rice or Caribbean flavored stews. You can add a handful to a vegetable soup recipe for instant protein. Try the *Caribbean aduki bean stew* during the fall or winter months; or the *aduki bean squares*.

ADUKI BLACK CANNELLINI GARBANZO

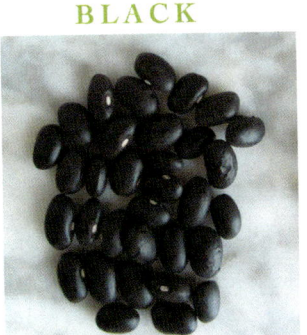

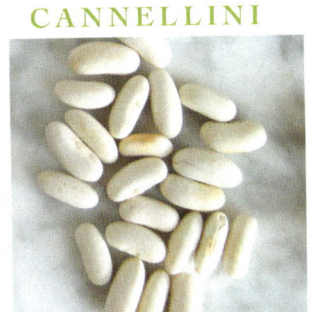

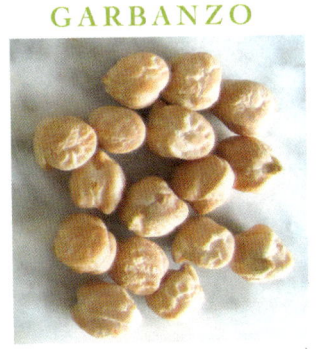

Black beans (or black turtle beans or Mexican beans) – Black beans are astringent, cooling and hard to digest so best for pitta and kapha. They are popular with Caribbean (i.e., allspice, cinnamon, nutmeg, cloves, ginger, etc.) and Mexican seasonings (i.e., cilantro, oregano, chilies, cumin, lime, etc.) and are often used in burritos, salads and stews. They can also be combined with garbanzo beans and puréed to make hummus by adding desired seasonings.

Cannellini beans (white kidney or Italian kidney) – Cannellini beans are astringent, cooling and hard to digest; best for pitta and kapha. They are used frequently with Italian seasonings (i.e., basil, oregano, marjoram, garlic, sage, rosemary, thyme, parsley, bay leaves, etc.) and are nice additions to soups, stews and salads. They can also be puréed to make a hummus.

Garbanzo beans (chickpeas) – Garbanzo beans are astringent, cooling and hard to digest; best for pitta and kapha. They are used frequently with Mediterranean seasonings (i.e., bay leaves, basil, cardamom, lemon, mint, cilantro, cloves, cumin, cinnamon, fennel, oregano, paprika, thyme, etc.) and are nice additions to soups, stews and salads. They are puréed with sesame seeds, lemon juice and garlic to make a traditional hummus dip.

Table 11 - Lentils, Dals & Beans

	LENTILS		**DALS**			**BEANS**			
	Puy or French	Red	Split Mung (yellow)	Split Tur (Pigeon Peas)	Split Urad (white)	Aduki	Black	Cannellini	Garbanzo (Chickpeas)
Best for VPK	vata and kapha	pitta	VPK	vata and kapha	vata	pitta and kapha	pitta and kapha	pitta and kapha	pitta and kapha
Sorting & Rinsing	required	required	required	required	required	required	required	required	required
Soaking	2 hours	none	overnight	overnight	overnight	overnight	overnight	overnight	overnight
Retain Shape	yes	no	no	no	no	yes	yes	yes	yes
Cooking Time* (Boiling Method)	20 minutes	10 minutes	20 minutes	60 minutes	60-90 minutes	50-60 minutes	75-90 minutes	60-90 minutes	120-240 minutes
Digestion Aid	During cooking add one or more of the following: a bay leaf, a 4" strip of kombu, a pinch of hing; aspiring vegetarians can start by experimenting with beans in soups for highest digestibility factor.								
Tips	Soak beans in three times their volume of filtered water; do not add salt or acid (i.e., vinegar, lemons or tomato juice) while cooking as this increases cooking time; after soaking, drain and change the water for cooking; bring to a boil, then simmer until done; skim the foam from the top of the pan during cooking if desired. *High altitude (above 3,500) feet will require longer cooking times								

GRAINS & SEEDS

AMARANTH

Amaranth is an ancient plant that dates back to the Aztecs, who used it as a food staple and in religious ceremonies. It is a complete protein that contains all nine essential amino acids that our bodies do not produce and in the correct proportions that are necessary to support the repair of tissues and organs. Amaranth is high in protein, iron, calcium, B6 and magnesium. The slightly astringent and bitter tasting seed of the plant is harvested for consumption; it must be cooked to obtain the nutritional benefits. It can be popped to make puffed amaranth for cereals or sweets; it can be added to soups, cooked as a breakfast porridge or made into tabbouleh salad by replacing the bulgur. It is gluten-free. Store in an air-tight container in the refrigerator or freezer for up to 6 months.

MILLET

Millet is an ancient plant that has its origins in Africa and Asia. There are many varieties and pearl millet is what is typically found in US markets. The seed is harvested and must be cooked to obtain the nutritional benefits; it is rich in protein, calcium, iron and manganese. Those with thyroid disease should not consume millet in large quantities as it is a mild thyroid peroxidase inhibitor[17]. Millet is dry, light and heating, so it is ideal for a kapha constitution; best moistened for vata and cooled for pitta. You can use millet in porridge, soups, stews, or as a crunchy addition to muffins and breads. It is gluten-free. Store in an air-tight container in the refrigerator or freezer for up to 6 months.

QUINOA

Quinoa (pronounced "KEEN-wah") is a complete protein containing all nine essential amino acids in the correct proportions that are necessary to support the repair of tissues and organs. It is a good source of manganese, magnesium, iron, tryptophan, copper, phosphorus and riboflavin (vitamin B2). Quinoa is coated with saponins (naturally-occurring bitter-tasting plant chemicals) that can be removed by rinsing. Due to its high oil content, quinoa should be stored in the refrigerator or freezer to avoid becoming rancid. Quinoa is readily available in most markets and I recently found organic red and white quinoa online at WalMart®. All varieties have a light, nutty flavor, but I find the white to be the "lightest", the red is a little heavier and the black the most dense. The darker colors are better for vata as they are more grounding and warming. The price of quinoa seems to increases with the color (the white color being the least expensive and black the most), so if you are on a budget and want to try the red or black quinoa, you may substitute ½ white quinoa with ½ of the darker quinoa and still have a delicious tasting dish.

BARLEY

Barley is a cereal grain that is rich in fiber and selenium; it is a good source of phosphorus, copper and manganese. It is sweet, cooling and light with diuretic properties, making it ideal for kapha and pitta. It can be purchased in most grocery stores (check the bulk bin section) and typically comes in one of three forms: hulled – the outer hull has been removed; it is a whole grain that is brown in color and requires more soaking and cooking, but has more nutrients and is very chewy; pearl barley – refined and "polished", it has a white color, has a lower cooking time and is less chewy, but it has less nutrients; pot/scotch barley – is slightly refined/polished to remove the outer hull, so it is not technically a whole grain, but it maintains a lot of the nutrients (more so than the pearled barley). Barley has been labeled a "gluten-grain" so one should consider this if they have allergies to gluten. Barley will absorb a lot of water so if you make a soup, only put a small handful in the water, otherwise you will end up with thick barley porridge. If using whole grain barley, you should soak it overnight prior to cooking; it will require 1 hour of cooking time. To save time: soak the barley on Sunday night; on Monday morning, cover and place in the refrigerator until ready to use in a recipe anytime later in the week. Barley can be used in a breakfast porridge, in a soup with root vegetables or in a warm salad seasoned with heating spices.

RICE

White rice is sweet and cooling and generally best for vata and pitta; long grain rice is drier and short grain rice is moister, more starchy and softer (better for vata). White basmati rice is considered tri-doshic. Brown rice is heavy and heating, making it more suitable for vata. Purple rice (forbidden rice or black rice) and red Bhutanese rice are sweet and chewy with a nutty flavor; they are warming and best for vata, but pitta can cool things down with the addition of unsweetened shredded coconut or serve with a coconut curry sauce. Wild rice is actually a grass. It is dark brown in color and very chewy. It is high in protein and has a warm and rough energetic. It is quite dense on its own, and is usually balanced by mixing with other varieties of rice.

Table 12 - Rice Cooking Chart

	Basmati Rice	Bhutanese Red Rice	Brown Rice (long grain)	Brown Rice (short grain)	Forbidden (purple/ black rice)	White Rice (long grain)	White Rice (short grain)	Wild Rice
Uncooked	½ cup	½ cup	½ cup	½ cup	½ cup	½ cup	½ cup	½ cup
Soaking Time	15 minutes*	none	none	none	none	none	none	5 minutes
Water	1 cup	¾ cups	1⅛ cups	1 cup	¾ cup + 2 tablespons	¾ cup	1 cup	2 cups**
Cook Time	12-15 minutes	20 minutes	35-40 minutes	40-45 minutes	30 minutes	20-25 minutes	20-25 minutes	40-50 minutes
Rest Time	10 minutes	5 minutes	5 minutes	5 minutes	5 minutes	5 minutes	5 minutes	5 minutes
Yield	1 cup cooked	1 cup cooked	1 cup cooked	1 cup cooked	1 cup cooked	1 cup cooked	1 cup cooked	1½ cups cooked

*after soaking, drain the rice and discard the soaking water
**wild rice will not absorb all the cooking water; it will burst open when it is done; drain after cooking

Basic rice cooking instructions (absorption method)
Rinse and soak rice (if necessary). For ½ cup of uncooked rice: in a 1½-quart sauce pan, combine rice, water and seasonings; bring to a boil. Reduce heat to simmer and cook, covered with a tight fitting lid so steam does not escape. Follow cooking times indicated in **Table 12 - Rice Cooking Chart**. Remove from heat and check for doneness. If the rice is still crunchy, add a few tablespoons of water and continue to cook for a few minutes until soft. When done, remove from heat, cover and let "rest". Fluff and serve.

Basic rice cooking instructions (rice cooker method)

Same as the absorption method except combine the rice, water and seasonings into the rice cooker; cover and switch on. When the cooker switches to the warm setting, check for doneness. If the rice is still crunchy, add one or two tablespoons of water and stir the rice; cover and allow to finish steaming on the warm setting for 10 minutes or until the rice is the desired consistency. Fluff and serve.

ॐ Recipes - Midday Main Meals: Legumes, Grains & Seeds

- KITCHARI
- BANGALORE TUR DAL SAMBHAR
- KERALA INSPIRED TUR DAL
- GUJARATI WEDDING DAL
- URAD DAL WITH TAMARIND
- PURPLE COCONUT RICE
- SPANISH SAFFRON RICE
- MEXICAN RICE
- JASMINE COCONUT RICE
- PUY LENTIL ARTICHOKE IN PUFF PASTRY PIE
- MOROCCAN VEGGIE BURGER WITH TANGY TAMARIND SAUCE
- BAKED FALAFEL BALLS
- PITTA KAPHA CANNELLINI KALE ARTICHOKE SAUTÉ
- DRY FRY TOFU
- LIME GINGER TOFU
- LIME GINGER MARINADE
- RED QUINOA WITH ENDIVE & CRANBERRIES
- FLUFFY CINNAMON CURRANT MILLET (PITTA/KAPHA)
- MINTED APRICOT COUSCOUS
- MILLET MASH
- POLENTA WITH SHIITAKE SAUCE
- SHIITAKE SAUCE
- BARLEY SAUTÉ WITH SWEET POTATO, ASPARAGUS & BURDOCK ROOT
- MARCO'S PORCINI RISOTTO

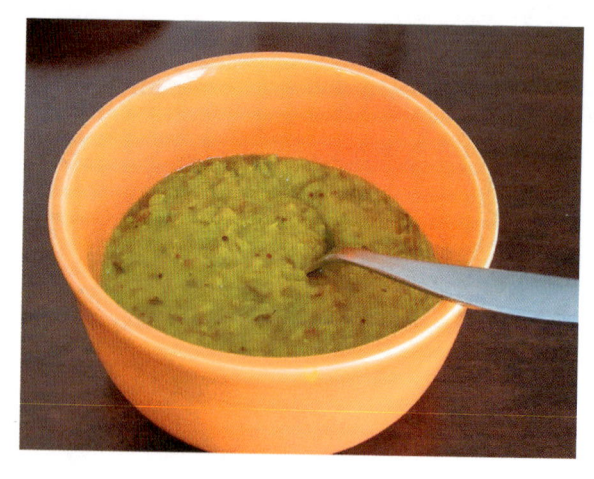

KITCHARI
GF/SF/V
Servings: 2

2 teaspoons ghee
1 teaspoon cumin seeds
¾ teaspoon fennel seeds
¾ teaspoon coriander seeds (lightly crushed with mortar and pestle)
¼ cup split peeled mung beans (soaked overnight to reduce cooking time)
¼ cup basmati rice
1½ cups water
½ teaspoon turmeric powder
½ teaspoon cumin powder
1 bay leaf
½ teaspoon Himalayan salt
¼ teaspoon pepper
1 tablespoon cilantro

Melt the ghee in a 2-quart sauce pan on medium low heat. Add cumin, fennel and coriander seeds. Cook until you hear the seeds "pop" (about 30 seconds). Then add the beans, rice, water, turmeric, cumin and bay leaf. Bring to a boil, stirring to combine. Reduce heat to low and simmer loosely covered until done. Check the pan after 20 minutes, then every few minutes until the beans are soft and the kitchari consistency is to your preference (from soupy to "dry"). You may need to add water if the beans don't cook fast enough, in which case, you may want to adjust (increase) the spices. Remove from heat and stir in the salt, pepper and cilantro.

SERVING SUGGESTIONS: Serve with steamed, seasonal vegetables.

VPK: If cooking solely for vata or kapha you can add ½ teaspoon black mustard seeds, ⅛ teaspoon ajwain, ½ teaspoon chopped ginger or ¼ teaspoon garlic when cooking the spices. You may sprinkle your *dosha-specific churna* on top.

ABOUT: This recipe is tri-doshic. It is intended to be a light dish that is easily digested. It can be eaten for breakfast, lunch and dinner to give the digestive system a rest for a day. If one's digestion is very sensitive, reduce the mung beans to ⅛ cup. If one has a strong digestion and appetite, substitute brown rice for the basmati rice.

Bangalore Tur Dal Sambhar
DF/GF/SF/V
Servings: 3

½ cup tur dal (stones removed, soaked overnight and drained)
3 cups water
1 bay leaf

1½ cups Yukon potatoes (peeled, cubed to ½ inch size)
1 cup tomato, peeled, seeded, chopped
½ teaspoon Himalayan salt
2 cups water
¼ cup coconut, shredded, unsweetened (fresh or frozen)
½ teaspoon thin, green chili, seeds removed, chopped
½ teaspoon garlic
1 teaspoon cumin powder
¼ cup cilantro, coarsely chopped

1 tablespoon ghee or safflower oil
1 teaspoon black mustard seeds
1 teaspoon urad dal

In a 3½-quart pan cook the dal with water and 1 bay leaf on medium heat until the dal is soft and creamy (about 1 hour). Watch the water level and add more water if it begins to dry out. When the dal is cooked, drain the water, discard the bay leaf and return the dal to the pan. Add the potatoes, tomato, salt and 2 cups of water to the pan of dal and bring to a boil. Reduce heat to low and simmer for 15-20 minutes until potatoes are soft. Remove from heat.

Place coconut, chilis, garlic and cumin in a blender with ¼ cup of water. Grind until smooth; add to the dal mixture and stir well. Add the cilantro and mix.

In an 8-inch fry pan, heat the ghee over low heat. Add the mustard seeds and urad dal. Fry until you hear the mustard seeds pop and the urad dal is golden about 30 seconds (be careful to not overcook the mustard seeds as they burn easily and will make the dal taste bitter). Stir this mixture into the dal and serve.

SERVING SUGGESTIONS: Serve with basmati rice, *cool coconut chutney* or *pitta cooling date chutney*, cucumbers, and steamed vegetables or salad of mixed greens.

VPK: Tur dal is ideal for vata as it is heavy and heating; the cool potatoes add balance for pitta; kapha benefits from the spices.

❁ Kerala Inspired Tur Dal
DF/GF/SF/V
Servings: 3

1 cup toor (or tur) dal (stones removed, soaked overnight, drained)
3 cups water
¾ teaspoon turmeric
1 bay leaf

2 cloves of garlic, peeled with skins removed
1 tablespoon ginger, peeled
⅛ teaspoon Himalayan salt
1 tablespoon ghee (or sunflower oil)
1 teaspoon cumin seed
½ cup tomato (peeled, seeds removed, finely chopped)
5 tablespoons chopped shallot (or red onion)
8 curry leaves (fresh or dried)
2 tablespoons shredded coconut (unsweetened), fresh or frozen
1 teaspoon green chili (seeded and diced) or ⅛ teaspoon cayenne pepper
¼ cup cilantro leaves, coarsely chopped

In a 2-quart pan, combine the dal, turmeric, bay leaf and water. Bring to a boil and cook until the dal is soft (about 50-60 minutes). Stir occasionally; monitor the water level while cooking and add more water if necessary to keep the lentils from drying out. The final product will be a thick porridge-like consistency. While the dal is cooking, prepare this spice sauce:

- Pound the garlic and ginger with the salt in a mortar to make a paste.
- In a 10" fry pan, melt the ghee over medium heat. Add the cumin seeds and cook until you hear them "pop" (about 30 seconds). Add the tomato, shallot, curry leaves, coconut and green chili, stirring until well combined. Cook for about 8 minutes then add the garlic-ginger paste and sauté for a few more minutes. Using your immersion blender or coffee-grinder, grind into a thick paste, adding a little water if necessary.

When the dal is done, remove and discard the bay leaf. Pour the spice sauce into the pan of dal; add the cilantro; stir to combine.

SERVING SUGGESTIONS: Serve with brown rice or chapattis and *cool coconut chutney* for pitta and *kapha hot onion chutney* for kapha; add a side of steamed greens for a balanced meal.

VPK: Tri-doshic with recommended chutneys and steamed greens.

ABOUT: Coconut is widely used in many forms (oil, milk, pulp, etc.) in southern Indian cooking. It is believed to have medicinal and therapeutic value including: increasing vitality; providing nourishment to the brain and nervous system; and anti-parasitic and anti-bacterial properties. Coconut has a cooling energetic and will offset the spicy taste of the chilies. This version of dal is quite mild in comparison to the fiery dals I had in Kerala, but I think it is more balancing to a western palate (and certainly if one is aiming for a tri-doshic dish).

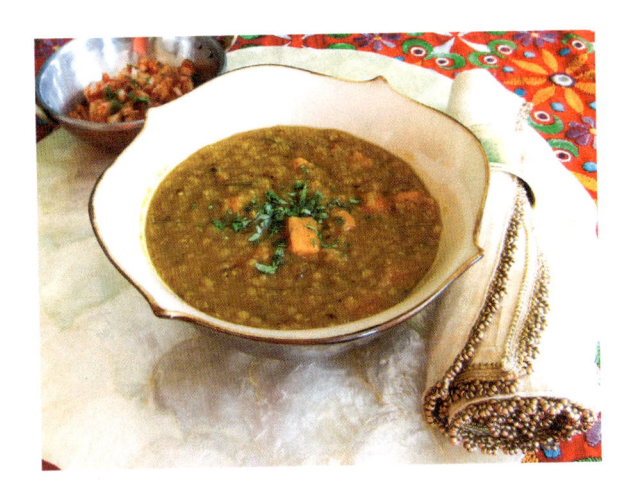

❀ Gujarati Wedding Dal
DF/GF/SF/V
Servings: 4

1 cup red lentils and 2½ cups water
½ cup yam, peeled and chopped
2 medjool dates, seeded, coarsely chopped
1½ cups water
1 tablespoon ghee (or sunflower oil)
¼ teaspoon cumin seeds

Spice Mix (combine in a small bowl):
- ¼ teaspoon fenugreek seeds
- 7 curry leaves
- 3 cloves
- 1 cinnamon stick (or 1 teaspoon cinnamon powder)
- 1 bay leaf
- 1 teaspoon green chili, seeded, chopped

1 cup water
½ teaspoon Neera's® tamarind paste
¼ cup tomatoes, peeled, seeded, finely chopped
2 teaspoons ginger, peeled, minced
¼ teaspoon chili powder
½ teaspoon turmeric powder
1 teaspoon Himalayan salt
2 tablespoons coriander, chopped

In a 2-quart sauce pan, cook the lentils in the water until soft (about 10 minutes). Drain and return the lentils to the pan. In a 1½-quart sauce pan, combine the yam and dates with 1½ cups water. Cover and cook until the yams are par-boiled (about 15 minutes). Transfer the contents (including the water) to the pan with the lentils and set aside. In a 10-inch fry pan, heat the ghee over medium heat. Add the cumin seeds. Listen for the seeds to pop (about 30 seconds), then add the spice mix; sauté for a few seconds. Add 1 cup of water, tamarind, tomatoes, ginger, chili powder, turmeric and salt. Mix well and bring to a boil. Reduce heat and simmer for 10 minutes, stirring constantly. Pour this spice sauce into the pan containing the dal mixture. Warm on low heat, stirring to combine; add the coriander and mix.

SERVING SUGGESTIONS: This sweet and slightly sour dal can be served with basmati rice, *fluffy cinnamon currant millet*, *GF corn bread* or roti and steamed green vegetables, and lime wedges. *kapha hot onion chutney* will balance for kapha.

VPK: The sweet, cooling dates make this dish ideal for vata and pitta; when served with above suggestions, it is also balancing for kapha.

VARIATIONS: If cooking for vata alone, add ⅛ cup of toasted cashews to the yams during cooking. For any dosha: substitute tur dal for red lentils (soak dal overnight and increase cooking time to 60 minutes).

ABOUT: This is an adaptation of a traditional sweet and sour dal recipe served at Gujarati weddings. I have modified the ingredients/spices due to availability and to be more balancing. Don't let the ingredient list put you off; the dish whips up quickly.

Urad Dal with Tamarind
DF/GF/SF/V
Servings: 4

2 cups split urad dal (soaked overnight)
4 cups water
1 bay leaf
¼ teaspoon cayenne

1 tablespoon coconut oil (or ghee)
½ teaspoon garlic, pressed
2 teaspoons cumin seed
2 teaspoons coriander seed, crushed
8 curry leaves (optional, but they add a really nice flavor if you use them!)
2 tablespoons Neera's® seedless tamarind concentrate
½ teaspoon turmeric powder
½ teaspoon Himalayan salt
2 tablespoons cilantro, chopped

Combine the soaked dal, cayenne and bay leaf with 4 cups of water in a 3-quart pan and bring to a boil. Reduce heat to medium and cook for 60-90 minutes, or until dal is soft and creamy and the lentils have started to lose their shape. Remove from heat and discard the bay leaf.

In an 8-inch fry pan, melt the coconut oil over medium-low heat. Add the garlic, cumin seeds, coriander seeds and curry leaves. Sauté for a few minutes then reduce heat to low and add the tamarind sauce, turmeric and salt. Stir until combined and remove from heat. Pour the spice mixture into the dal mixture. Purée with an immersion blender. Add cilantro; stir to combine.

SERVING SUGGESTIONS: Serve with basmati rice and steamed vegetables and *dosha specific chutneys*.

VPK: This mildly spiced dish is suitable for all doshas. Urad dal is heavy and warm; pitta can eat on occasion with extra cilantro or a side of *cool coconut chutney*. Kapha can add extra cayenne and a side of *kapha hot onion chutney*.

VARIATIONS: Add 1 teaspoon of chopped chili and/or 2 teaspoons of fresh chopped ginger to the spice mixture for additional flavoring.

Rice Variations:

Purple Coconut Rice (**vata and pitta balancing**) – Follow directions for making ½ cup of purple rice, adding 5 teaspoons shredded coconut to the pan before cooking. For vata only: may also add toasted nuts (pecans, almonds, walnuts) after cooking. Pitta (or vata) can also add cilantro or serve with *pitta cooling date chutney*.

Spanish Saffron Rice (**vata and pitta balancing; kapha can eat on occasion**) – Follow directions for making ½ cup of white long-grain rice, adding the following ingredients to the pan before cooking: a few strands of saffron, ¼ teaspoon paprika, ¼ cup chopped onion, ½ teaspoon olive oil and ¼ teaspoon Himalayan salt. Stir until well combined then cook; optional: toss with ¼ cup of steamed peas after cooking.

Mexican Rice (**vata and kapha balancing; pitta can eat on occasion**) – Follow directions for making ½ cup of white or brown long-grain rice, adding the following ingredients to the pan before cooking: ¼ cup tomatoes (peeled, chopped, seeded), ¼ cup chopped onion, ½ teaspoon jalapeno chili (seeded and diced), ¼ teaspoon sunflower oil, ¼ teaspoon Himalayan salt. When the rice is done, add 2 tablespoons chopped cilantro.

Jasmine Coconut Rice (**vata and pitta balancing**) – In a rice cooker combine: ¼ teaspoon sunflower oil, 3 tablespoon minced onion, ⅛ teaspoon salt, 6 tablespoon coconut milk, ¾ cup water, 1 tablespoon shredded coconut with ½ cup of jasmine rice. Turn on the cooker.

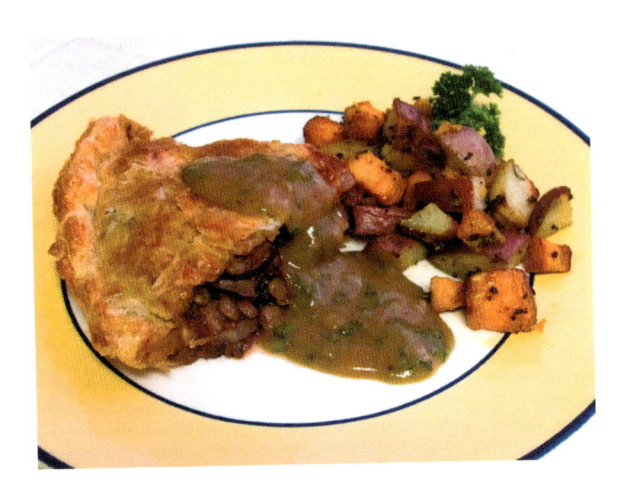

🍀 Puy Lentil Artichoke in Puff Pastry Pie

SF/V
Servings: 4

14-ounce can artichoke hearts packed in water, drained, thinly sliced
⅓ cup shallots, peeled, chopped
1½ tablespoons ghee (or olive oil)
2½ cups Portobello mushrooms, chopped
½ teaspoon fresh rosemary, chopped fine
¼ teaspoon dried tarragon
4 ounces water
1 tablespoon lemon juice
1 cup tomatoes, peeled, seeded, minced
1 tablespoon tomato paste
½ cup Puy lentils (or French green lentils), cooked
18 ounce puff pastry, thawed*
1 medium egg (to glaze pastry)
¼ teaspoon Himalayan salt
¼ teaspoon pepper

Preheat the oven to 400°F. In a 3-quart sauté pan, sauté the artichokes and shallots in ghee over medium-heat until softened and slightly golden. Add the mushrooms, rosemary and tarragon, stirring to combine. Add the water, lemon juice, chopped tomatoes and tomato paste. Reduce heat and simmer until sauce has thickened. Add the cooked lentils, salt and pepper, stirring to combine. Remove from heat and set aside.

Roll the pastry sheets into two circles ⅛ inch thick - one with a diameter of 10-inches and one with a diameter of 8½ inches. Place the smaller circle in an 8-inch, ungreased pie plate, and add the filling. Cover with the larger circle, pressing the edges neatly together and crimping with a fork. Slice a small hole in the center and brush the pastry with the egg. Bake for 20 – 25 minutes until puffed and golden.

SERVING SUGGESTIONS: Serve with steamed, seasonal vegetables or a green leaf salad; for a midday meal serve with *puréed parsnips with thyme* or *rosemary roasted root vegetables* or *ginger pumpkin soup*.

VPK: The buttery puff pastry wouldn't be the first choice for kapha, but the filling is kapha-friendly; kapha should eat in moderation and combine with a salad.

VARIATIONS: You may substitute artichoke hearts with jicama, water chestnuts or sliced potatoes.

ABOUT: *Puff pastry can be purchased in the freezer section of the supermarket. To use, thaw in the refrigerator overnight, then remove from refrigerator 10 minutes prior to using in the recipe; alternatively, you can thaw at room temperature for 45 minutes. Unfold the dough onto a smooth, lightly floured surface. With a paper towel, blot any beads of moisture. If the dough has cracks from trying to unfold before it was completely thawed, press it back together. Flour the rolling pin. Roll from center to edges to desired shape. If dough starts sticking to counter, lift and throw some flour underneath.

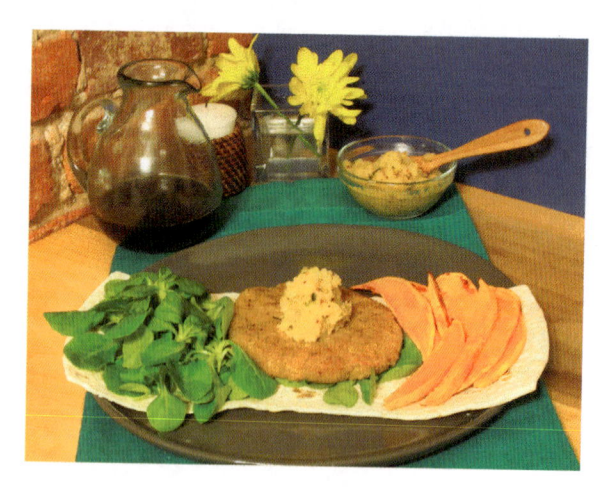

Moroccan Veggie Burger with Tangy Tamarind Sauce
DF/GF/SF/V
Yield: 6 burgers

½ cup long grain brown rice (or 1 cup cooked long grain brown rice)
¾ cup red lentils (or 1½ cups leftover/cooked red lentils)
¼ cup pumpkin seeds, coarsely chopped
½ cup onion, peeled, minced
2 tablespoons sunflower oil
¾ teaspoon *Moroccan spice blend*
1 teaspoon Neera's® tamarind paste
¾ teaspoon Himalayan salt
⅛ cup cilantro, coarsely chopped
6 tablespoons *tangy tamarind sauce*

Prepare the *tangy tamarind sauce* and set aside. Cook the rice in a rice cooker with 1 cup of water. In a 1½-quart sauce pan, cook the lentils with 3 cups of water over medium heat until done (about 10 minutes; the lentils are done when they are soft and mushy). Drain any excess water. In a food processor, combine the cooked rice, cooked lentils and remaining ingredients; pulse until the rice is well chopped and all the ingredients are combined. Form into 6 patties. (Patties can be wrapped in plastic wrap and frozen in Ziploc® baggies at this point.)

In an 8-inch fry pan, heat 1 tablespoon of oil over low heat. Do not use high heat or the burgers may burn. Place one burger in the pan and cook until browned on the first side (about 5 minutes) then flip and brown the second side.

SERVING SUGGESTIONS: Serve on lavash bread with a side of mixed salad greens and sweet potato fries; drizzle *tangy tamarind sauce* on top; serve with *vata sweet onion chutney* or *pitta cooling date chutney* or *kapha hot onion chutney*.

VPK: Well balanced for all doshas. Kapha could use mustard (or honey mustard) instead of the tamarind honey sauce.

VARIATIONS: Vata and kapha could add a pinch of cayenne or ¼ teaspoon of paprika.

ABOUT: These veggie burgers are easy to form into patties, and they don't fall apart during cooking. The brown rice keeps them moist making them well-tolerated by delicate digestive systems.

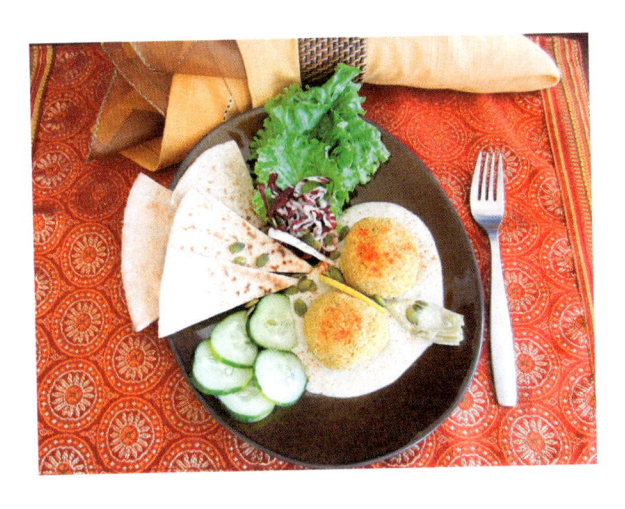

❀ Baked Falafel Balls
DF/GF/SF/V
Servings: 2 (6 balls)

¾ cup dry chickpeas (soaked overnight in kombu for 24 hours; 1¾ cups after soaking)
4 tablespoons cooked/leftover short grain brown rice
½ cup onion, coarsely chopped
2 teaspoons *Moroccan spice mix*
4 tablespoons olive oil
1 tablespoon lemon juice
¼ teaspoon garlic
2 tablespoons cilantro, coarsely chopped
½ teaspoon Himalayan salt

Preheat oven to 350°F. Place all the ingredients in a food processor. Pulse about 30 times until it's a sticky, chunky paste consistency; do not purée to a smooth texture. Transfer to a large mixing bowl and stir to even out the spices, removing any chickpeas that did not get chopped. Form into 6 balls then transfer to an ungreased bakingsheet; cook until the center is solid, about 20-25 minutes. These will keep in the refrigerator for 3 or 4 days.

SERVING SUGGESTIONS: Serve in a pita pocket with *vata sweet onion chutney* or *artichoke lemon cream sauce* and sprinkle pumpkin seeds on top; Pitta and kapha may opt to top with some fresh squeezed lime juice or sprouts. Serve as part of a *Mediterranean salad plate*.

VPK: The brown rice and oil in this recipe will balance the dryness of the chickpeas and will greatly assist vata in digestion; do not reduce oil if vata will be consuming. Vata or pitta can top with yogurt sauce (dilute whole, plain yogurt with water to desired consistency and add a grating of lemon peel and chopped cilantro). Kapha can add some fresh lime juice or *kapha wasabi dressing* or *kapha hot onion chutney*.

VARIATIONS: Try substituting parsley for cilantro; substituting lime juice for lemon juice; omit the garlic.

ABOUT: I recommend that you do not use canned chickpeas for this recipe. Canned chickpeas are pre-cooked and the additional baking in this recipe will create a falafel ball with a soggy consistency.

In a 3-quart sauté pan, heat the oil over medium-low heat. Add onions and garlic and cook until fragrant (about 1 minute); add the tomatoes and cook for 3 minutes, stirring frequently. Remove from heat and add the remaining ingredients, gently mixing to evenly distribute the spices.

SERVING SUGGESTIONS: Serve with a side of couscous or quinoa; pita bread or *GF corn bread*.

VPK: This is well balanced for pitta and kapha. It is too dry for vata

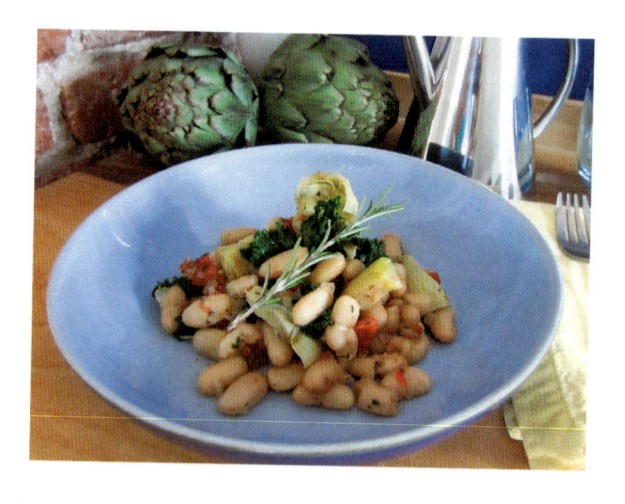

Pitta Kapha Cannellini Kale & Artichoke Sauté
DF/GF/SF/V
Servings: 3

3 tablespoons olive oil
½ cup onion, chopped fine
¼ teaspoon garlic, pressed
½ cup artichoke hearts (canned, packed in water), quartered
1½ cups kale, leaves torn from vein and coarsely chopped
½ cup plum tomatoes (peeled, seeded, coarsely chopped)
15-ounce can cannellini beans, rinsed, drained
¼ cup water
½ teaspoon fresh oregano leaves, finely chopped
1¼ teaspoons rosemary leaves (not the stem), finely chopped
½ teaspoon Himalayan salt
¼ teaspoon pepper
2 tablespoons lemon juice

❁ Dry Fry Tofu

DF/GF/V
Servings: 4

1 16-ounch container extra-firm tofu

Drain the tofu and slice into desired shape (for use in a main-dish meal, cut into triangles that are a ½-inch thick; for use in a salad or curry, cut into ½ inch cubes). Put the tofu pieces between two absorbent cotton towels and gently press to remove additional water. Place the tofu in a single layer in a 10-inch non-stick fry pan or well-seasoned cast-iron fry pan. Cook on low heat to allow additional water to evaporate. Press the tofu down gently with the back of a spatula. Once the bottom side is firm and golden, flip and fry the other side until golden. Remove from pan.

Once the tofu has been fried, you can marinate and use in stir fry recipes or curries; the dry-frying prevents the tofu from crumbling during cooking.

VPK: Tofu is cooling and heavy. It is suitable for pitta; vata and kapha can tolerate it with appropriate seasonings.

❁ Lime-Ginger Tofu

DF/GF/V
Servings: 4

16-ounce package extra firm tofu, cut into triangles and dry fried

Lime Ginger Marinade
2 tablespoons lime juice
2 tablespoons tamari
1 tablespoon ginger, chopped
¼ cup sesame oil

Whisk all ingredients together and a non-metallic bowl; add the tofu and marinate in the refrigerator for 30 minutes. Remove the tofu from the marinade and reserve the liquid. Sauté tofu in a 10-inch, non-stick fry pan over medium heat; Add 2 tablespoons of the marinade and bring to a boil. Reduce heat to low and simmer, covered for 2 minutes.

SERVING SUGGESTIONS: Serve with Asian vegetables and purple rice with toasted pecans or jasmine coconut rice.

VPK: Tofu is generally best tolerated by pitta; the lime ginger marinade provides some balance to vata and kapha.

VARIATIONS: You can substitute boneless chicken or shrimp for the tofu.

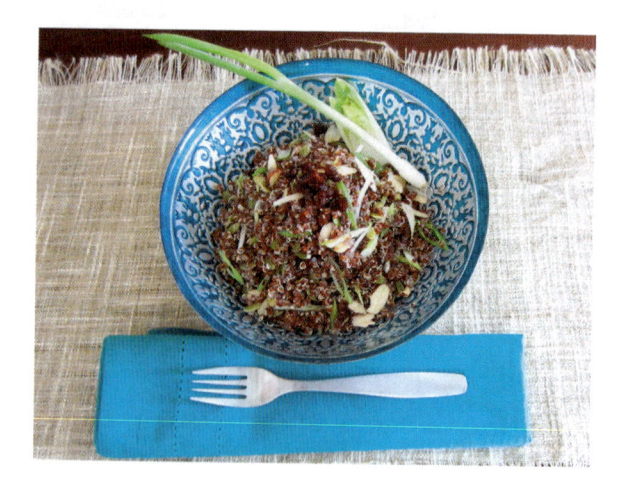

❀Red Quinoa with Endive and Cranberries
DF/GF/SF/V
Servings: 2

¾ cup red quinoa, rinsed (or ⅓ cup red and ⅓ cup white)
1½ cups water
⅛ cup scallions, ends removed, thinly sliced on the diagonal
⅓ cup almonds, slivered and toasted
½ cup Belgian endive (or fennel), coarsely chopped
⅛ cup dried cranberries (fruit juice-sweetened), coarsely chopped
⅛ cup pumpkin seeds (or sunflower seeds)
½ teaspoon Himalayan salt
¼ teaspoon ground black pepper
2 tablespoons sunflower oil (or avocado oil, olive oil)
2 tablespoons white balsamic vinegar
2 tablespoons apple cider vinegar (or lime juice)

Add the quinoa and water to a 2-quart saucepan and bring to a boil. Reduce the heat to low and simmer, covered tightly until the quinoa is tender but still delicately crunchy, about 10 minutes. Drain the quinoa and return it to the pot. Cover and let rest for 5 minutes (the heat should be off at this point). Remove cover and fluff it with a fork. Allow to **cool to room temperature**. Transfer quinoa to a 2½-quart mixing bowl; add the scallions, endive, almonds, cranberries, pumpkin seeds, salt and pepper; gently combine with a wooden spoon.

Vinaigrette
Whisk together the oil with the vinegars. Pour the dressing over the salad and gently toss. Let rest 10 minutes.

SERVING SUGGESTIONS: Serve with *ginger pumpkin soup*, *rosemary roasted root vegetables*, steamed asparagus or French green beans with lemon.

VPK: Quinoa is a little drying and is great for kapha and pitta; vata should apply liberal amounts of the oil vinaigrette; vata may also substitute *vata tamarind honey dressing*.

ABOUT: I recommend that you do not substitute 100% white quinoa; it will be very bland. The white balsamic vinegar adds sweetness (and sour). If you substitute with another vinegar, you will need to add a sweetener to the dressing such as honey, maple syrup, or coconut sugar.

VARIATIONS: You can vary the ingredients by season or dosha (using the *dosha diet aids* in the appendix). Here are some examples:

Replace	Summer	Spring	Fall & Winter
endive	fennel	asparagus	roasted sweet potato or pumpkin
dried cranberries	golden	dried apricots	dried sour cherries
scallions	fresh mint	chives	parsley

❀ Fluffy Cinnamon Currant Millet (Pitta/Kapha)
DF/GF/SF/V
Servings: 2

¾ cup millet
1¾ cups water
1 teaspoon ghee or sunflower oil
⅛ teaspoon Himalayan salt
1 tablespoon currants
½ teaspoon cinnamon

Rinse the millet then spread over the bottom of a 10-inch skillet. On medium heat, toast the millet, gently stirring to cook evenly (about 4 minutes). The millet will dry out and turn slightly golden brown. In a 2½-quart saucepan, bring the water to a boil. Add the toasted millet, ghee and salt. Then reduce heat to low; cover and simmer for 20-25 minutes until the liquid is absorbed and the grain is soft. Turn off the heat and let stand, covered for 10 minutes. Stir in the currants and cinnamon then fluff with a fork.

SERVING SUGGESTIONS: Serve with *Gujarati wedding dal* and steamed greens. Leftovers can be added to a salad of leafy greens for pitta and kapha or added to vegetable soup for vata. Leftovers may also be used for *millet breakfast patty*.

VPK: Millet is dry, light and heating and is ideal for kapha; too dry for vata. Vata can tolerate if they pour some melted ghee on their serving or top with *tri-doshic southwest pumpkin seed citrus dressing, vata lemon cashew cream sauce*, tahini sauce or *vata plum compote*. Pitta can add chopped cilantro or *creamy yogurt* to cool the dish.

VARIATIONS: You can omit the cinnamon and currants if you want a simple grain. You could make a sweeter dish by replacing ½ cup of the water with apple or pear juice.

❀ Minted Apricot Couscous
DF/GF/SF/V
Servings: 2

1¾ cup water
½ teaspoon Himalayan salt
1 tablespoon dried apricots, chopped
1 cup couscous (substitute white quinoa for GF)
1 tablespoon fresh mint, chopped

In a 1½-quart saucepan, bring the water to a boil. Add the salt and stir to dissolve. Add the apricots and couscous, stirring to combine; remove from heat and cover, then let set for 5 minutes. Remove the cover add the mint and fluff with a fork. Serve.

SERVING SUGGESTIONS: Serve with *Moroccan lamb meatballs* or *summer vegetable soup*.

VPK: This is balanced for all doshas.

VARIATIONS: Add ½ teaspoon of grated orange, lemon or lime peel; replace ¾ cup of the water with pear juice or apple juice; substitute the dried apricots (which are warming) for other dried fruit (cranberries, sour cherries, raisins, etc.); add ½ cup roasted sweet potato.

ABOUT: Couscous is made from durum wheat or semolina. It is sweet and cool, balancing to pitta and vata.

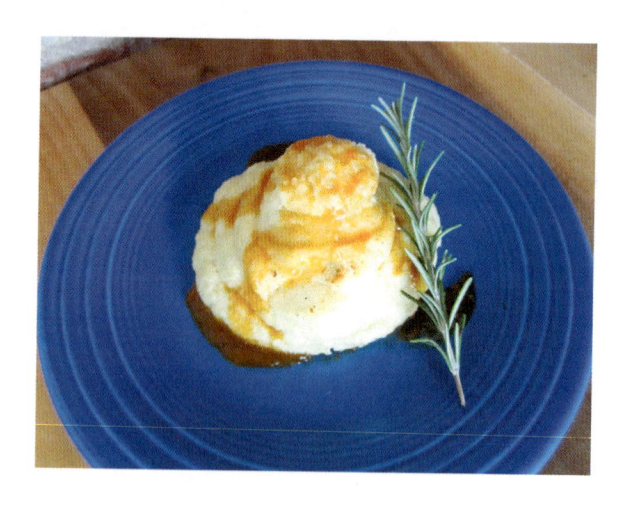

❁ Millet Mash
GF/SF/V
Servings: 2

¼ cup of millet
1¼ cups water
⅛ cup almond milk (or rice, soy, cow)
1 tablespoon butter
¼ teaspoon Himalayan salt
¼ teaspoon crushed black pepper

In a 2-quart saucepan, toast the millet over low heat for 5-10 minutes, stirring frequently. Add the water and bring to a boil. Reduce heat to low; simmer covered for 30 minutes, until the millet is soft and it is a porridge-like consistency. You may need to add a little more water, so keep an eye on it while cooking to ensure it doesn't dry out. Remove from heat and add the remaining ingredients. Purée with immersion blender.

SERVING SUGGESTIONS: Serve with *bison meat loaf* and steamed vegetables.

VPK: The millet is warm, dry and light, so adding the butter and milk will bring balance to the dish. Vata can add more butter and salt on their serving.

VARIATIONS: For vata or kapha: garnish with chives or parsley; add a clove of garlic during cooking and a squirt of lemon juice; after cooking flavor with ¼ teaspoon cumin or ¼ teaspoon cinnamon and/or ⅛ teaspoon cayenne.

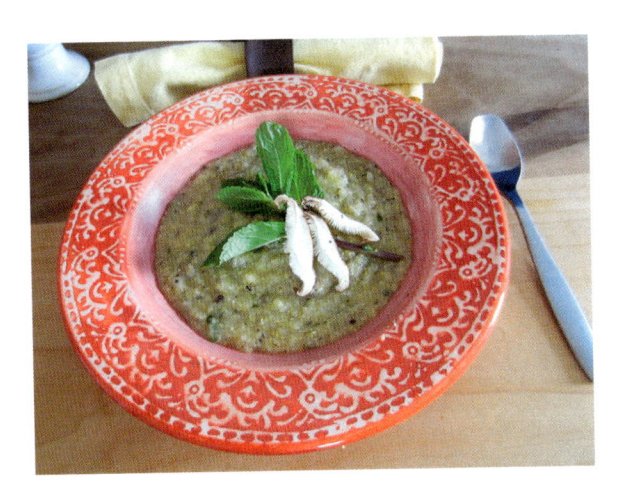

❁ Polenta with Minted Shiitake Sauce
DF/GF/SF/V
Servings: 4

18 ounces polenta ("Food Merchants"® Pre-cooked Organic Polenta)
1½ cups water

Shiitake Sauce
¼ cup dried shiitake mushrooms, stems removed and discarded
½ cup boiling water
¼ cup crimini (or baby bella) mushrooms, stems removed and discarded
2 tablespoon sunflower oil
½ cup onion, chopped
2 teaspoons coconut sugar
⅛ teaspoon Himalayan salt
⅛ teaspoon crushed black pepper
¼ cup water
½ cup rice milk
4 teaspoons fresh mint, chopped

For the Sauce
Rehydrate the dried mushrooms in ½ cup of boiling water for about 30 minutes; strain reserving the liquid. Coarsely chop the shiitake and crimini mushroom tops. Heat the oil in a 1½-quart saucepan over medium-low heat. Add the re-hydrated shiitake and crimini mushrooms; cook for 1 minute, stirring constantly. Add the onion; cook for 2 minutes, stirring constantly. Add the sugar, salt and pepper stirring to evenly distribute. Add the reserved mushroom water and ¼ cup of water and bring to a boil; deglaze the pan, scraping up brown bits off the bottom of the pan. Whisk for five minutes or until the mixture has reduced 25%; remove from heat and add the milk and mint. Use an immersion blender to blend into a chunky sauce. Cover to keep warm while the polenta is cooking.

For the Polenta
In a heavy 2-quart saucepan, combine 1½ cups water with the pre-cooked polenta. Whisk over low heat about five minutes until the mixture is a thick, porridge consistency. Add the shiitake sauce and mint, stirring until well combined.

SERVING SUGGESTIONS: Serve immediately. The polenta will firm up as it cools. Serve with steamed bok choy or asparagus and *tri-doshic arugula radicchio cherry salad*.

VPK: This dish is ideal for kapha as it is light and warm. Vata will benefit from the moist, soupy consistency of the dish. Substituting coconut milk for the rice milk will not impart any coconut flavor. If cooking solely for vata, substitute the mushroom sauce for *vata lemon cashew cream sauce*. Pitta and kapha can garnish with mung bean sprouts and/or cilantro.

ABOUT: The shiitake mushrooms (astringent, dry, heating) and polenta (sweet, dry and heating) are ideal for kapha. Cooked in this manner, however, it is tolerated by all doshas, in moderation.

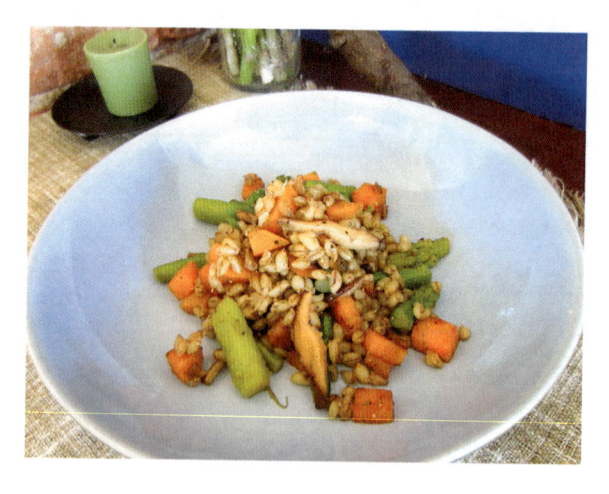

❀ Barley Sauté with Sweet Potato, Asparagus & Burdock Root
DF/GF/SF/V
Servings: 2

¼ cup whole grain barley, soaked overnight, drained
4 cups water
1 tablespoon sunflower oil
½ cup sweet potatoes, peeled, chopped into ½-inch cubes
2 tablespoons burdock root, peeled, diced into ¼-inch cubes
2 tablespoons shiitake mushroom caps, sliced
½ cup asparagus, chopped into 1-inch slices
¼ teaspoon crushed black pepper
¼ teaspoon Himalayan salt
2 tablespoons *tri-doshic Asian tamari dressing*

Prepare the *tri-doshic Asian tamari dressing* recipe. Cook the barley: In a 2-quart sauce pan, combine the barley and water; bring to a boil and cook, uncovered until tender (about 1 hour); drain and return to the pan; cover to keep warm while you prepare the vegetables. In a 2½-quart sauté pan, warm the oil over medium heat. Add the sweet potatoes and burdock root. Using a wooden spoon, stir continually for 5 minutes. Do not stop stirring or the vegetables will burn. Add the shiitake mushrooms and continue to stir for another 5 minutes. Add the asparagus and continue cooking and stirring until the asparagus are just tender (about 1 minute). Remove from heat. In a 2½-quart mixing bowl, combine the barley, vegetables, salt, pepper and the *tri-doshic Asian tamari dressing*. Gently stir to evenly coat with the dressing. Serve.

SERVING SUGGESTIONS: Serve with *ginger pumpkin soup*.

VPK: Tri doshic; vata should eat in moderation; kapha can sprinkle cayenne or chili peppers on their serving.

VARIATIONS: Vata can add ¼ pound grilled beef tips for additional grounding.

❁ Marco's Porcini Risotto
GF/SF/V
Servings: 4

1½ tablespoons olive oil
2 ounces dried porcini mushrooms (soak for 30 minutes in ½ cup boiling water; then chop +strain; RESERVE the soaking water)
½ cup onion, finely chopped
1 teaspoon garlic, pressed
1¼ cups abborio rice
½ cup red wine
~4-6 cups of simmering water
¼ cup parsley, coarsely chopped
¼ cup grated parmesan cheese
½ teaspoon Himalayan salt
¼ teaspoon crushed black pepper

In a heavy 3-quart pan, heat the oil over medium heat. Add the mushrooms and cook for 5 minutes. Add the onions and garlic and sauté until translucent (about 2-4 minutes). Add the rice and stir to combine with all the flavors. Increase the heat to medium-high and add the wine, stirring constantly so the rice does not stick to the bottom of the pan. When the rice has absorbed 90% of the wine, add the reserved water from the mushrooms. Stir until 90% of the liquid has been absorbed. Add a cup of simmering water and stir continually until the rice has absorbed 90% of the water. Repeat with the remainder of the water, stopping when the rice is done (it will be soft and chewy).

TIPS: Keep enough liquid in the pan so the rice doesn't stick to the bottom of the pan. Stir slowly and constantly. Observe the appearance of the rice as it absorbs the water. The exact amount of water that you need will vary. Risotto making is more art than science. If you add too much water, the rice will be soggy…too little, and the rice will be crunchy. When rice is done, remove from the heat and stir in the parsley, parmesan cheese, salt and pepper. Serve Immediately.

SERVING SUGGESTIONS: Serve with *tridoshic arugula radicchio cherry salad* with *tridoshic white balsamic vinaigrette* and steamed vegetables.

VPK: The dry, warm mushrooms compliment the moist, cooling rice making the dish suitable for all doshas.

VARIATIONS: Add 1 tablespoon fresh rosemary; add ½ cup of asparagus during the last 5 minutes of cooking.

ABOUT: I learned how to make risotto from my friend Marco. He learned with his dad as a child, while living in Bolzano, Italy. Marco didn't cook from a recipe, he just tasted and adjusted seasonings as I watched and took notes. The original version had about ½ cup of parmesan cheese and ¼ cup whipping cream – it was quite delicious! This adaptation is a bit more balancing from an ayurvedic perspective and perhaps only slightly less tasty. *Mangia*!

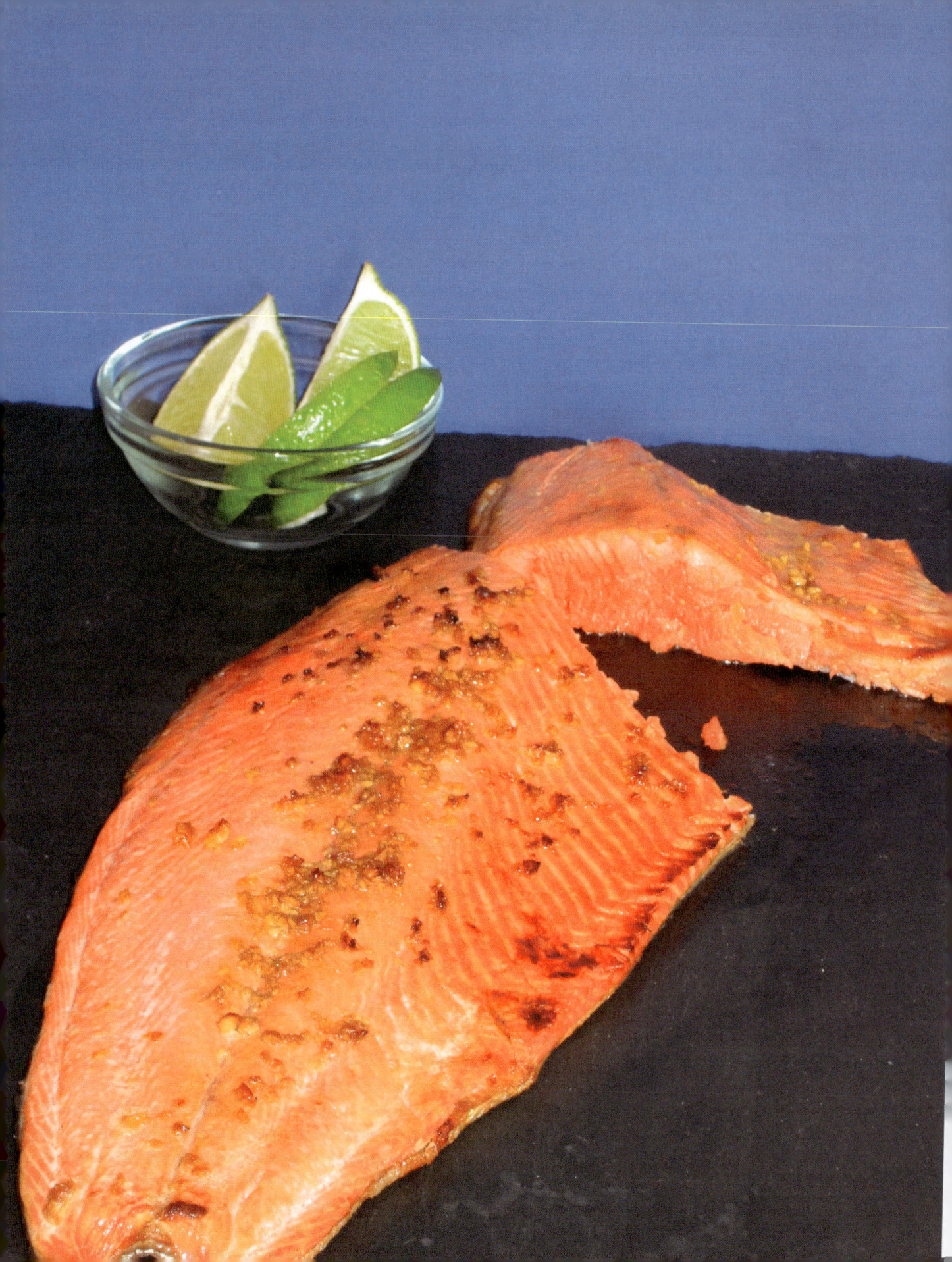

Animal & Dairy

In general, animal protein is heating and heavy, making it least suitable for pitta and kapha, but beneficial for vata, as it can be very grounding. Ayurveda asserts that ingested animal flesh creates the feelings of heaviness, dullness, depression and sleepiness; opposite to the qualities that ayurveda is trying to cultivate. Ayurveda recommends a diet of light and easily digestible foods. Light foods promote clarity and perception and are believed to have the ability to unfold compassion and love – the qualities of meat are the exact opposite.

Nonetheless, ayurveda is practical and animal protein is recommended in certain cases where the body is depleted or emaciated. Specific meat is prescribed for certain conditions (i.e., rabbit for menstrual issues, mutton for anemia) and for building strength. For medicinal purposes, meat is generally prepared in soups or stews that have been cooked for many hours (sometimes days) with appropriate herbs for optimal assimilation of the nutrients and to balance the energetics. The recommended portion of meat in ayurveda is small relative to typical portions in America. When I was anemic in India, an ayurvedic doctor in Kerala had her cook prepare me a stew of mutton and pomegranate (seeds and peel!); it provided instant energy after months of exhaustion and taking ineffective herbs. Pomegranate is loaded with vitamin C and combined with the mutton helps aid the absorption of the iron.

If you're feeling the need for red meat, try the *bison meatloaf* which is a lean alternative to eating beef. Darker meats tend to be heavier and more heating than white meats, qualities that are generally aggravating to pitta. But in this recipe, I have added some quinoa which will lighten and cool the overall energetic. Bison meat promotes strength so pitta can benefit with moderate intake. Vata can benefit because of its warming and grounding effect; it is lean and easier to digest than other fatty meats. Bison is least suitable to kapha (due to its heavy quality); but the mixture with quinoa provides some balance. Kapha would be more suited to lean, light meats (white turkey meat, white chicken meat, rabbit and venison) in small portions. Pitta can benefit from the cooling meats (white chicken, rabbit, white turkey and venison). Cooked in stews and properly spiced, meats can be tolerated by all doshas.

Most fish (especially fish from the ocean which have a warming energetic due to living in salt water) are heating and should be avoided by pitta. Shrimp and freshwater fish are generally tri-doshic to all the doshas. Vata does well with all fish.

When purchasing fish, choose fillets that are firm and bright with a fresh smell – fish should not smell "fishy". The skin should be firmly attached to the meat. Ask the vendor when it was caught – eating it the same day it was caught is ideal, more than 3 days old is not. If using frozen fish, thaw overnight by placing the fish (in its original plastic packaging) in a dish in the refrigerator; alternatively, you can thaw in 10 minutes by placing the fish (that is in its original packaging) into a bowl of cold water. If you are not using immediately, place the defrosted fish in the refrigerator. Once thawed, the fish should be cooked that same day.

Rabbit is cooling (pungent post digestive), drying and astringent, making it most suitable for pitta and kapha; vata does well with rabbit in a stew.

Lamb (sheep less than 1 year old) and mutton (adult sheep) meat are heating, strengthening and heavy. Cooked in stews, they are ideal for gaining weight after an illness.

Ayurveda recommended only eating meat of animals which have been just killed, which are pure (uncontaminated) and of adult animals[18]. Today, this is unrealistic unless you live near a farm. The main point is that you will be consuming the energetics of the animal when you eat meat. Ethical considerations notwithstanding, that should be your minimum motivation for seeking out organically raised and humanely treated animals for consumption.

In India, the cow is considered sacred and is symbolic of the bounty of mother earth, the giver of life. Traditionally, cows were not eaten and in fact people would go out of their way to make sure not to cause them harm. Today, thin cows can be found roaming the streets eating garbage in smaller Indian towns. While this doesn't fit the image of one who is revered, it more likely reflects lack of financial resources for caring for the cow than the loss of respect. This can be supported by the fact that a cow taking a nap in the middle of a street will be left unharmed as rickshaws, pedestrians, autos and buses carefully navigate around the animal so as not to disturb him.

The milk from a happy cow (allowed to graze in the grass and who is humanely treated) is considered light and easily digestible, as is everything made from its milk – yogurt, cheese, paneer, butter, buttermilk and ghee. Understanding the Indian culture, one can appreciate why ayurveda praises dairy products in general and ghee in particular.

In the west, the status of the cow is generally much lower and we mostly equate dairy products with high cholesterol and gaining weight. Many cows are kept in over-crowded feed-stalls with inadequate space for resting and without access to pasture. The cows from these farms are not cherished and the resultant mass-produced milk does not have a light, easily digestible energetic.

If you are consuming dairy products, you should look for the organic label at a minimum and ideally "certified humane raised and handled"[19]. Toxins tend to settle in body fat, and especially mammary glands, which makes it important to choose organic animal products like milk and butter, to minimize the impurities caused from pesticides, herbicides and toxins.

Ghee is a type of clarified butter that is commonly used in Indian cooking due to its high melting point, ability to be stored long-term without refrigeration and amazing taste. The best ghee is said to come from cows that have been grazing in pastures. You should expect seasonal variation in the taste if the cows switch to eating hay, legumes and silage (such as in the winter months).

The traditional method of ghee preparation in India entails: fermenting the cream from whole milk into yogurt; churning the yogurt into butter; then cooking the butter over low heat until all the moisture evaporates, and brown milk solids drop to the bottom. The golden liquid is strained through a fine mesh strainer and stored in a dry glass jar.

Ghee is highly regarded in ayurveda and is considered to both detoxify and rejuvenate at the same time. It lubricates the joints and muscles and is generally indicated for vata conditions. It should be avoided if there is high cholesterol or high ama.

ॐ Recipes - Midday Main Meals: Animal & Dairy

- GHEE
- PANEER
- FENNEL CRUSTED PANEER WITH BALSAMIC REDUCTION
- BALSAMIC REDUCTION SAUCE
- BROILED SALMON IN MAPLE LIME MARINADE
- MAPLE LIME MARINADE
- GINGER SALMON TEMAKI (HAND ROLL)
- BROILED LIME GINGER SHRIMP
- LIME GINGER MARINADE
- SPANISH CHICKEN
- MOROCCAN LAMB MEATBALLS
- ROASTED TURKEY BREAST WITH TARRAGON CREAM SAUCE
- RABBIT COCONUT FENUGREEK STEW
- BISON MEATLOAF WITH MAPLE TAMARIND SAUCE
- MAPLE TAMARIND SAUCE

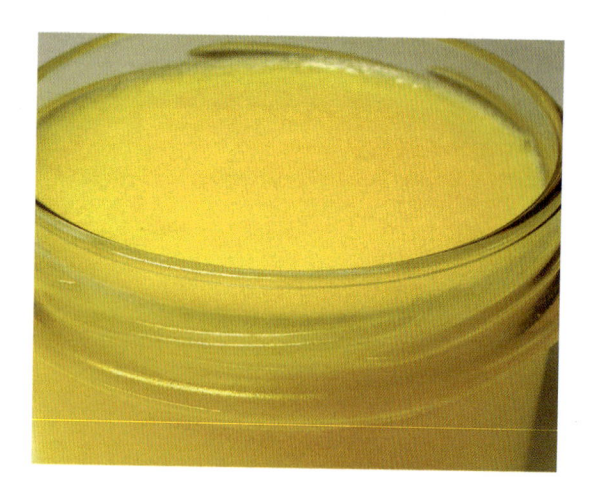

Ghee
GF/SF/V
Yield: 16 ounces

1 pound organic unsalted butter
2 quart, heavy bottom sauce pan
16-ounce clean, DRY glass container with lid
1 fine mesh sieve
1 large spoon, clean and DRY
Cheese cloth

In the saucepan over medium heat, melt the butter and bring to a boil. Immediately reduce heat to low and gently simmer uncovered; the water content will evaporate. Milk solids (small white curds) will form and fall to the bottom of the pan and begin to turn brown. Skim the froth from the top using a dry spoon and discard. The ghee is done in about 25-30 minutes when:
1. the sputtering ceases;
2. the ghee is clear;
3. the color is golden; and
4. it smells like popcorn.

Immediately remove the ghee from the heat and allow to cool (~ 15 minutes). Place a sieve lined with cheesecloth over the glass jar. Slowly pour the ghee into the sieve, straining out the curds. Cool to room temperature. Cover and store at room temperature.

VPK: Ghee is considered tri-doshic; it is especially good for vata who can benefit immensely from the lubricating qualities; its cooling energetics make it suitable for pitta; kapha can tolerate in moderation if cholesterol levels are normal.

VARIATIONS: Try using cultured butter to approximate the traditional Indian preparation.

ABOUT: Ghee gives a distinctive flavor to Indian cooking. Because the milk solids have been removed, it has a higher smoking point than butter. Ghee should not be used when there is high ama, high cholesterol, obesity or fever.

Ghee is the most refined end product of milk. When making ghee, there is a concentration of all the qualities of the milk (including antibiotics, hormones (rGBH), chemical pesticides, etc.). So it is best to use organic butter when making your ghee.

Moisture allows for bacteria to grow and will spoil the ghee. Be sure to use clean, dry utensils when scooping out the ghee and avoid moisture contacting the ghee. If you store ghee in the refrigerator, condensation may form from bringing the jar in and out of the refrigerator; this condensation can spoil the ghee.

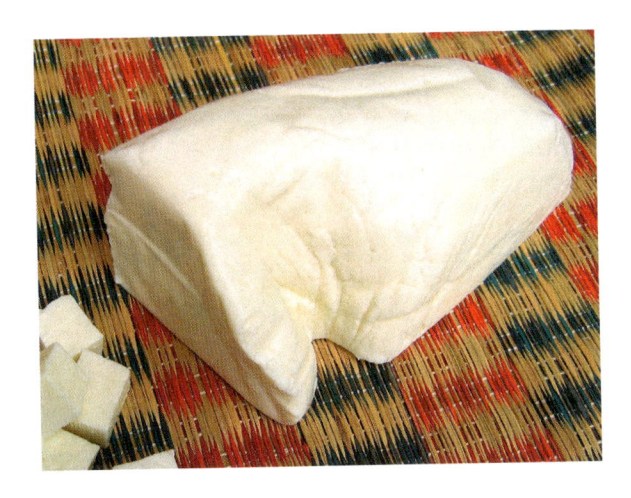

❁ Paneer
GF/SF/V
Yield: 8 ounces

½ gallon milk, full cream
3 ounces plain yogurt
1-4 tablespoons lime juice (or lemon juice)

- thin cotton cloth (do not use a colored cloth because the colors may bleed onto the cheese)
- 6-inch fine mesh sieve
- a heavy weight (i.e., a pan, dish, etc.)

In a 4-quart pan, bring the milk to a boil over medium heat. Add yogurt and stir gently, bringing back to a boil; add lime juice. When the milk splits, immediately remove from heat; let rest for 2 minutes.

Strain through a sieve lined with the cotton cloth. Lift the cloth (with the cheese) from the sieve and fold the cloth around the cheese, squeezing out more liquid as you fold; set the cloth containing the cheese on a plate. Place a weight on top of the cheese and transfer to the refrigerator. The weight will press the moisture out of the cheese. Refrigerate until most of the liquid has drained and the cheese has firmed (about ½ hour). At this point, the cheese will keep refrigerated for up to 1 week if it is tightly wrapped in plastic.

SERVING SUGGESTIONS: Cut into cubes and add to curries; crumble and add to main dish salads; cut into triangles and use for *fennel crusted paneer* recipe; add to *tri-doshic red lentil hummus*.

ABOUT: Fresh made paneer is considered tri-doshic; it is sweet, light and cooling. Discard any unused portion after a week as the properties will change to sour, heating and heavy as it ages. You may be thinking back to the food combining table and wondering why I am combining lime (citrus) with milk here. Well the food combining table refers to foods that are raw. So if you drank a glass of milk and then a tablespoon of lime/lemon juice, it would curdle in your stomach and create potential digestive issues (sour stomach). However, by cooking the milk and lime together, the curdling occurs outside of the stomach (during the cooking process); so when you ingest the cooked product, it does not create as much of a digestive burden on your system.

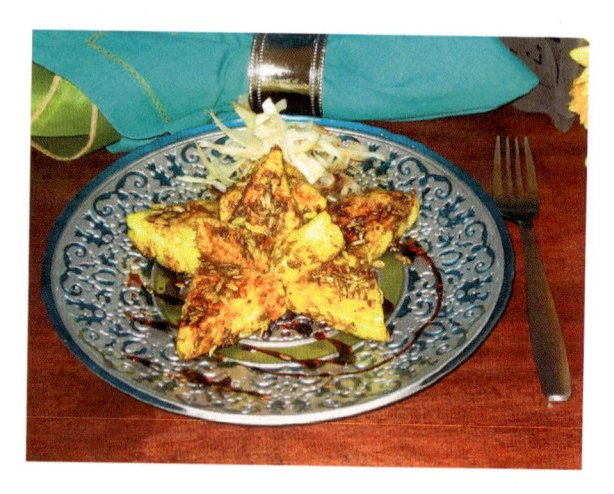

❁ Fennel Crusted Paneer with Balsamic Reduction
GF/SF/V
Servings: 2

Fennel Crusted Paneer
3 tablespoons ghee (or sunflower oil)
2 teaspoons cumin seeds
3 teaspoons fennel seeds
1½ teaspoons coriander powder
¼ teaspoon garlic, pressed
¼ teaspoon crushed black pepper
¼ teaspoon turmeric
24 ounces of paneer, cut into 2-inch triangles or squares
cilantro, garnish
lemon peel, garnish

Make the balsamic reduction sauce first (recipe to the right). Melt the ghee in a 3-quart sauté pan over medium heat. Add the cumin seeds and fennel seeds. Heat until the seeds pop (about 30 seconds) and then immediately reduce heat to low so the seeds don't burn. Add the coriander powder, garlic, pepper and turmeric and stir fry for 1 minute. Add the paneer in a single layer on top of the mixed spices. Add more ghee as needed.

Cook until browned and gently flip to cook the other side. The seeds will stick to the paneer and make a crunchy coating. Place onto a serving plate and drizzle with the balsamic reduction. Garnish with cilantro and lemon peel.

SERVING SUGGESTIONS: Serve with *kapha hot onion chutney*, steamed vegetable or *Brussels sprout sweet potato sauté* and saffron basmati rice.

VPK: This dish is well balanced, especially with the recommended serving suggestions. Fresh paneer is tri-doshic.

VARIATIONS: Try *tangy tamarind sauce* or *tri-doshic pomegranate orange reduction sauce* in lieu of the balsamic reduction. This can also be made with halibut or tofu in place of the paneer.

Balsamic Reduction Sauce:
1 cup balsamic vinegar
1 small garlic clove (cut in half)

Pour balsamic vinegar into a 1-quart saucepan, and add the garlic; stir over **medium-high** heat until it comes to a boil. Reduce heat to **medium-low**, and simmer until the vinegar has reduced (about 15 minutes). Shut off the heat and remove the garlic; cool to room temperature.

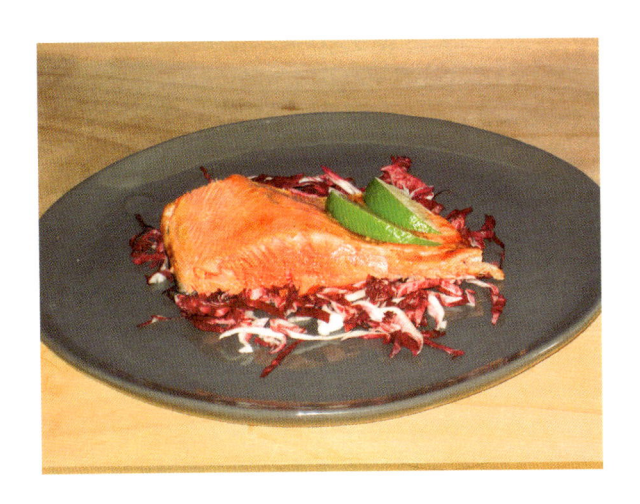

❋ Broiled Salmon in Maple Lime Marinade
DF/GF
Servings: 2

½ pound of wild salmon filet, rinsed, skin intact, pin bones removed

Maple Lime Marinade:
6 tablespoons sunflower oil
3 tablespoons lime juice
2 tablespoons maple syrup
1 tablespoon tamari

Prepare the marinade: Whisk together all the ingredients in a small, non-metallic bowl. Place the salmon (skin-side down) in a shallow non-metallic dish and pour the marinade on top, then flip the fish so it is skin-side up and allow the marinade to absorb into the meat. Cover with plastic wrap and marinate for 20 minutes in the refrigerator.

Place the salmon in a pre-heated broiler and cook with the skin side down for 3-4 minutes per 1-inch thickness of fish. Flip and cook the other side until internal temperature reaches 145°F (start checking after 2 minutes to ensure you don't overcook the fish). You will know the fish is done when: the color lightens; it is firm to the touch; the center is a little rare (it will continue cooking once removed from the heat); the meat separates easily from the skin. If it is flaky, then it is overdone and will be dry. Remove from the broiler and let the salmon set for a few minutes before serving.

SERVING SUGGESTIONS: Serve with steamed vegetables (asparagus, string beans, carrots, kale, bok choy, etc.) or a salad of mixed greens and purple (forbidden) rice.

VPK: Vata can add 1 tablespoon of sesame oil and reduce the sunflower oil by the same amount. If cooking solely for vata or kapha, you can add 1 teaspoon grated orange rind and ½ teaspoon cinnamon to the marinade. The oily salmon skin is beneficial for vata (less so for pitta and not for kapha). If cooking solely for kapha, you could skip the marinade and broil with a little sesame oil, then top with *kapha wasabi dressing*.

ABOUT: Wild salmon is lean and heating – ideal for vata. Pitta and kapha will benefit from the lean protein source when eaten in moderation (note the serving size of this recipe) and served with the green vegetables (i.e., bok choy, kale and salad). For easy clean-up, line the broiler tray with aluminum foil prior to pre-heating the oven.

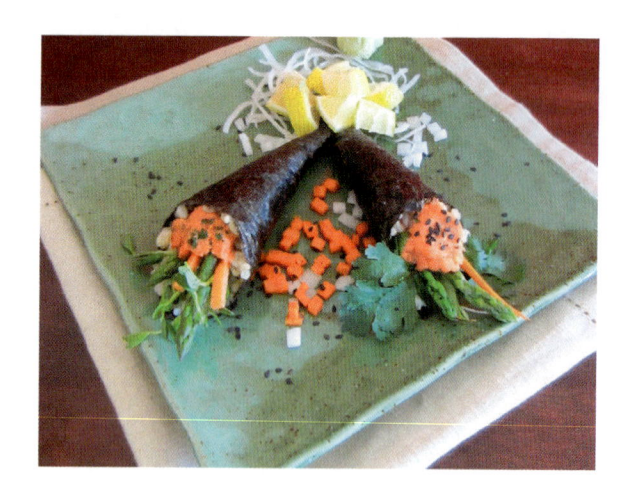

❋ Ginger Salmon Temaki (Hand Roll)
DF/GF
Yield: 6 hand rolls / 2 servings

¼ pound salmon filet, skin removed, pin bones removed
1 heaping teaspoon ginger, peeled, minced
2 teaspoons apple cider vinegar
1 tablespoon tamari
3 teaspoons sesame oil
2 tablespoons cilantro, coarsely chopped
1 cup cooked brown rice
3 toasted nori sheets, cut in half (you will have two 4½ x 7½ sheets)
12 asparagus stalks, gently steamed, trimmed to 5½ inches long
Sesame seeds (for garnish)

Poach the salmon: Add 5 cups of water to a 3-quart sauté pan (the pan should be about ½ filled with water, adjust accordingly). Bring the water to a boil and then reduce heat to low (water should be slightly simmering. Add the salmon filets and cook until done (about 4-5 minutes each side for a 1-inch thick filet). Using a slotted spoon transfer the salmon to a plate lined with a paper towel.

In a mini food processor, combine the salmon, ginger, apple cider vinegar, tamari and sesame oil. Pulse until the ingredients are ground into a sticky mixture. Transfer to a small bowl and add the cilantro.

With dry hands, place one of the ½ sheets of nori, shiny side down, on a clean, dry work surface (position it so the longer edges of the rectangle are parallel to you. Spread ¼ cup of the rice along the left (vertical) edge of the nori sheet. Moisten your fingers with water and gently press, while spreading the rice toward the right until it is covering one-third of the sheet. Position 2 asparagus stems on the rice diagonally, overhanging the top left corner. Place one tablespoon of the salmon mixture, diagonally on top of the asparagus. Bring the bottom left corner to the upper right corner where the rice ends to make a cone shape. Press tightly then begin to roll in the shape of an ice cream cone. Seal the edge of the hand roll with a few drops of water or a few grains of the cooked rice. Allow the seal to dry for 5 minutes prior to serving. Repeat with the remaining nori sheets to make 6 hand rolls.

SERVING SUGGESTIONS: Serve with *dashi clear broth* (or miso soup) in the winter; with *wakami daikon salad* in the summer. Kapha or vata could top with *kapha wasabi dressing*; tamari and/or lime juice is best for pitta.

VARIATIONS: Keep the fillings simple (only one or two per roll) and vary as per the *dosha diet aids* in the appendix. Traditional fillings include: watercress, cucumber, avocado, sprouts, lettuce, pickled daikon, scallions, shrimp, cilantro, etc.

ABOUT: You can substitute smoked salmon for the poached salmon, as long as it does not contain added salt or strong flavorings which will overpower this dish.

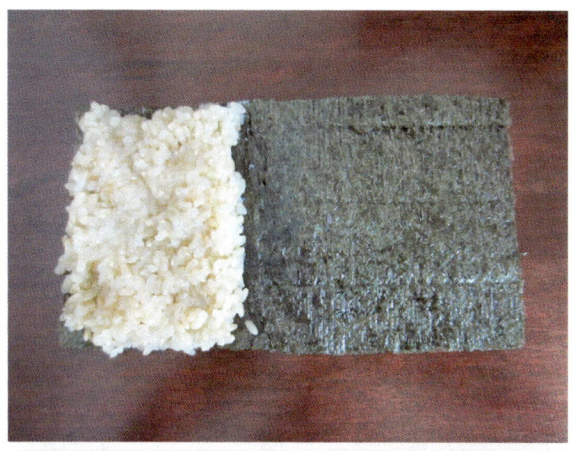

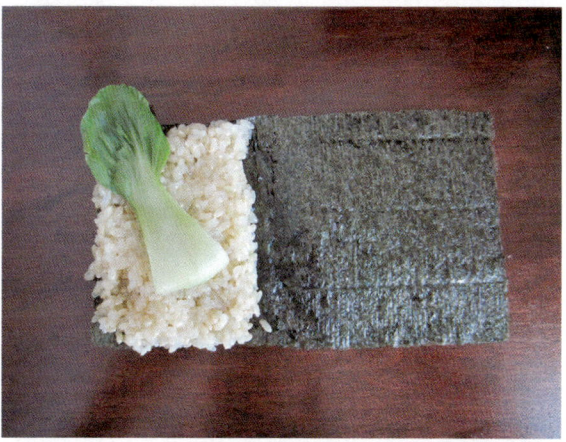

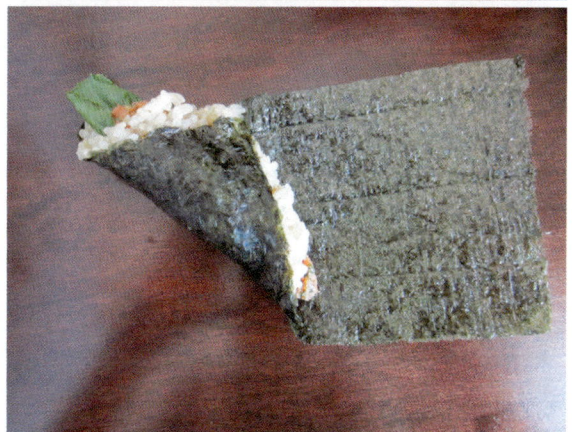

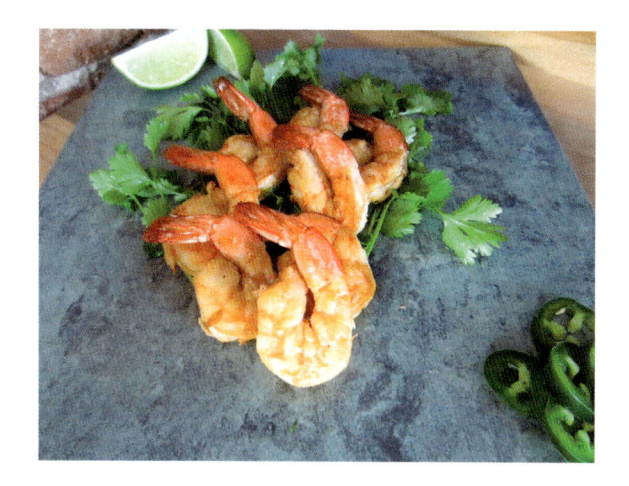

🌼 Broiled Lime Ginger Shrimp

DF/GF
Servings: 2
½ pound large shrimp, peeled and deveined

Lime Ginger Marinade
Yield: ¼ cup
**2 tablespoons lime juice
2 tablespoons tamari
1 tablespoon ginger, chopped
1 teaspoon coconut sugar
¼ cup sesame oil**

Whisk all ingredients together in a non-metallic bowl; add the shrimp and marinate in the refrigerator for 1 hour. Remove shrimp from marinade and discard the marinade.

Broil the shrimp until they are done (about 1-2 minutes each side). You will know they are done when they turn light pink in color and start to curl into a circle shape.

SERVING SUGGESTIONS: Serve with *Asian vegetables* and *coconut forbidden rice* or with *summer Israeli couscous salad*.

VPK: If cooking for kapha only, you can add chilies and garlic to the marinade.

VARIATIONS: You can substitute boneless chicken breast or extra-firm tofu for the shrimp.

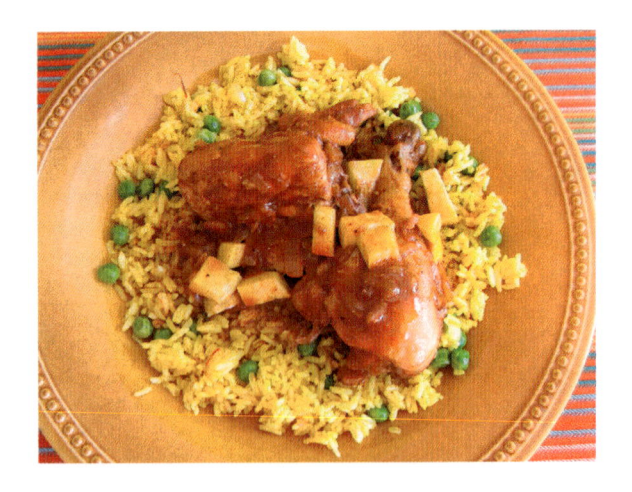

🌸 Spanish Chicken
DF/GF/SF
Servings: 4

1 tablespoon butter (if you substitute oil here, the chicken will not brown)
3 tablespoons sunflower oil
1 pound chicken, skin removed, quartered (or shrimp)
½ cup onion, chopped fine
2 tablespoons tomato paste
1 teaspoon garlic, pressed
2 teaspoons grated orange rind
1 teaspoon cinnamon powder
1 teaspoon cumin powder
½ teaspoon chili powder
1 teaspoon paprika
1 bay leaf
1 teaspoon coconut sugar
½ teaspoon Himalayan salt
¼ teaspoon crushed black pepper
½ cup orange juice
1 teaspoon apple cider vinegar
1½ cups water
2 teaspoons arrowroot powder (mixed with 2 teaspoons water)
¾ cup summer squash

In a 3-quart sauté pan, heat the oil and butter over medium low heat. Add the chicken and sauté until browned. Remove chicken from the pan and reserve. Add the onion and garlic; sauté for 2 minutes. Add the tomato paste, orange rind, cumin, chili, paprika, sugar, salt and pepper; sauté for 1 minute. Add the orange juice, vinegar and water; bring to a boil. Add the chicken then reduce heat to simmer. Cook covered until done (check after 10 minutes). Remove from heat; add the squash. Cover and steam for 5 minutes until the squash is tender.

SERVING SUGGESTIONS: Serve with *Spanish Saffron Rice* with steamed peas.

VPK: This is a mild dish that is suitable for all doshas in moderation. Kapha can sprinkle extra paprika or cayenne onto their serving.

VARIATIONS: Substitute shrimp for the chicken (use 1 pound of large shrimp, peeled and deveined, "tails" removed; add the shrimp at the end of the recipe and cook until it turns pink and "curls up" (about 3-5 minutes).

🌸 Moroccan Lamb Meatballs
GF/SF
Servings: 2 (makes 6 meatballs)

½ pound ground lamb (you may substitute ground chicken, but you should omit the garlic with this variation)
1 egg, beaten
¼ cup onion, minced
½ teaspoon garlic, pressed
1 teaspoon *Moroccan spice blend*
2 teaspoons fresh mint, chopped fine
2 teaspoons cooked white quinoa
¼ teaspoon Himalayan salt

Preheat oven to 350°F. In a 2-½ quart bowl, combine all the ingredients. Form into 6 balls.

Assemble on a baking sheet so they are not touching; bake until internal temperature is 160°F (about 20 minutes).

SERVING SUGGESTIONS: Serve with minted apricot couscous (substitute white quinoa for gluten-free), steamed green vegetables and pitta cooling date chutney. Kapha could add a side of kapha hot onion chutney.

ABOUT: The quinoa lightens and cools the heavy, heating lamb. The meatballs can be made ahead and frozen prior to cooking; when ready to use, remove from freezer and place directly in the oven without thawing.

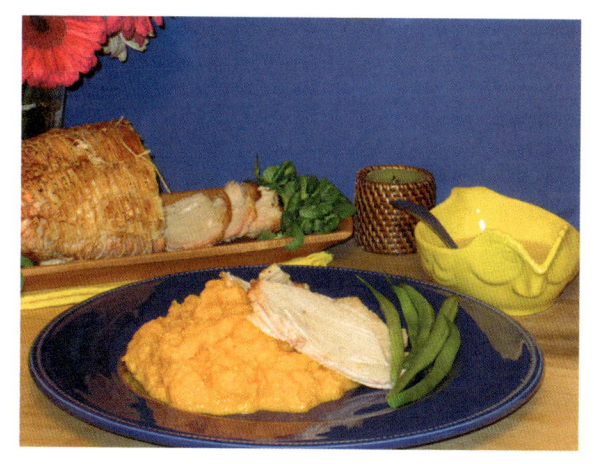

❀ Roasted Turkey Breast with Tarragon Cream Sauce
GF/SF
Servings: 4

2 tablespoons melted ghee (or sunflower oil)
1½ pounds organic turkey breast, boneless with skin
½ cup shallots, peeled and coarsely chopped
1 cup water
1 bay leaf
½ teaspoon Himalayan salt
¼ teaspoon crushed black pepper
1 teaspoon tarragon, dried
3 tablespoons lemon juice
½ teaspoon grated lemon rind
3 tablespoons whipping cream
¾ teaspoon tarragon, fresh, chopped

Aluminum foil
Meat thermometer

Preheat oven to 400°F. In 3½-quart oven proof sauté pan, melt the ghee over medium heat. Add the turkey breast and brown both sides. Remove turkey and set aside. Add the shallots and sauté for 1 minute. Add the water and stir to scrape up any brown bits that are on the bottom of the pan. Return the turkey to the pan and add the bay leaf. Sprinkle with salt, pepper and the tarragon. Place the pan in the oven and cook (uncovered) for 30 minutes; baste the turkey with pan juices after 30 minutes and check the internal temperature with a meat thermometer. Continue cooking until internal temperature is 155°F (another 10-20 minutes). If the skin is getting too crispy, you can "tent" it with aluminum foil at this point to inhibit additional browning. Remove from oven and transfer turkey breast to a serving platter. Remove bay leaf and discard. Cover the turkey with foil and let rest for 15 minutes as it continues to cook. Prepare the cream sauce.

Tarragon Cream Sauce
Place pan with drippings on the stove top on medium heat. Add lemon juice and grated rind; whisk, scraping any brown bits from the bottom of the pan. Remove from heat. Add the whipping cream and tarragon; whisk to combine.

VPK: Tri-doshic; kapha should use minimal amount of the cream sauce or omit. The cream sauce in this recipe is very light; moderation and balance are the key. Alternatively, you could substitute the cream for rice milk for an even lighter version.

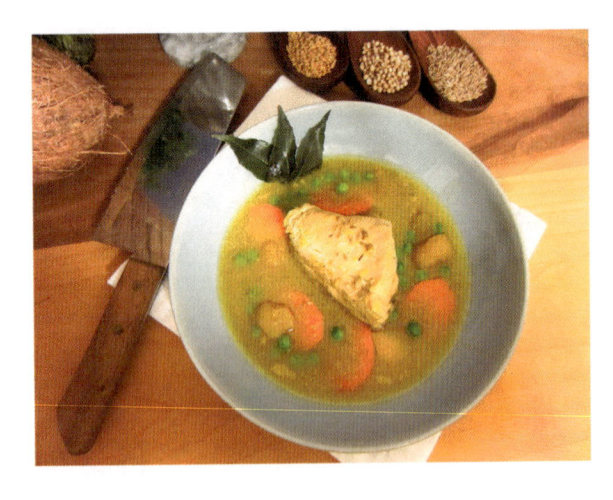

Rabbit Coconut Fenugreek Stew
DF/GF/SF
Servings: 4

1 pound rabbit, cut into parts, bone included
14-ounce can coconut milk
1 cup water
1 cup onion, chopped
1-2 tablespoons black sesame seed oil
1 teaspoon fenugreek seeds (methi), crushed
½ teaspoon coriander seed, crushed
½ teaspoon cumin seeds
2 teaspoons ginger, peeled and minced
5 curry leaves
½ teaspoon Himalayan salt
¼ teaspoon crushed black pepper

Vegetables:
1½ cups sweet potatoes, peeled, cut into ½-inch cubes
1 cup peas
2 tablespoons cilantro

In a 3-quart pan, combine all the ingredients except the vegetables and bring to a boil. Reduce heat to low and simmer, uncovered for 1 hour; the meat will begin to fall off the bones. Add the sweet potatoes and cook for another 20 minutes. Remove from heat and stir in the peas and cilantro; cover and let set for 5 minutes while the peas steam.

SERVING SUGGESTIONS: Serve with *GF corn bread* or wheat chapatti.

VPK: This is relatively balanced for all doshas. Kapha can add some chili peppers to their serving.

VARIATIONS: Your can substitute a chicken for the rabbit. The photo shown here is with chicken.

ABOUT: The rabbit is cool and dry, so the coconut sauce balances this energetic. The fenugreek is heating; it reduces vata and kapha and kindles the digestive fire. The black sesame oil gives the dish a rich, distinct flavor. Add the amount that suits your taste. You can purchase black sesame oil at Asian markets and international stores.

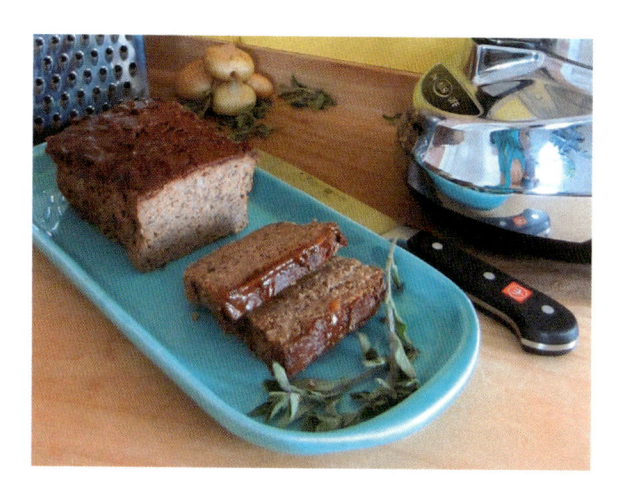

🌸 Bison Meatloaf with Maple Tamarind Sauce
DF/GF
Servings: 5

Maple Tamarind Sauce
4 tablespoons tomato paste
1½ teaspoons apple cider vinegar
3 teaspoons tamari
½ teaspoon tamarind sauce
1 teaspoon maple syrup (or molasses or coconut sugar – do not use honey)

Combine all ingredients in a small bowl. Set aside for meatloaf preparation.

Bison Meatloaf
¾ cup onion, shredded with box grater
1 teaspoon dried oregano
1 teaspoon dried tarragon
1 teaspoon dried summer savory
½ cup white quinoa, cooked
1 pound bison, ground
2 tablespoons parsley, coarsely chopped
½ teaspoon Himalayan salt
½ teaspoon crushed black pepper

Preheat oven to 350°F. In a food processor, combine all the meatloaf ingredients plus 2 tablespoons of the maple tamarind sauce; pulse to combine. Transfer to an 8" non-stick loaf pan and pat down into the pan using the back of a spoon. Top with a layer of the remaining tamarind sauce and bake for 1 hour or until a thermometer inserted two inches into the center registers 160°F. Transfer meat loaf to a platter and let stand 10 minutes. **Optional**: Reserve the juices if you desire to make gravy (see recipe below).

SERVING SUGGESTIONS: With basmati rice or *millet mash* with gravy and asparagus; with *puréed parsnips with thyme* and steamed summer squash. Make extra tomato sauce and serve leftovers on a corn tortilla with steamed swiss chard for a gluten-free lunch the next day.

VPK: Bison is a lean red meat that is heavy, heating and strengthening. The tarragon and quinoa will lend some coolness and lightness to bring some balance. All doshas should eat in moderation. Kapha and pitta can add a side of sprouts.

VARIATIONS: Reduce the bison by half and replace with ground turkey or chicken for kapha or pitta.

Gravy (optional)
While meat loaf is standing, make the gravy: In a small bowl combine 2 teaspoons of water with 2 teaspoons of crushed kuzu root starch. Place a fine mesh sieve over a 1-quart sauce pan and strain the juices from the meatloaf pan into the sauce pan. Add the kuzu root mixture to the pan. Bring to a boil, then reduce heat to simmer, whisking constantly until desired thickness.

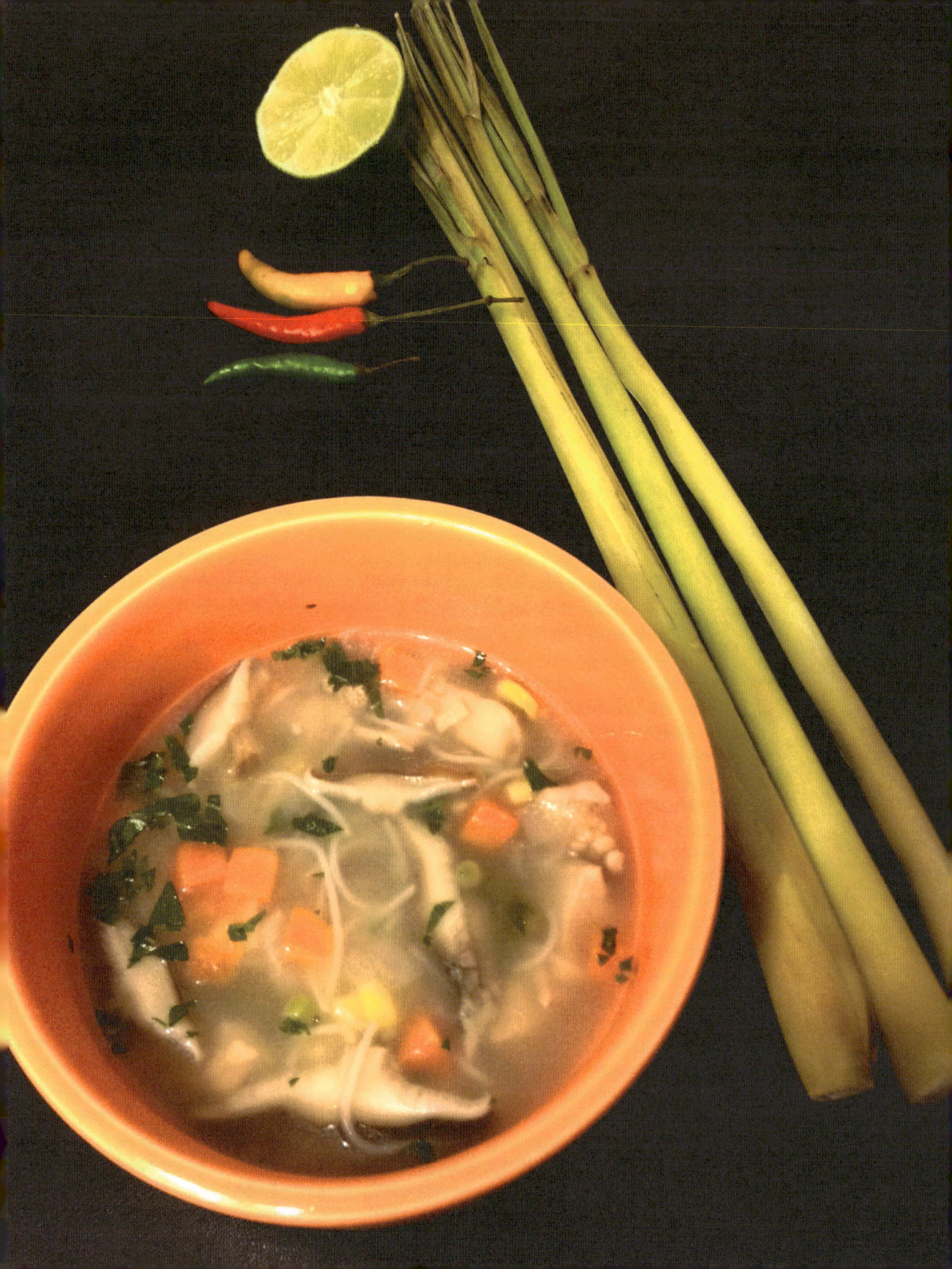

Chapter 11: Any Time Soups & Stews

Soups and stews are a great meal any time of the day. They are the easiest food to make for tri-doshic cooking, because when foods are cooked together the qualities will tend to mellow and balance each other.

I like to purée soups to give them a creamy texture, without adding the fat or calories of cream or dairy. It's a healthy way to eat a rich tasting soup.

Commercially prepared vegetable broths, stocks and bouillion cubes are generally high in sodium. As a healthier and lower cost option, the recipes here for soups and stews use water as their base. The flavor will come from the herbs and vegetables that comprise the soup, rather than salt.

ॐ Recipes - Any Time Soups & Stews

- Brazilian Black Bean Stew
- Caribbean Aduki Bean Stew
- Puréed Lemon Garbanzo Soup
- Creamy Corn Soup
- Summer Vegetable Soup
- Creamy Beet Leek Soup with Minted Yogurt
- Beet Sweet Potato Soup
- Borscht Lentil Soup
- Winter Chestnut Soup
- Ginger Pumpkin Soup
- Thai Lemongrass Vermicelli Soup
- Mung Dal Cilantro Soup
- Dashi Clear Broth
- Dashi Puy Lentil Soup
- Miso Soup
- Dashi Noodle Soup
- Turkey Cilantro Meatballs for Dashi Broth
- French Lentil Soup with Pork
- Kapha Pitta Barley Kale Soup
- Mushroom Tarragon Purée

❁ Brazilian Black Bean Stew
DF/GF/SF

Servings: 3

2 tablespoons sunflower oil
½ cup onion, peeled and chopped
½ teaspoon ginger, peeled, minced

1 cup tomatoes, peeled, seeded, minced
¾ cup water
1 cup sweet potatoes, peeled, cut into ½-inch cubes
15-ounce can black beans, rinsed and drained
½ teaspoon Himalayan salt
½ teaspoon crushed black pepper
2 teaspoons maple syrup
¾ cup frozen corn
½ cup frozen string beans, ends trimmed, chopped
2 tablespoons cilantro, chopped
2 tablespoons lime juice

In a 2-quart pan, warm the sunflower oil over medium heat. Add the onion and ginger and sauté for 2 minutes. Add the tomatoes, water, sweet potatoes, black beans, salt, pepper and maple syrup and bring to a boil. Reduce heat to low and simmer, covered until the potatoes are done (about 15 minutes). Add the corn and string beans and cook, uncovered for 3 minutes. Remove from heat and add the cilantro and lime juice.

SERVING SUGGESTIONS: Serve with basmati rice or *jasmine coconut rice* and salad of mixed greens with *tri-doshic white balsamic vinaigrette*.

VPK: Vata can eat this on occasion. Beans in general are best for pitta and kapha, due to their cold, dry qualities and astringent taste.

VARIATIONS: Add ¼ pound chorizo sausage (or linguica), broiled and cut into ¼ inch slices. Chorizo and linguica are spicy Portuguese sausages; purchase a brand that is nitrate-free. Otherwise, substitute with any spicy sausage that does not contain nitrates.

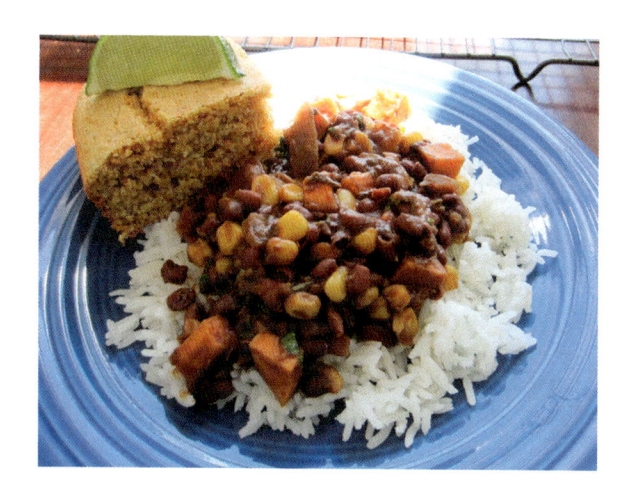

❀ Caribbean Aduki Bean Stew
DF/GF/SF/V
Servings: 3

3 tablespoons sunflower oil
½ cup onion, diced
2 tablespoons fresh ginger, minced

Spice Mix (combine in a small bowl):
¼ teaspoon allspice
⅛ teaspoon nutmeg
⅛ teaspoon cayenne pepper
¼ teaspoon ground cinnamon
¼ teaspoon ground cumin
¼ teaspoon thyme

1 cup yam, peeled, cut into ½-inch cubes (or squash or pumpkin)
2 tablespoons molasses (or coconut sugar)
1½ cups water
¼ teaspoon Himalayan salt
¼ teaspoon crushed black pepper
15-ounce can aduki beans
¾ cup frozen corn
2 tablespoons cilantro, chopped
2 tablespoons lime juice

Heat the oil in a 2-quart pan over medium heat. Add the onions and ginger and cook until the onions are soft and translucent (3-5 minutes). Add the spice mix and cook about 1 minute, stirring to infuse the flavor of the spices. Add the yam, molasses, water, salt and pepper and bring to a boil. Reduce heat and simmer, uncovered until the yams are tender (about 15 minutes). The liquid will cook down to a thick sauce. Add the beans and stir; cook for an additional minute. Remove from heat and add the corn; cover and let the corn steam for 5 minutes. Stir in the cilantro and lime juice and serve.

SERVING SUGGESTIONS: Serve with *jasmine coconut rice* or with *GF corn bread* or corn tortillas and a green leaf or spinach salad.

VPK: This is ideal for kapha and pitta; vata can eat in moderation.

❁ Puréed Lemon Garbanzo Soup
DF/GF/SF/V
Servings: 4

1 tablespoon avocado oil (or sunflower or grapeseed)
½ cup chopped onion
15-ounce can garbanzo beans (chickpeas)
4 cups water
1 bay leaf
1 teaspoon oregano, dried
2 tablespoons lemon juice
½ teaspoon Himalayan salt
¼ teaspoon pepper

In a 3-quart pan, warm the oil over medium-low heat. Add the onion and sauté until translucent. Add the remaining ingredients and cook for 30 minutes. Remove the bay leaf and discard. Purée with an immersion blender.

SERVING SUGGESTIONS: Serve with blue corn chips or pita bread; or serve with *Moroccan veggie burgers* or *wild rice with acorn squash & Brussels sprouts in sweet balsamic dressing*.

VPK: Vata and kapha can add ½ teaspoon pressed garlic or ½ teaspoon cayenne pepper when sautéing the onion; vata and pitta can serve with *avocado cucumber salad* (vata can add *tahini dressing*); kapha can serve with a chicory and mixed greens salad with lime juice.

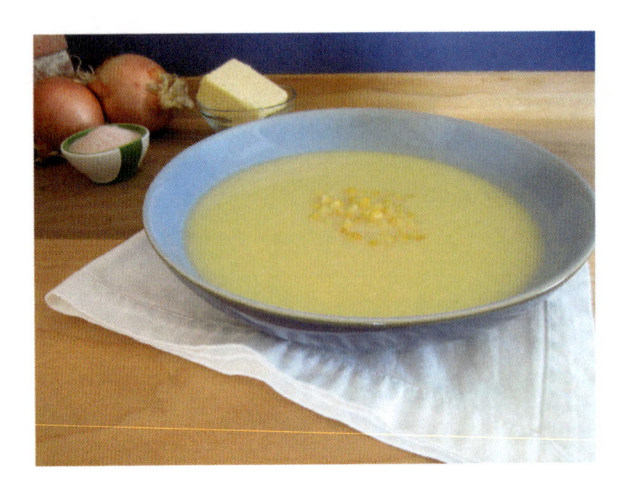

❁ Creamy Corn Soup
GF/SF/V
Servings: 2

2 teaspoons butter or ghee (do not substitute)
1 cup onions, chopped
4 cups water
½ teaspoon Himalayan salt
1 cup Yukon potato, peeled and chopped
10-ounce bag frozen corn, steamed

In a 2-quart pot, warm the butter over medium-low heat. Add the onions and cook for 3 minutes, stirring continually. Add the water, salt and potato and bring to a boil. Reduce heat to low and simmer until the potatoes are soft (about 15 minutes). Add half the corn. Remove from heat and purée with an immersion blender. Add half of the remaing corn to the pan and stir to combine. Ladle into individual serving bowls and garnish with the remaining corn.

SERVING SUGGESTIONS: Serve with *Moroccan veggie burgers* or *bison meat loaf* or *warm beet salad with beet greens*.

VPK: Well balanced for pitta and kapha; vata can add extra ghee or butter on their serving.

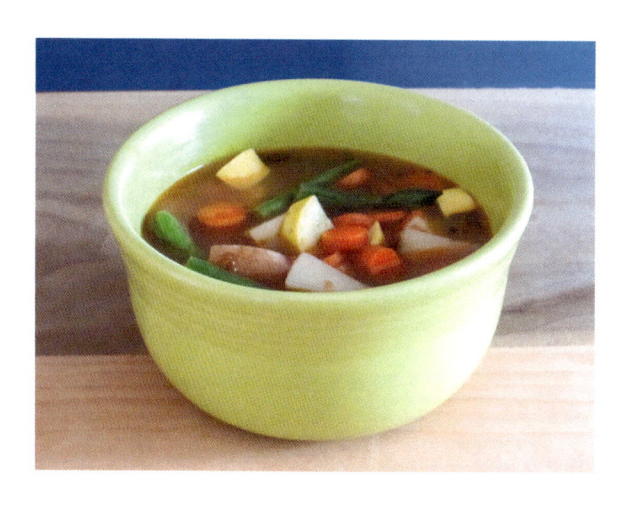

❀ Summer Vegetable Soup
DF/GF/SF/V
Servings: 3

1½ tablespoons sunflower oil
½ cup leeks* (outer tough stems removed, washed, coarsely chopped)
¼ teaspoon tarragon, dried
¼ teaspoon savory, dried
½ teaspoon Himalayan salt
¼ teaspoon crushed black pepper
¼ cup tomatoes, peeled, seeded, coarsely chopped
1 cup red potato, skin scrubbed, chopped into ¾-inch pieces
½ cup carrots, scrubbed, coarsely chopped
3 cups water
½ cup string beans, rinsed, chopped
¼ cup summer squash, coarsely chopped
¼ teaspoon apple cider vinegar

In a 2½-quart pan, warm the oil over low heat. Add the leeks and sauté for a few minutes until fragrant. Add the tarragon, savory, salt and pepper, stirring until combined. Add the tomatoes, potatoes, carrots and water; bring to a boil. Reduce heat to simmer; cook covered until the potatoes and carrots are almost done (about 10 minutes). Add the remaining ingredients and simmer until the vegetables are soft (about 5 minutes).

Serving suggestions: Serve with a salad of mixed greens or *minted apricot couscous* or Bhutanese red rice.

VPK: Tri-doshic.

VARIATIONS: You may add ½ cup of cooked cannellini beans or chickpeas for a heartier soup. If you use fresh herbs, add them during the last few minutes of cooking. You may substitute 1 tablespoon of lemon juice for the apple cider vinegar.

ABOUT: *Leeks have a sweet, mild oniony taste. If you can't find leeks, you may substitute an onion. To prepare leeks, remove the tough, outer stalks. Slice about ¼ inch from the bottom (white) end and discard; slice the tops (dark green) off and discard. Cut the leek in half lengthwise then rinse under cold water, spreading apart the layers to remove any dirt. Coarsely chop.

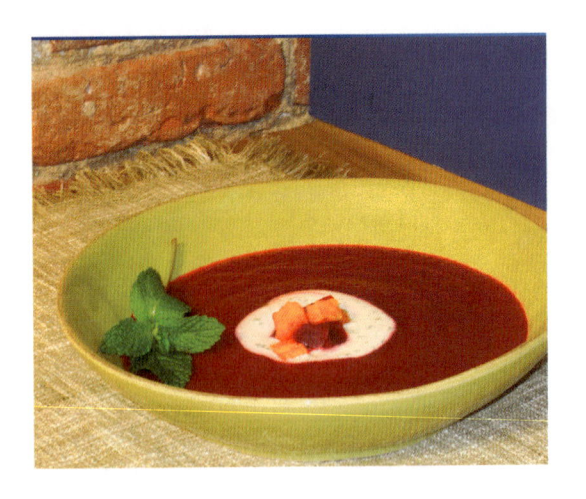

❁ Creamy Beet Leek Soup with Minted Yogurt
GF/SF/V
Servings: 4

1 tablespoon ghee or butter (or sunflower oil)
1 cup leeks, chopped
1½ cups carrots, chopped
3 cups beets, peeled, chopped
1 teaspoon coriander powder
1 teaspoon Himalayan salt
½ teaspoon ground pepper
2 teaspoons orange zest
4 cups water

Minted Yogurt (vata/pitta)
1 cup plain yogurt (soy or coconut yogurt for dairy free)
2 teaspoons mint, chopped
1 teaspoon rice syrup (or coconut sugar or maple syrup)

For the minted yogurt, combine the ingredients in a 2-cup container and whisk to blend.

In a 3-quart sauce pan, warm the butter over medium low heat. Add the leeks and sauté until translucent (about 3 minutes). Add the remaining ingredients and bring to a boil. Reduce heat, cover and simmer until the vegetables are tender (about 25 minutes). Purée with immersion blender. Transfer to serving bowls; top with 1 tablespoon of minted yogurt. Optional garnish: using a spoon, transfer a few beets to a cutting board before you purée the soup; chop the beets into half-inch cubes and spoon into the middle of each serving dish.

SERVING SUGGESTIONS: This can be served with *Moroccan veggie burgers*, *baked falafel balls*, *lime-ginger tofu* or *Marco's porcini risotto*.

VPK: Tri-doshic; kapha can omit the yogurt topping.

ABOUT: Leeks are tri-doshic; beets are sweet with a warming energy, making them suitable for vata and kapha. When cooked, the flavor mellows. Some of my pitta friends feel that peeling the beets reduces their pungency. I have found that beets vary significantly depending on where they were grown. So experiment for yourselves and follow your intuition.

❁ Beet Sweet Potato Soup
GF/SF/V

Modify the *Creamy Beet Leek Soup* recipe as follows: substitute 2 cups peeled, sweet potato for the carrot and reduce the beets to 1½ cups to create a cooler energetic with a beautiful magenta-color!

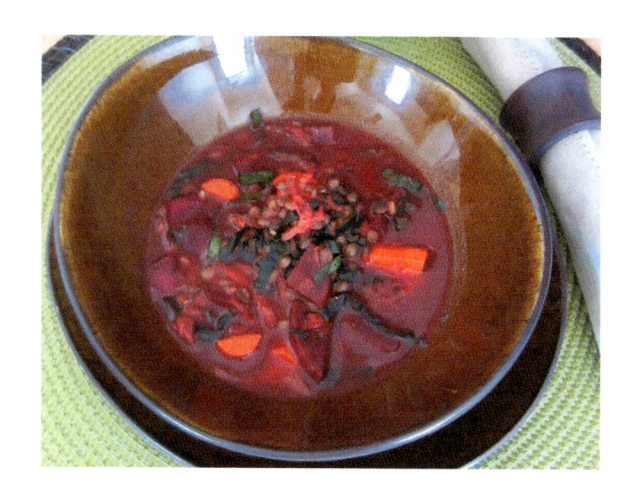

❀ Borscht Lentil Soup

DF/GF/SF/V
Servings: 3

1 tablespoon sunflower oil
½ cup onion, chopped
5 cups water
½ cup carrots, skins scrubbed, diced
2 cups beets, peeled, chopped into ½ inch cubes
Reserve the leafy tops from the beets: wash, leaves torn from inner stem, chopped into 1-inch pieces (tough stalks discard)
½ cup French lentils
1 cup napa cabbage, shredded
½ teaspoon dried dill
1 tablespoon white balsamic vinegar
2 tablespoons lemon juice
½ teaspoon Himalayan salt
¼ teaspoon crushed black pepper
½ cup plain yogurt (optional)

In a 3-quart pan, warm the oil over medium heat. Add the onion and sauté for 3 minutes. Add water, carrots, beets, lentils and cabbage and bring to boil. Reduce heat to low; simmer uncovered until the beets and lentils are tender (about 20 minutes). Remove from heat and add the beet greens, dill, balsamic vinegar, lemon juice, salt and pepper. Cover and allow the beet greens to wilt (about 5 minutes). Stir and serve.

SERVING SUGGESTIONS: Garnish with plain yogurt for vata or pitta. Serve with *fennel crusted paneer* or plain paneer.

VPK: This combination of vegetables and lentils in a soup is easy for all digestive systems, while providing a hearty, balanced meal. The warm, pungent beets are cooled by the bitter beet greens. Napa cabbage is mild and the easiest cabbage for vata to tolerate, especially here in a soup.

❀ Winter Chestnut Soup

DF/GF/SF/V
Servings: 4

3 tablespoons sunflower oil
1 bay leaf
1 cup onion, peeled, finely chopped
15-ounce jar of chestnuts, peeled, roasted
½ teaspoon Himalayan salt
½ teaspoon crushed black pepper
½ teaspoon dried sage
1 cup water
¼ cup cream (or almond milk or cashew cream sauce)

Heat the sunflower oil in a 3-quart pan over medium heat. Add the bay leaf and onions and sauté until lightly golden (about 3 minutes). Add the chestnuts salt, pepper and sage; cook for two minutes. Add the water and bring to a boil. Reduce heat and simmer until the chestnuts are soft (about 10 minutes). Remove from heat and add the cream. Purée with an immersion blender.

SERVING SUGGESTIONS: Serve with *ginger almond squash pie*.

VPK: This creamy soup is balancing for vata; pitta and kapha can eat on occasion.

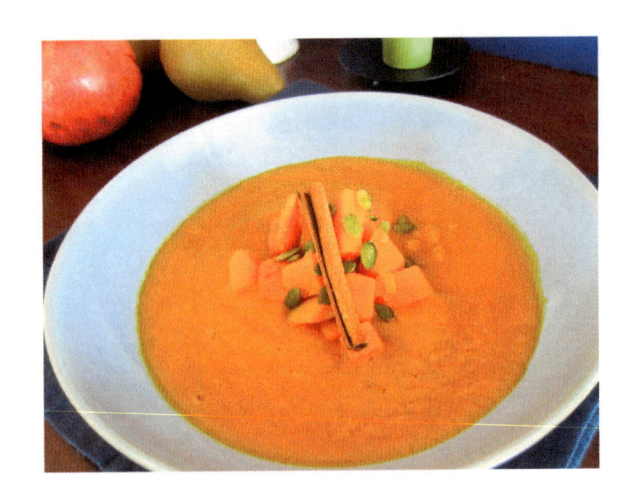

🌸 Ginger Pumpkin Soup
DF/GF/SF/V
Servings: 2

1 tablespoon butter or ghee (or sunflower oil)
1 teaspon fresh ginger, peeled, chopped
½ cup brown onion, peeled, chopped

Spice Mix (combine in a small bowl):
- ½ teaspoon coriander powder
- ½ teaspoon cinnamon
- ⅛ teaspoon paprika
- 1 teaspoon coconut sugar (or maple syrup)
- ½ teaspoon Himalayan salt

2 cups pumpkin, peeled, seeded, chopped
1 cup sweet potato, peeled, chopped
3-4 cups water (enough to just cover the vegetables)
2 tablespoons pumpkin seeds (for garnish)

In a 2½-quart sauce pan, melt the butter over medium heat. Add the ginger and onions and sauté for two minutes. Add the spice mix and stir until combined. Add the pumpkin, potato and water; bring to a boil. Reduce heat to low and simmer, uncovered until the vegetables are soft (15-20 minutes).

SERVING SUGGESTIONS: Serve with *Brazilian black bean stew* or *Puy lentil artichoke in puff pastry pie, French lentil salad, fennel crusted paneer* or *Moroccan meatballs*.

VPK: Tri-doshic.

VARIATIONS: You can substitute acorn or butternut squash for the pumpkin; try garnishing with some grated orange rind; add a star anise or add a pinch of mace during cooking. For a heartier dish, add some leftover quinoa (about a half cup) when you add the pumpkin.

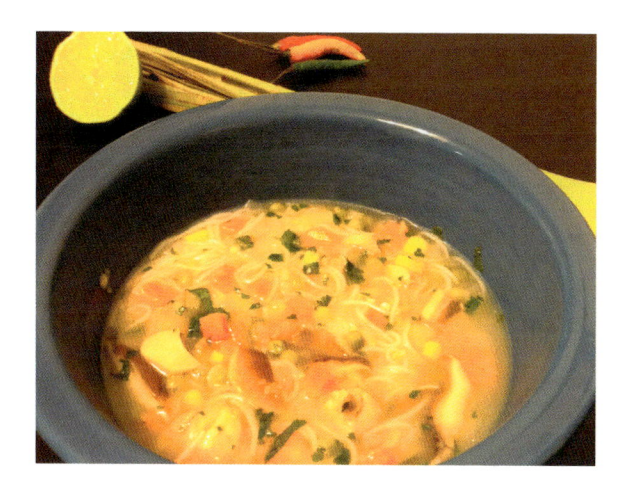

❀ Thai Lemongrass Vermicelli Soup
DF/GF/SF/V
Servings: 2

2 ounces vermicelli rice noodles
1 lemongrass stalk, outer tough layers removed
2 large (or 4 small) kaffir limes leaves (fresh or frozen)
¼ cup shiitake mushroom caps, sliced thin
3 cups water
1 tablespoons ginger, finely chopped
1 teaspoon garlic, pressed
½ teaspoon thin green chili, minced, (or ½ teaspoon cayenne)
¼ cup shallots, minced (or red onion)
1½ tablespoon fish sauce (omit for vegetarian)
1 teaspoon coconut sugar
2 ounces coconut milk
½ cup chopped vegetables of your choice (napa cabbage, carrots, summer squash, bok choy)
½ pound chicken thigh meat, boneless, skinless, diced (optional)
2 tablespoons cilantro, chopped
2 tablespoons basil, chopped
1 tablespoon tamari
1 tablespoon lime juice

Pour 5 cups of water into a 2-quart sauce pan and bring to a boil. Add the vermicelli and cook for 2-3 minutes until tender. Drain; rinse under cold water and set aside.

Place the lemongrass stalk onto a cutting board and trim an inch from both ends. Using the back of a knife blade, bruise the lemongrass (or pound with a mallet). Place the lemongrass, lime leaves and shitake into a into a 4-quart pot with 3-cups water. Bring to a boil. (The lemongrass stalks will stick out of the pan.) Add the ginger, garlic, chili and shallots. If you are using chicken, add it at this point; cook for a few minutes (or until the meat is almost done). Reduce heat to simmer and add the fish sauce, coconut sugar, coconut milk and vegetables, stirring to mix. Cover and cook for a few minutes until the vegetables are lightly steamed. Remove from heat. Remove lemongrass stalk and lime leaves. Stir in the vermicelli, cilantro, basil, tamari and lime juice. Serve.

SERVING SUGGESTIONS: Serve with *GF corn bread* or corn tortillas.

VPK: This is great for vata. Vata could also add a splash of sesame oil and/or additional coconut milk for more grounding; pitta can add additional coconut milk and cilantro to cool things down; kapha can omit the coconut milk entirely and add additional chilies if desired.

Variations: Shrimp can be substituted for chicken; *turkey cilantro meatballs* can be added; extra firm tofu can be added.

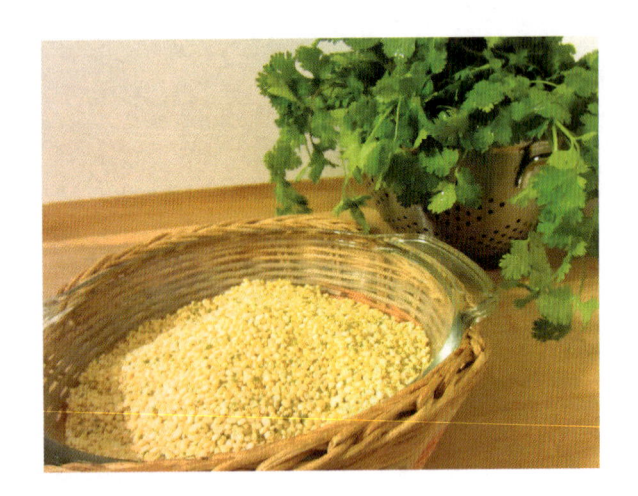

Mung Dal Cilantro Soup
DF/GF/SF/V
Servings: 3

1 cup mung dal, soaked overnight and drained
2½ cups water
¼ teaspoon turmeric
1 bay leaf
1 tablespoon grape seed oil
2 teaspoons ghee (sunflower oil for dairy free)
1 teaspoon cumin seeds
½ teaspoon coriander seeds, crushed
½ teaspoon black mustard seeds
1 teaspoon garlic, crushed
4 curry leaves
½ teaspoon Himalayan salt
⅛ teaspoon crushed black pepper
3 tablespoons cilantro, coarsely chopped

In a 2-quart pan, combine the dal, water, turmeric, bay leaf and grapeseed oil and bring to a boil. Reduce heat to simmer and cook uncovered until the dal is soft (about 20 minutes). Remove and discard the bay leaf. Purée, cover and set aside.

In an 8-inch fry pan, warm the ghee or sunflower oil over medium low heat. Add the cumin, coriander and black mustard seeds and sauté briefly until the mustard seeds pop. It will be quick (30 seconds or so). Be careful not to burn the mustard seeds or they will impart a bitter taste on your dish. Add the garlic and curry leaves, stirring to combine. Remove from heat and pour the spice mixture into the dal; add salt and pepper and top with cilantro. Stir to combine and serve.

SERVING SUGGESTIONS: Serve with steamed green vegetables and roti or corn tortilla. For a midday meal, add a serving of brown rice and steamed vegetables.

VPK: The lentils are well-soaked making them more balancing to vata; the mild spices are suitable for pitta; kapha can add some chili pepper on their serving

ABOUT: This is my recreation of a dish I would eat at The Tandoori Grill in Boulder, Colorado. When I was working late hours and too tired to cook, I would pair this with naan smothered in ghee and call it dinner! It is my Indian "comfort" food.

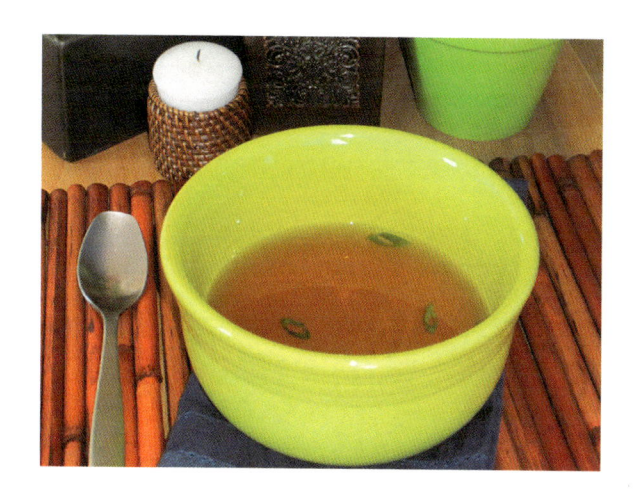

❀ Dashi Clear Broth
DF/GF/V

Yield: 4 cups of broth concentrate

4 cups of water
5 inch stick of kombu/dried kelp (gently wipe the kombu with clean cloth)
2 dried shiitake mushrooms
½ ounce tororo-kombu seaweed (optional)
2 teaspoons mirin (or coconut sugar)
2 tablespoons sake (rice wine)
2½ tablespoons tamari

Place the water kombu and shiitake in a 3-quart saucepan; place a small plate on the mushrooms to keep them submerged. After 4 hours, remove the plate and place on stover; bring water to just below a boil. Remove the kombu and shiitake. Cut off the shiitake stems and discard. Thinly slice the caps and return the caps to the water. Add tororo-kombu (if using) to the shiitake mushrooms and bring to a boil. Reduce heat and simmer for 5 minutes. Add remaining ingredients and stir to combine. Return to a boil and simmer for 2 minutes. Drain through a sieve lined with a paper towel (or thin cloth) into a spouted measuring cup. You now have a concentrated broth. To make a soup, dilute 50% with water and follow the recipe instructions.

You may store the concentrated broth in the freezer for later use. Transfer to a 1-cup air-tight freezer containers (for making *dashi Puy lentil soup* or *miso soup*, etc.) or use ice cube trays (to use as a flavoring to soup broths).

SERVING SUGGESTIONS: Use as a base for *dashi Puy lentil soup*, *miso soup* or *dashi noodle soup*.

VPK: Tri-doshic.

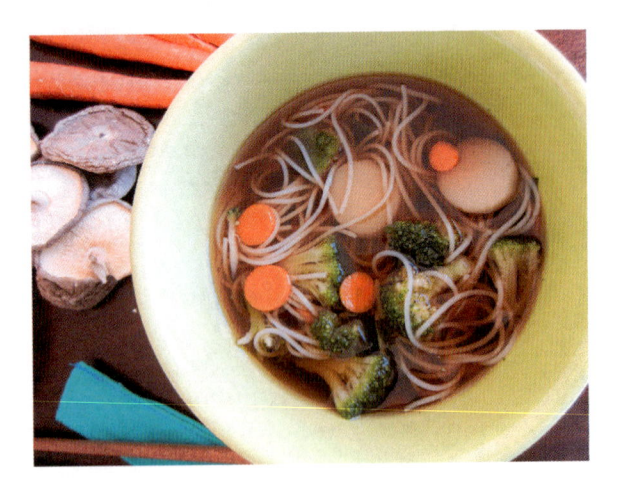

✿ Tri-doshic Dashi Clear Broth Soup Variations
DF/GF/V
Serves: 2

Dashi Puy lentil soup
2 cups *dashi clear broth*
2 cups water
½ cup puy lentils
½ cup carrots, sliced thin

Combine all ingredients in a 2-quart pan. Simmer on medium heat until carrots and lentils are tender (about 20 minutes). Serve.

Miso Soup
2 cups *dashi clear broth*
2 cups water
1 tablespoon white miso, dissolved in 1 teaspoon water
1 tablespoon scallions
1 tablespoon cilantro, chopped
½ teaspoon wakame, soaked for 15 minutes, drained, chopped

Combine the broth and water in a 2-quart pan and warm over medium heat. Remove from heat and add remaining ingredients. Stir and serve.
Variation: Add ⅛ cup cooked barley for pitta or kapha.

Dashi Noodle Soup
2 cups *dashi clear broth*
2 cups water
½ cup carrot, sliced thin
1 cup broccoli crowns, sliced like thin trees
4 water chestnuts
8 ounces fine rice vermicelli noodles (cooked for 2 minutes in boiling water; rinsed under cold water, then drained)

Combine the broth, water, carrot, broccoli and water chestnuts in a 2-quart pan and cook over medium heat until the vegetables are tender (about 15 minutes). Remove from heat; add the noodles; garnish with cilantro and lime. Serve.

Turkey Cilantro Meatballs – for Dashi broth
¼ pound of ground turkey
4 teaspoons cilantro (finely chopped)
1½ teaspoons bread crumbs, or gluten free bread crumbs
⅛ teaspoon crushed black pepper
⅛ teaspoon Himalayan salt
1 teaspoon grated lemon rind (optional)

Combine ingredients in a 2-quart mixing bowl. Shape into 18 mini meatballs (¾-inch in diameter). Cook for 15-20 minutes at 350°F. Add to dashi broth (diluted 50% with water) with vegetables and cooked lentils (or noodles); warm and serve. Prior to cooking, these can be frozen in Ziploc® freezer baggies for later use.

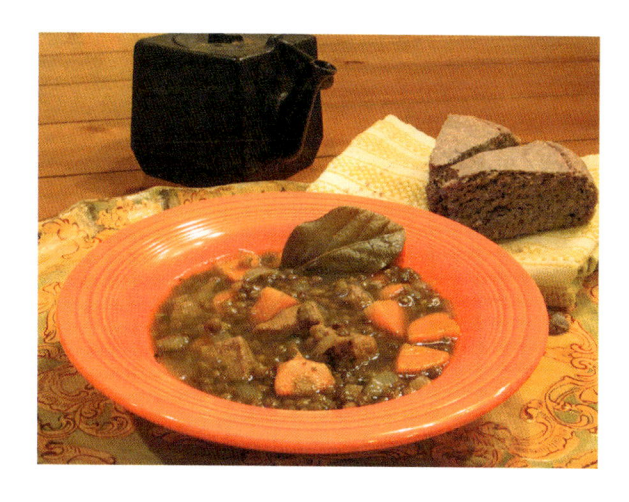

🌸 French Lentil Soup with Pork

DF/GF/SF
Servings: 3

1 tablespoon butter (or sunflower oil)
½ pound of pork sausage, sliced into 1-inch pieces
½ cup onion, peeled and chopped
1 bay leaf
4 cups water
1 cup Puy lentils (or French lentils)
¾ cup carrots, sliced thin
2 whole cloves
¼ teaspoon Himalayan salt
⅛ teaspoon dried tarragon
⅛ teaspoon dried thyme
½ teaspoon fresh rosemary, finely chopped
¼ teaspoon crushed black pepper

In a 3-quart pan, warm the butter over medium heat. Add the pork and sauté until browned; remove from pan and reserve. Add the onion and bay leaf and sauté for one minute. Add the water, lentils, carrots, cloves, salt and reserved pork and bring to a boil. Reduce heat to low and simmer, uncovered until the lentils are soft (about 20 minutes). Add the tarragon, thyme, rosemary and pepper and stir to combine. Remove from heat and serve.

SERVING SUGGESTIONS: Serve with crusty French bread or *GF corn bread* and *tri-doshic arugula radicchio cherry salad*.

VPK: Tri-doshic.

VARIATIONS: This can be made vegetarian by omitting the pork. Try adding ¼ teaspoon organic dry lavender.

ABOUT: If you are new to lentils or are serving them to people unaccustomed to eating lentils, this dish is a nice introduction. French lentils are relatively easy on the digestive system and, prepared with the well spiced broth makes them even more so; the small amount of pork in the dish provides some heaviness and grounding which carnivores generally seek in their meals.

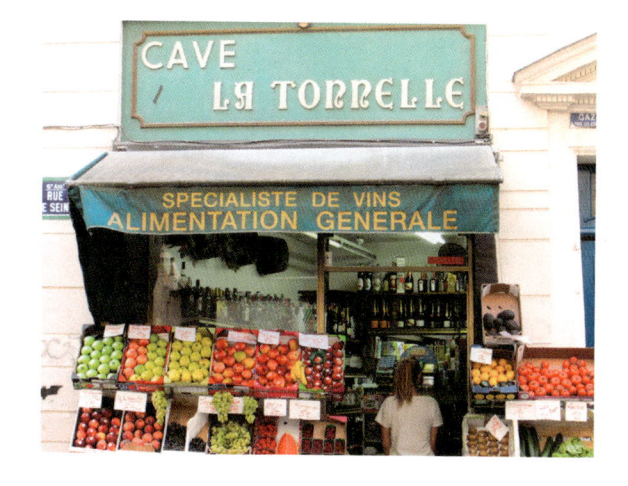

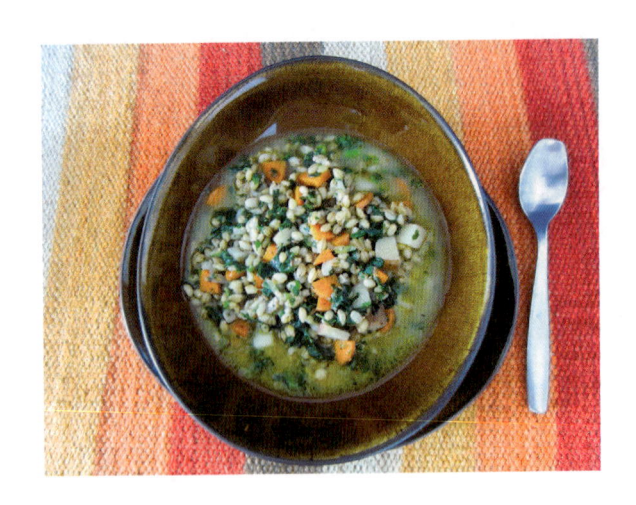

🌸 Kapha Pitta Barley Kale Soup
DF/GF/SF/V
Servings: 2

½ tablespoon sunflower seed oil
1 teaspoon cumin seed, coarsely ground
½ teaspoon dried savory
½ cup onion, chopped
½ teaspoon garlic, pressed
4 cups water
¼ cup water chestnuts, sliced in half
⅜ cup barley, uncooked, soaked overnight, drained
⅛ teaspoon cayenne powder
½ teaspoon Himalayan salt
¼ teaspoon pepper
½ cup carrots, slice into ¼-inch pieces
½ cup red potatoes, skin scrubbed, cut in ½-inch cubes
1 cup kale, rinsed, chopped into 1-inch pieces
1 teaspoon lemon juice

Add oil to a 2½-quart sauce and warm over medium heat. Add the cumin seeds and savory, stirring until fragrant (about 30 seconds). Add the onion and garlic and sauté for one minute. Add the water, water chestnuts, barley, cayenne, salt and pepper and bring to a boil. Reduce heat and simmer, uncovered for 40 minutes. Add the carrots and potatoes and cook until the barley and vegetables are tender (about another 20 minutes). Remove from heat and stir in the kale and lemon juice; cover and let set for 5 minutes for the kale to wilt. Serve.

SERVING SUGGESTIONS: This is a hearty one-dish meal.

VPK: This is balancing for pitta and kapha. If serving for vata, substitute the red potatoes for sweet potatoes and substitute the kale for asparagus.

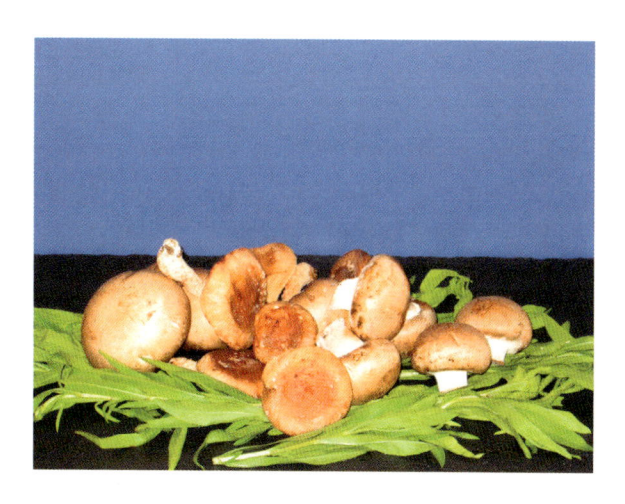

✿ Mushroom Tarragon Purée
DF/GF/SF/V
Servings: 2

2 tablespoons sunflower oil
½ tablespoon minced shallots
½ cup button mushroom caps, sliced
¼ cup dried shiitake mushroom caps, rehydrated in 1 cup water, liquid reserved, sliced
½ cup portobello (or baby bella) mushroom caps, sliced
¾ cup red potato, peeled, chopped
⅛ teaspoon dried tarragon
1¼ cups water
¼ teaspoon Himalayan salt
⅛ teaspoon pepper
¼ cup coconut milk
1 tablespoon lemon juice

In a 2-quart sauté pan, warm the oil over medium-low heat. Add the shallots and cook for 2 minutes, gently stirring; add the sliced mushroom caps and cook for another 2 minutes, stirring constantly. Add the potato, tarragon, water, reserved mushroom liquid, salt and pepper and bring to a boil. Reduce heat to low and simmer until the potatoes are soft (about 15-20 minutes); remove from heat and add the coconut milk and the lemon juice. Purée with an immersion blender.

Serving suggestions: Serve with a salad of mixed greens and *red quinoa with endive & cranberries* or *wild rice with acorn squash & Brussels sprouts*.

VPK: The coconut milk (and tarragon) helps cool the energetics of the warm mushrooms; the small amount does not impart any coconut taste. If cooking solely for pitta, increase the potatoes to one cup and reduce the lemon juice to one teaspoon.

Radishes $2

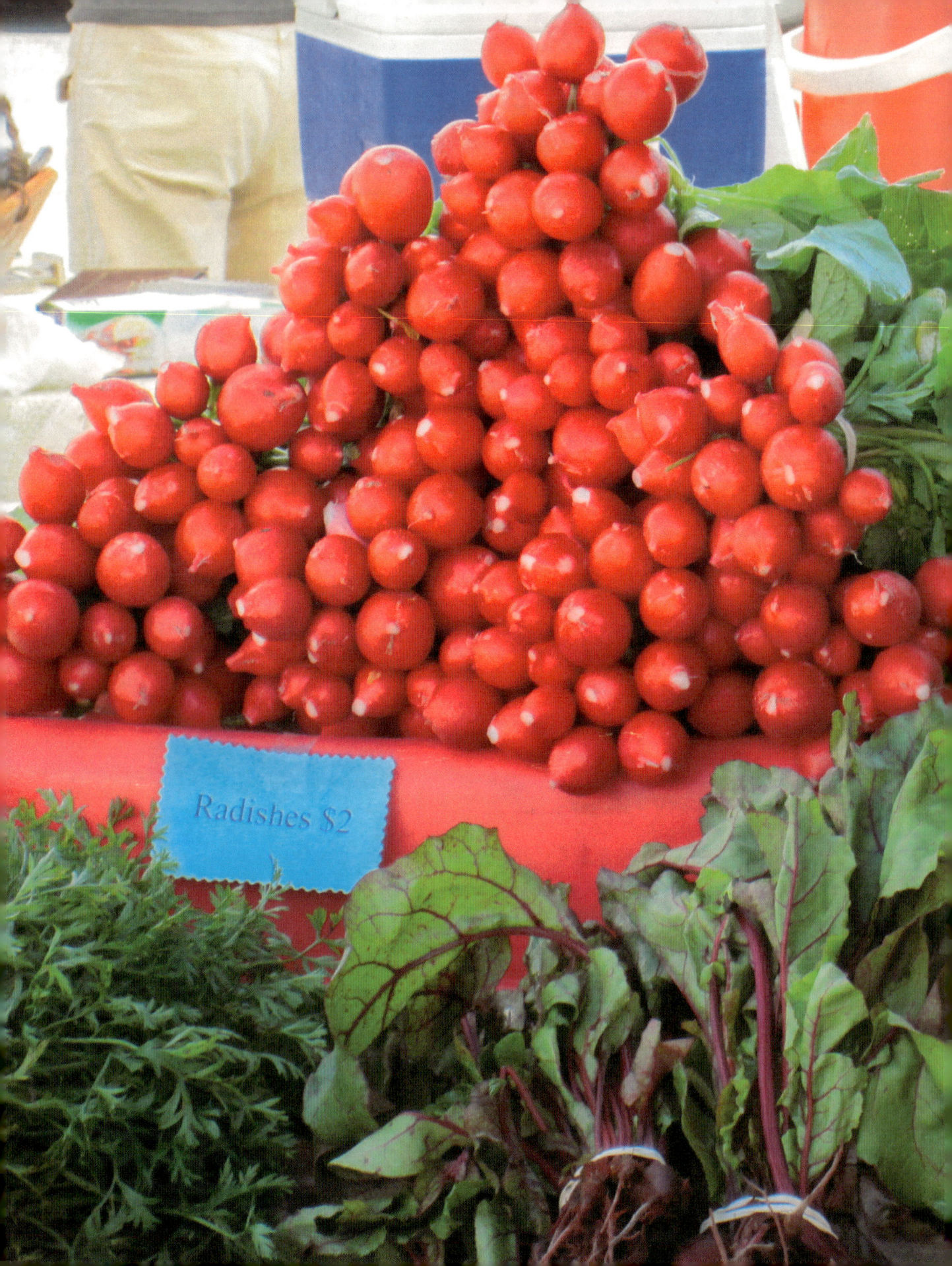

Chapter 12: Vegetables

If you are using fresh, seasonal and local vegetables, then preparation should be simple to allow the natural flavors of the vegetables to fully awaken. I always keep some organic frozen vegetables in my freezer; because sometimes, I don't have time to make it to the supermarket.

For pitta and kapha, gently steam some greens; for vata purée root vegetables with almond, cashew or coconut milk. Garnish with wedges of lemon or lime and top with toasted nuts. Leafy greens tend to be cool and bitter, so vata does best when these are cooked in a soup or covered in a creamy sauce (such as a nut butter sauce) to bring warmth and grounding.

ॐ Recipes - Vegetables

- **GINGER ALMOND SQUASH PIE**
- **ROSEMARY ROASTED ROOT VEGETABLES**
- **ZUCCHINI PASTA**
- **ASIAN VEGETABLES**
- **PURÉED ORANGE GINGER YAMS**
- **PURÉED PARSNIPS WITH THYME**
- **BRUSSELS SPROUT SWEET POTATO SAUTÉ**
- **KELP NOODLES WITH ALMOND SAUCE**
- **ALMOND SAUCE**
- **SHAVED FENNEL IN ORANGE SAUCE**
- **SWEET POTATO FRIES**

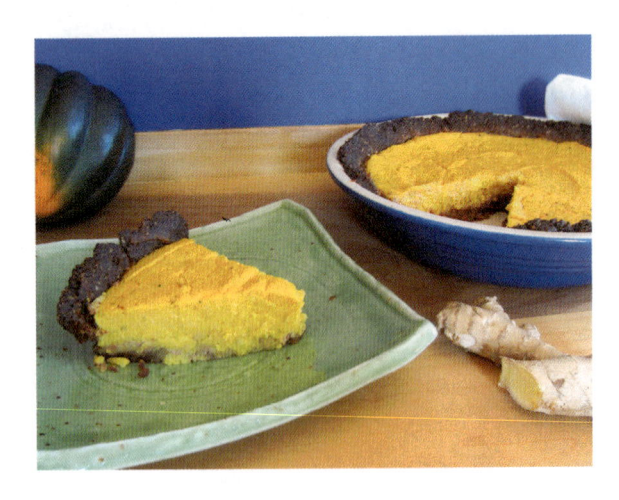

🌸 Ginger Almond Squash Pie

DF/GF/SF/V
Yield: one 9-inch pie

2 cups acorn squash, peeled, cubed
2 cups sweet potato, peeled, chopped
1 cup Yukon potato, peeled, chopped
1 tablespoon ghee (or sunflower oil)

Spice Mix (combine in a small bowl):
- 1 tablespoon ginger, peeled and minced
- ½ teaspoon cinnamon powder
- 1 teaspoon coconut sugar
- ½ teaspoon Himalayan salt
- ¼ teaspoon crushed black pepper

1 egg, beaten
¼ cup almond milk
½ teaspoon grated orange rind
One 9-inch *GF Macadamia Nut Pie Crust*

Preheat the oven to 300°F. Prepare the Macadamia Nut Pie Crust.

Place the squash and potatoes in a 3-quart saucepan; add 4 cups of water and bring to a boil. Cook until the vegetables are par-boiled (about 10 minutes). Drain and transfer to a 3-quart mixing bowl. Set aside. Heat the ghee in an 8-inch fry pan over low heat. Add the spice mix and cook for 1 minute, stirring to combine. Pour over the vegetables and add the egg, almond milk and orange rind; purée with immersion blender until just combined. Transfer to the prepared pie crust and bake in the oven until the pie is firm to the touch (about 45-60 minutes).

SERVING SUGGESTIONS: For a mid-day meal, serve with *tri-doshic arugula radicchio cherry salad* and *French lentil soup with pork* (or vegetarian version); or serve with *wild rice with acorn squash & Brussels sprouts in sweet balsamic dressing* topped with *dry fry tofu*.

VPK: Nicely balanced for all doshas.

VARIATIONS: Add 2 drops of rose water and ½ teaspoon cardamom; substitute a 9-inch ready-made organic pie crust.

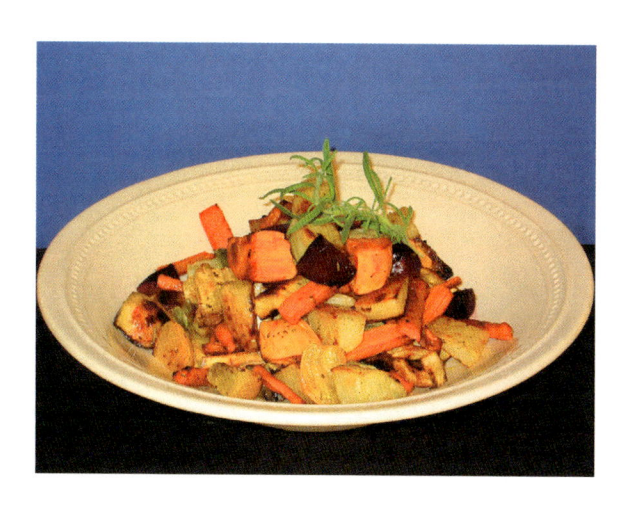

❁Rosemary Roasted Root Vegetables
DF/GF/SF/V
Servings: 4

1 cup red potatoes
1 cup yams
½ cup turnips
½ cup parsnips
1 cup red or yellow beets
4 Brussels sprouts, sliced in quarters

Seasoning:
2 tablespoons sunflower oil
1 tablespoon dried rosemary
½ teaspoon Himalayan salt
¼ teaspoon crushed black pepper
1 tablespoon lemon juice

Preheat oven to 400°F and grease a 13x9x2 pan with sunflower oil. Prepare the vegetables by scrubbing them with a vegetable brush under cold running water. Remove any stems/ends and cut into 1-inch pieces. Transfer to a large bowl. Add "seasoning" ingredients and toss with the vegetables until evenly coated. It's easiest to do with your hands. Transfer the veggies into the prepared pan and bake until they are soft (about 1 hour).

VARIATIONS: You can substitute ½ tablespoon of oregano for the rosemary; add ⅛ cup of coarsely chopped parsley. Leftovers can be added to soup the next day or added to couscous salads or rice salads.

ABOUT: Turnips are part of the same family as radishes; they are balancing to kapha. Parsnips are related to carrots and when cooked, are balancing to vata and pitta. Brussels sprouts are part of the cabbage family so they are best tolerated by pitta and kapha.

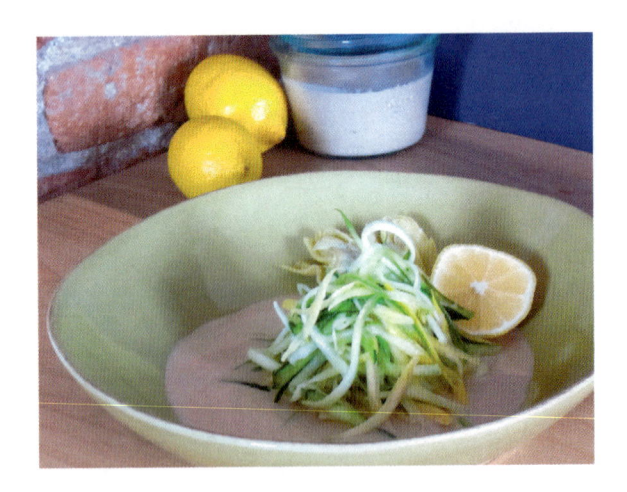

🌸 Zucchini Pasta
DF/GF/SF/V
Servings: 2

½ pound of zucchini (about 2 small zucchinis), washed
½ pound of summer squash, washed
1 tablespoon sunflower oil
Box grater*

Cut the ends off of the zucchini and summer squash. On a clean cutting surface, place the box grater on its side with the largest holes on top. Hold the zucchini lengthwise and slide it across the box grater, making long, thin strands. Don't grate the seeds in the middle; when you reach the seeds at the core, flip the zucchini over and start grating the opposite side. Continue working your way around the zucchini. Discard the inner seeds. Repeat with the summer squash.

In a 10-inch non-stick fry pan, dry fry the vegetables over low heat until they are slightly wilted (about 3 minutes). Transfer to a paper towel to drain excess moisture.

SERVING SUGGESTIONS: Serve with *artichoke lemon cream sauce* and broiled chicken, shrimp or tofu (marinated in *tri-doshic lime-cumin vinaigrette* or *lime ginger marinade*) and *borscht lentil soup*.

VPK: Balancing to all three doshas. The dry frying removes some of the moisture to make the vegetables suitable for kapha. If serving for vata only, sauté the zucchini with sunflower oil instead of dry-frying.

*You can also use a mandolin or food processor with a julienne blade; or a spiral vegetable slicer; or a knife.

🌸 Asian Vegetables
DF/GF/V
Servings: 2

½ cup red cabbage, thinly shredded
½ cup carrot, thinly sliced
½ cup zucchini, thinly sliced

Pour 1 cup water into a 10-inch fry pan and bring to a boil. Add the cabbage and cook until the cabbage is wilted (about 5 minutes); remove the cabbage, drain and cool on a paper towel-lined plate (the red/purple will bleed onto everything it touches so handle with care). Pour 1 cup of fresh water into the fry pan and again bring to a boil; blanch the carrots and zucchini in the same fashion. Strain and cool on a paper towel-lined plate; transfer all the vegetables to a 2½-quart mixing bowl; Add ¼ cup *tri-doshic Asian lime dressing* and toss gently with a wooden spoon.

SERVING SUGGESTIONS: Serve with *broiled lime ginger shrimp*, chicken or tofu.

VPK: Well balanced for all doshas.

❁ Puréed Orange Ginger Yams
DF/GF/SF/V
Servings: 3

2 cups yams, peeled, diced
4 cups water
1 tablespoons fresh ginger, grated
2 tablespoons ghee (or sunflower oil)
¼ teaspoon each: nutmeg, mace, cinnamon
1 teaspoon grated orange peel
½ - 1 cup yogurt or almond milk
1 tablespoon honey (optional)
3 tablespoons toasted almonds (optional)

Place the yams and water in a 3-quart sauce pan. Bring to a boil over medium heat; cook until tender (about 20 minutes). Drain the water and transfer yams to a bowl; set aside. Add ghee to the pan and warm over medium heat. Add the ginger and sweat until aromatic (about 30 seconds). Add the nutmeg, mace, cinnamon and orange peel and sauté for 1 minute. Remove the pan from the heat and return the yams to the pan and stir. Add the yogurt or almond milk and purée to desired consistency. Add honey (optional) and garnish with toasted almonds (optional).

SERVING SUGGESTIONS: Serve with *bison meatloaf* or broiled fish or chicken. Leftovers can be added to a soup broth (in lieu of tomatoes) for a sweet cooling energetic or can be used to make *millet breakfast patties*.

VPK: Tri-doshic.

❁ Puréed Parsnips with Thyme
DF/GF/SF/V
Servings: 2

1 cup parsnips, peeled, chopped
2 cups water
1 tablespoon sunflower oil (or organic butter)
¼ teaspoon garlic, pressed
¼ cup *cashew cream sauce* (or cream)
¼ teaspoon fresh thyme
½ teaspoon Himalayan salt
¼ teaspoon crushed black pepper

Place the parsnips in a 2-quart sauce pan with the water. Bring to a boil; reduce heat and simmer until tender (about 15 minutes). Drain the parsnips (reserving ¼ cup of the cooking water), then return parsnips to the pan.

In an 8-inch fry pan, warm the oil over low heat. Add the garlic and sauté for a few seconds until the garlic becomes fragrant. If the garlic turns brown, it will taste bitter, so discard and start fresh. Whisk in the cashew cream sauce and thyme and gently simmer for a few minutes. Add this mixture to the drained parsnips with the reserved cooking liquid, salt and pepper; purée with an immersion blender.

SERVING SUGGESTIONS: Serve as a side dish with fish, poultry or *bison meatloaf* or *wild rice salad with acorn squash & Brussels sprouts in sweet balsamic dressing* or *French lentil salad*.

VPK: Parsnips are in the carrot family, so share similar energetics: sweet, cooling and mildly astringent; they are most balancing for vata and pitta. The garlic and thyme balance the dish for kapha.

VARIATIONS: Add one tablespoon minced shallots (sauté with the garlic) or chives or scallions; if serving solely for kapha or pitta, you can substitute white potatoes for the parsnips.

Brussels Sprout Sweet Potato Sauté

DF/GF/SF/V
Servings: 2

1 tablespoon sunflower oil (or butter)
½ teaspoon cumin seeds, lightly crushed
¼ teaspoon fennel seeds, lightly crushed
1½ cups sweet potato, peeled, chopped into ½-inch cubes
1 cup Brussels sprouts, ends removed, and wilted leaves trimmed
2 tablespoons lemon juice
½ teaspoon grated lemon peel
¼ teaspoon Himalayan salt

Cut the Brussels sprouts into wedges (i.e., first cut them in half lengthwise from the stem, then in half again, lengthwise). Pour the oil into a 2-quart sauté pan; it should be just enough to make a thin layer on the bottom of the pan (adjust – more or less oil - if necessary). Warm the oil over medium heat. Add the cumin and fennel and sauté for 30 seconds. Add the sweet potato and sauté, stirring constantly for 5 minutes. Add additional oil if the pan is drying out. Add the Brussels sprouts and sauté an additional 2 – 3 minutes until tender. Be careful not to overcook the Brussels sprouts or they will taste bitter. Remove from heat and add the lemon juice, lemon peel and salt. Stir to combine. Serve.

SERVING SUGGESTIONS: Serve with *mushroom tarragon purée* soup and brown rice; serve with *creamy beet leek soup with minted yogurt* and brown rice or *minted apricot couscous*. For non-vegetarian, this goes well with a broiled white fish such as halibut (fennel crusted) or *fennel crusted paneer*.

VPK: Brussels sprouts are very drying, so vata may want to add extra butter on their serving (or a nut butter sauce, a seed butter sauce or a vinaigrette); if serving for vata or kapha only, add ½ cup peeled, chopped beets.

ABOUT: Brussels sprouts are astringent and mildly heating and diuretic; ideal for pitta and kapha. Here they are combined with sweet potatoes to bring some balance and grounding for vata without upsetting pitta.

TOPPING OPTIONS

Cilantro (VPK)
Fresh fennel, raw, finely chopped (VPK)
Steamed cabbage, chopped fine (PK)
Steamed carrots, cut in match sticks (VPK)
Scallions (VK)
Sesame Seeds (V)
Pumpkin seeds (VPK)

VPK: This is balancing for pitta and kapha; vata needs liberal use of the almond sauce.

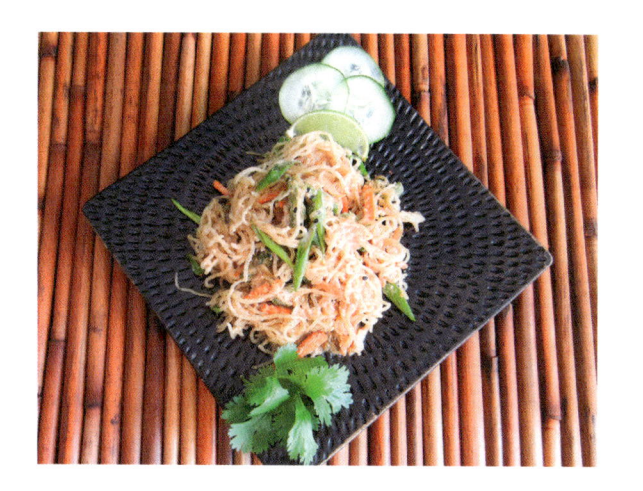

❁ KELP NOODLES WITH ALMOND SAUCE
DF/GF/V
Servings: 3

12 ounces kelp noodles, rinsed [Tangle Noodle Co®, San Diego, CA]
Almond Sauce
3 tablespoons almond butter
½ teaspoon jalapeño chili, minced, seeds removed
½ cup water
2 teaspoons tamari
1 teaspoon apple cider vinegar
1 tablespoon maple syrup (or coconut sugar)
⅛ teaspoon chili powder

In a 3-quart sauté pan, combine the almond butter, chili, water, tamari, apple cider vinegar, maple syrup and chili powder. Stir over low heat for 5-10 minutes until the consistency thickens, but do not let it boil; add the kelp noodles and stir. Warm over low heat to soften the noodles and infuse the flavors.

SERVING SUGGESTIONS: Top with any of the following toppings and serve with *miso soup*.

🍽 **Tangle Noodle Company** says, "We use sun-dried kelp minus the green outer layer, which is a skin. What is left is white and looks very much like our noodles. The dried kelp is made into a powder, which is then added to water and sodium alginate (sodium salt extracted from a brown seaweed), and then made into the noodles. No heat is used in the process of making the noodles."

Kelp noodles are low in fat and a good source of iron, calcium, iodine and other trace minerals. They are gluten-free, low in calories and carbohydrates with a neutral taste. The drying process and removal of the outer skin, makes them suitable for kapha and pitta, even though they contain the salty taste/energetics. While it is possible to eat these raw (they are dry and crunchy), I recommend slightly sautéing them so as to moisten the texture and aid digestion. For vata, these noodles must be cooked, served with a heavy, grounding sauce or in a soup and eaten in moderation.

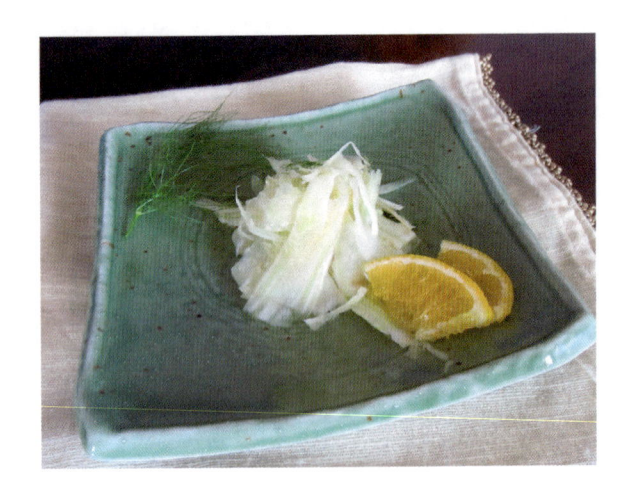

Shaved Fennel in Orange Sauce
DF/GF/SF/V
Servings: 2

1 large Fennel
Sauce:
2 tablespoons sunflower oil
1 tablespoon white balsamic vinegar
½ cup orange juice
½ teaspoon grated orange rind
1 teaspoon fennel fronds, chopped

Trim the base of the fennel; remove the top stalks (with the fronds) at their base of attachment. Hold the fennel in your hand and run a vegetable peeler lengthwise down one side. Repeat on this side for several more times. Then flip and shave the opposite side. Repeat this until all four sides have been shaved and all that is remaining is the inner core. Place in a 2-quart mixing bowl and set aside.

Make the dressing by whisking all the ingredients in a small, non-metallic bowl. Pour over the shaved fennel and gently toss. Transfer to a 10-inch fry pan and cook over medium-low heat for 1 to 2 minutes, stirring constantly. Remove from heat when the fennel is tender, but has a slight crunch in the middle. Sprinkle the fronds on top and serve.

SERVING SUGGESTIONS: Serve with *Moroccan veggie burger, red quinoa with endive and cranberries, polenta with shitake mushroom sauce, minted apricot couscous, Marco's porcini risotto, mushroom tarragon purée*.

VPK: Fennel is tri-doshic.

Sweet Potato Fries
DF/GF/SF/V
Servings: 2

2 cups sweet potatoes, skins scrubbed
3 tablespoons sunflower oil
¼ teaspoon Himalayan salt
¼ teaspoon crushed black pepper

Line your broiler with aluminum foil and preheat. Cut the potatoes into thick wedges: slice the potatoes in half, lengthwise; then slice lengthwise one or two more times until you have several wedges about ¾-inch thick. In a 3-quart mixing bowl, combine the oil, salt and pepper. Add the potatoes and toss until lightly coated. Transfer to the broiler. Cook until the first side is just starting to turn golden - check after 3 minutes; broiler settings will vary. Flip and cook the other side for about 2 minutes until just starting to brown.

SERVING SUGGESTIONS: Serve with *Moroccan veggie burgers*.

VPK: Ideal for vata; pitta can eat in moderation; kapha can eat on occasion and should add crushed garlic or cayenne pepper.

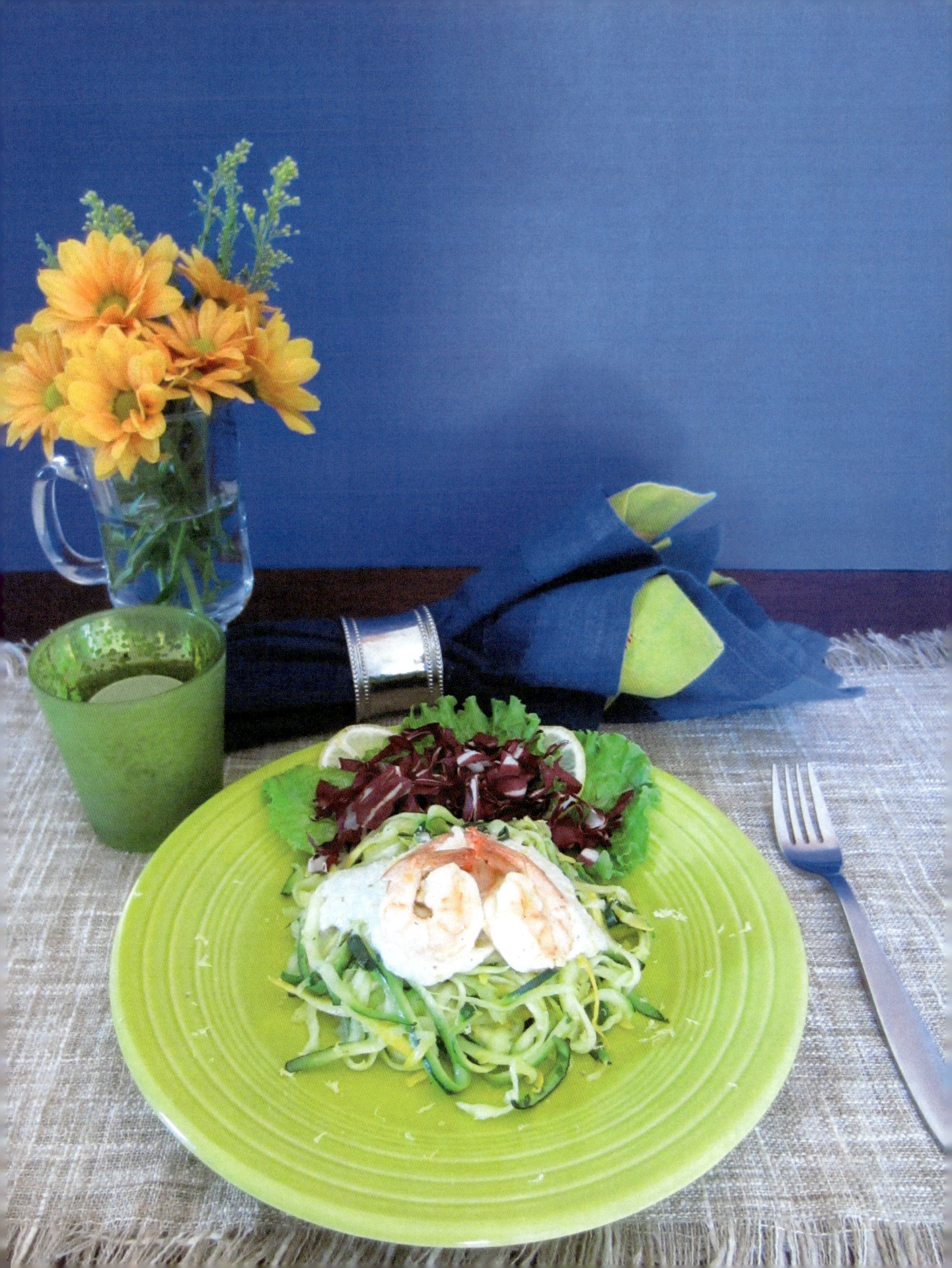

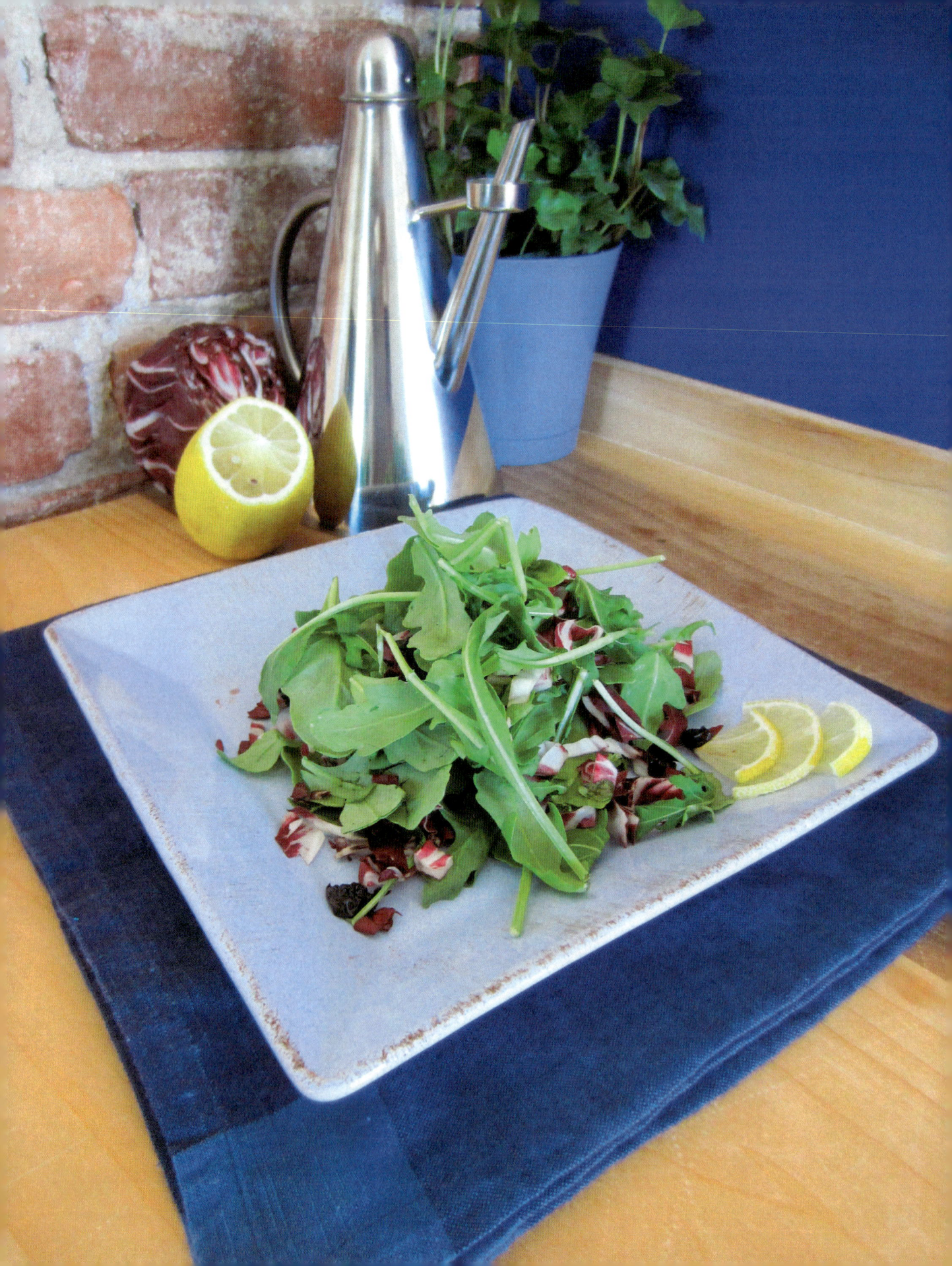

Chapter 13: Salads & Vinaigrettes

As has been discussed earlier, ayurveda recommends that foods be cooked prior to eating in order to make the food easier to digest. While it is true that raw foods have more enzymes than their cooked counterparts, one must have a very strong digestive fire to unlock the energy of the enzymes and receive their benefits. Understanding this logic, one should try to minimize raw, foods. To the extent that one partakes in uncooked foods, one can assist the digestion, absorption and assimilation by: adding warming herbs, sauces and dressings; consuming at midday when the digestive fire is strongest; and letting moderation and balance be one's guide

Vata can eat softer salads with a base of baby arugula or baby spinach. Vata should avoid rough vegetables (i.e., cabbage, cauliflower, kale, corn, radish, etc.), and apply liberal amounts of oils and lemon; or top with a warming dressing (tahini dressing, umeboshi vinaigrette, etc.).

Fiery pitta can benefit from the cool salads, in moderation. Pitta can add some lime juice to aid digestion or tamari for flavoring.

If the salad is strictly for kapha, then a spicy dressing (such as *kapha wasabi dressing*) will balance the salad for kapha. Dressings prepared with a small amount of high quality corn oil or sesame oil are also beneficial for balancing kapha.

ॐ Recipes - Salads & Vinaigrettes

- BLACK BEAN AVOCADO SALAD
- WILD RICE WITH ACORN SQUASH & BRUSSELS SPROUTS IN SWEET BALSAMIC DRESSING
- SWEET BALSAMIC DRESSING
- SUMMER ISRAELI COUSCOUS SALAD
- WAKAME DAIKON SALAD
- VATA PITTA AVOCADO CUCUMBER SALAD
- SOBA NOODLE SALAD
- TRI-DOSHIC ARUGULA RADICCHIO CHERRY SALAD
- WARM BEET SALAD WITH BEET GREENS
- FRENCH LENTIL SALAD WITH LEMON VINAIGRETTE
- LEMON VINAIGRETE
- TRI-DOSHIC MEDITERRANEAN SALAD PLATE
- OREGANO VINAIGRETTE
- MIZUNA MIXED GREENS SALAD
- BUILD YOUR OWN SALAD
- BASIC VINAIGRETTE
- TRI-DOSHIC ASIAN LIME VINAIGRETTE
- TRI-DOSHIC ASIAN TAMARI DRESSING
- TRI-DOSHIC LIME-CUMIN VINAIGRETTE
- TRI-DOSHIC WHITE BALSAMIC VINAIGRETTE
- VATA TAMARIND HONEY DRESSING
- PITTA KAPHA POMEGRANATE VINAIGRETTE
- KAPHA WASABI DRESSING

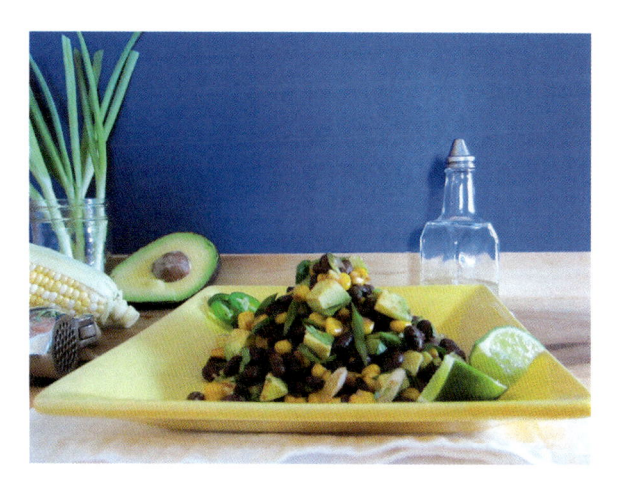

❁Black Bean Avocado Salad
DF/GF/SF/V
Servings: 4

2 teaspoons sunflower oil
½ teaspoon green chili, seeded, chopped fine
½ teaspoon garlic, pressed
15-ounce can black beans, rinsed, drained
8 ounces frozen sweet corn, thawed
½ teaspoon chili powder
4-6 tablespoons *tri-doshic lime cumin vinaigrette*
¼ cup scallions, chopped
2 tablespoons cilantro, chopped
1 avocado, peeled, chopped
lime wedges for garnish

In a 2-quart sauté pan, warm the oil over medium-low heat. Add the garlic and chili and cook for 30 seconds, stirring constantly so as not to let the garlic brown. Add the beans, corn and chili powder, stirring gently; cook for 3 minutes to warm all the ingredients. Remove from heat and transfer to a 2½-quart mixing bowl; add dressing and mix well to evenly coat the beans. Add the scallions, cilantro and avocado; toss together and serve. Garnish with lime wedges.

SERVING SUGGESTIONS: Serve with *creamy corn soup*.

VPK: This is best for pitta; the avocados are a little heavy for kapha, but the lightness of the beans and heat of the spices make this dish OK in moderation; vata can eat on occasion with liberal amounts of the lime cumin vinaigrette dressing.

ABOUT: Avocado is astringent, cooling, oily and heavy so it provides balance to pitta and vata. The black beans are astringent (dry) and cooling, providing balance to pitta and kapha.

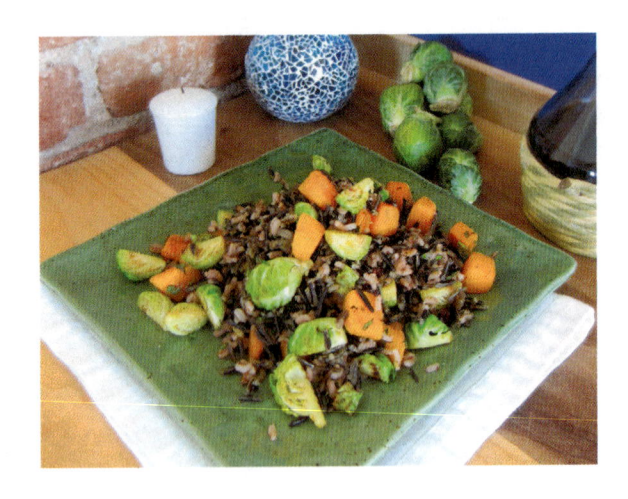

🌸 Wild Rice
with Acorn Squash & Brussels Sprouts in Sweet Balsamic Dressing
DF/GF/SF/V
Servings: 2

½ cup wild rice, cooked (will yield 1½ cups)
¼ cup brown rice, cooked (will yield ½ cup)
1 tablespoon sunflower oil (for sautéing)
1 cup acorn squash, peeled, seeded, cut into ½-inch cubes
1 cup Brussels sprouts, ends and outer leaves trimmed, cut into small wedges (quartered)
2 tablespoons chives, finely chopped
4 tablespoons dried cranberries, chopped
¼ teaspoon Himalayan salt
¼ teaspoon crushed black pepper
2 tablespoons mint, chopped

Sweet Balsamic Dressing:
2½ teaspoons white balsamic vinegar
4½ teaspoons sunflower oil
½ teaspoon honey

Cook the rice separately, following the individual instructions as per the rice cooking chart (Table 12); set aside. Prepare the *sweet balsamic dressing* by combining all the ingredients in a jar and shaking vigorously until completely blended. Warm a 10-inch fry pan over medium heat and add the oil; it should just coat the bottom of the pan in a very thin layer. Add the squash and sauté (stir constantly) for 5 minutes until the outer edges are browned and the inside is tender; remove the squash from the pan. Add additional oil if necessary. Add the Brussels sprouts and sauté until tender (about 2-3 minutes, depending on the size of the Brussels sprouts; do not overcook or they will taste bitter). Allow the ingredients to cool to room temperature. Place the rice, chives, cranberries, salt, pepper and mint in a 2½-quart mixing bowl. Shake the sweet balsamic dressing again then add to the salad. Add the squash and Brussels sprouts, stirring to combine. Serve.

SERVING SUGGESTIONS: For a main dish salad, top with ¾ cup crumbled *paneer* or cubes of *dry-fry tofu*; serve with *beet sweet potato soup*.

VPK: Vata can top with toasted nuts. Pitta and kapha could add ½ cup of cooked chickpeas or steamed cauliflower.

VARIATIONS: Substitute the acorn squash for pumpkin or sweet potato; substitute the Brussels sprouts for asparagus or string beans; substitute the dried cranberries for other cooling, dry fruits such as dates or currants. You can substitute the brown rice for red rice or short-grain white rice. Vata can substitute the sweet balsamic dressing for *vata tamarind honey dressing*.

ABOUT: This dish is light and warming. The earthy flavor of the wild rice is balanced by the sweet (and sour) balsamic dressing.

❁ Summer Israeli Couscous Salad
DF/SF/V
Servings: 2

¾ cup Israeli couscous
1½ cups water
¼ teaspoon Himalayan salt

½ cup water
¼ cup carrot, diced into ¼-inch squares
¼ cup peas
½ cup kale, leaves torn from the veins and chopped into ½-inch pieces
2 tablespoons sultanas, raisins or dried apricots (chopped)
2 tablespoon chives, chopped
¼ cup fresh mint, chopped
¼ teaspoon Himalayan salt
2 tablespoons lime juice

Make the couscous: In a 1½-quart saucepan, bring 1½ cups water to a boil. Add the couscous and salt then reduce heat, cover and simmer for about 10 minutes (stirring occasionally) until the couscous is done. The couscous is done when: the water is completely absorbed and the couscous is tender. Remove from heat and fluff with a fork; let rest, covered while preparing the other ingredients.

In a 10-inch fry pan, bring ¼ cup water to a boil. Add the carrots, peas and kale and cook until they are tender (about 1 or 2 minutes). Remove from heat and strain; transfer to a plate lined with a paper towel and pat dry. In a 2½-quart mixing bowl, combine the cooked vegetables, couscous, dried fruit, chives, mint and salt. Transfer to individual serving plates and sprinkle lime juice over the top.

SERVING SUGGESTIONS: Top with *tri-doshic southwest pumpkin seed citrus dressing*. As a main dish, serve with a side of *vata sweet onion chutney* and grilled polenta; as a side dish, serve with *lime ginger shrimp*.

VPK: The couscous is a little heavy for kapha, so they can add some cayenne to their serving and add lime juice in addition (or instead of) the tri-doshic southwest pumpkin citrus seed dressing.

VARIATIONS: You can vary the vegetables according to the seasons or your dosha (using the **dosha diet aids** in the appendix).

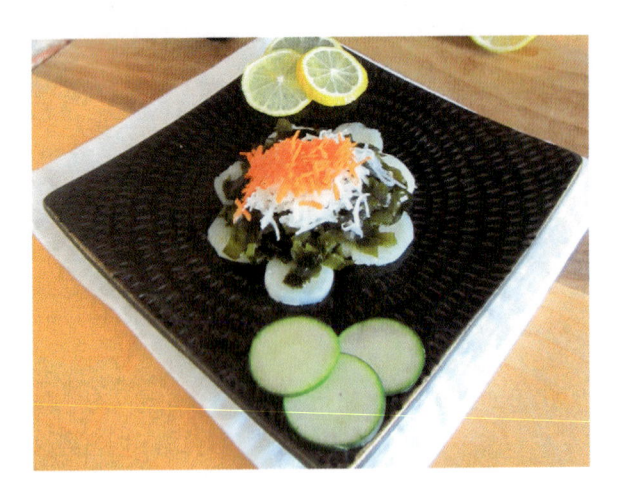

❁ Wakame Daikon Salad
DF/GF/V
Servings: 2

½ cup wakame, cut into small strips, soaked in warm water for 15 minutes, drained
¼ cup carrot, shredded
½ cup daikon, shredded
2 teaspoons *tri-doshic Asian tamari dressing*
12 water chestnuts
2 teaspoons sesame seeds

In a 2-quart mixing bowl, toss the wakame with the *tri-doshic Asian tamari dressing*; mix to coat evenly. Divide the water chestnuts onto two serving plates, arranging in a single layer. Layer half of the ingredients on top of each plate, starting with the wakame, then the daikon, then the carrots. Sprinkle the sesame seeds on top.

SERVING SUGGESTIONS: Serve with *dashi noodle soup*.

VPK: Vata or pitta can add chopped cucumbers and/or avocado slices; kapha could add some sprouts.

❁ Vata Pitta Avocado Cucumber Salad
DF/GF/SF/V
Servings: 2

1 cup cucumbers, peeled, chopped into ¾-inch squares
1 avocado, pitted, peeled, chopped into ½-inch squares
2 cups mizuna (or baby spinach)
2 tablespoons pumpkin seeds

Layer the mizuna on a serving plate and top with the avocado and cucumbers. Sprinkle with pumpkin seeds.

SERVING SUGGESTIONS: Dress with *tri-doshic Asian tamari dressing* or *tri-doshic white balsamic vinaigrette*.

VPK: Balancing for vata and pitta.

ABOUT: Avocados are astringent, cooling and sweet, making them ideal for pitta. They are also heavy, oily and soft, which is balancing to vata. Kapha should avoid avocados. Cucumbers are sweet and cooling – ideal for pitta; and are also soft and liquid which balances vata. Kapha should avoid cucumbers.

❀ Soba Noodle Salad
DF/GF/V
Servings: 3

12 ounces soba noodles
3 tablespoons *tri-doshic Asian lime vinaigrette*
1 cup cucumber, peeled, seeded, diced
½ cup frozen peas, thawed
4 tablespoons basil, chopped
4 tablespoons mint, chopped
½ cup toasted black sesame seeds
1 tablespoon pumpkin seeds
lime wedges

Cook noodles in a 3-quart sauce pan of boiling salted water until tender (3-6 minutes); stir occasionally. Drain well. Rinse under cold water; drain again. Transfer noodles to paper towel-lined plate to drain. Transfer noodles to 2½-quart bowl. Add dressing and toss to coat. (At this point, you can place in the refrigerator overnight if you want to serve the recipe the next day; otherwise, continue with the recipe.)

Add the cucumber, peas, basil and mint and toss gently. Arrange salad on a platter. Sprinkle with black sesame seeds and pumpkin seeds; garnish with lime wedges.

SERVING SUGGESTIONS: Serve with *lime ginger tofu* or shrimp and *miso soup*.

VPK: Vata can add roasted cashews; kapha can add a chili.

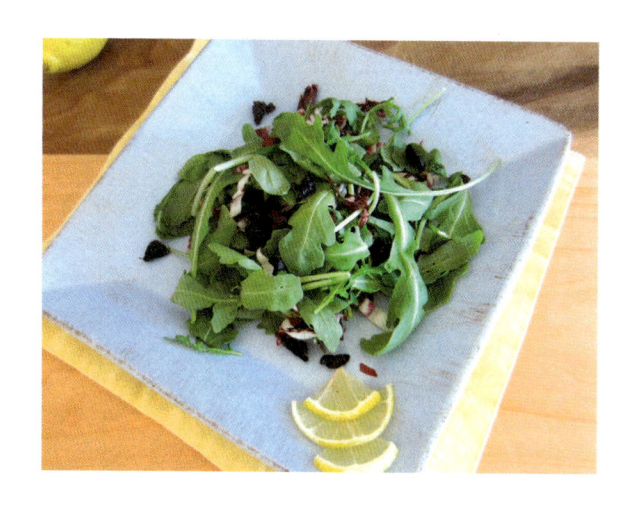

❀ Tri-doshic Arugula Radicchio Cherry Salad
DF/GF/SF/V
Servings: 3

2 cups baby arugula, rinsed and dried
1 cup curly green leaf lettuce, chopped
1 cup radicchio, chopped
⅛ cup dried unsweetened cherries, chopped

Combine the ingredients in a 2½-quart mixing bowl. Toss with salad dressing and serve.

SERVING SUGGESTIONS: Top with *tri-doshic white balsamic vinaigrette*. Serve with *summer vegetable soup* or *Marco's porcini risotto* or *ginger almond squash pie*. As a main dish salad, you could serve with *paneer* or *fennel crusted paneer*.

VPK: Vata can serve with *vata plum compote* or *sweet onion chutney*.

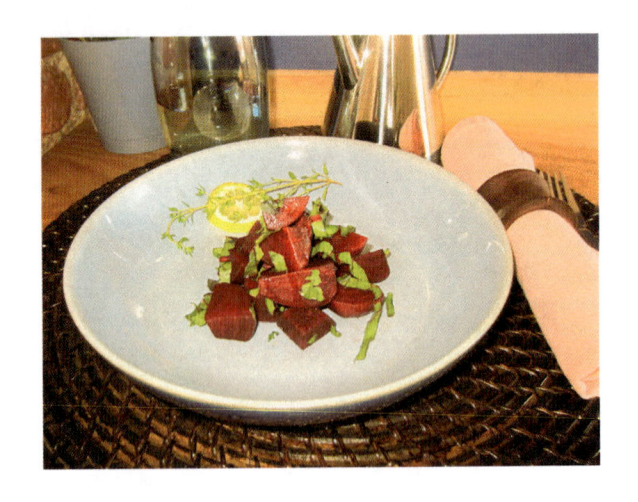

❀ Warm Beet Salad with Beet Greens
DF/GF/SF/V
Servings: 2

2 cups of beets (mixed colors: gold, red, etc.), peeled, chopped into 1-inch chunks
beet greens: trim stalks, wash, chop into ½-inch pieces
1 tablespoon chives, ends removed, chopped fine
2 tablespoons mint leaves (no stems), chopped
1 teaspoon thyme leaves (no stems), chopped
1 tablespoon lemon juice (or 1 teaspoon white balsamic vinegar)
⅛ cup *tri-doshic white balsamic vinaigrette*

Pour 2 cups of water in a 2-quart sauté pan and bring to a boil. Add the beets. Cook until tender (about 20 minutes). Drain the beets and cool on a paper towel-lined plate. Add the beet greens to the boiling water and cook until wilted (about 30 seconds). Remove from the pan with a slotted spoon and cool on a paper towel-lined plate.

In a 2½-quart mixing bowl, combine the beets and beet greens with the *tri-doshic white balsamic vinaigrette*; toss until evenly coated with the dressing.

SERVING SUGGESTIONS: This is a great salad to bring for lunch to work with a wrap made from *lemon cannellini bean spread* or hummus or *baked falafel balls*. Alternatively, you can serve as a salad plate with cannellini spread, artichoke hearts and chickpeas or broiled chicken (marinated in *tri-doshic lime cumin vinaigrette*).

VPK: Tri-doshic; the cool energetic of the beet greens balance the warm energetics of the beets.

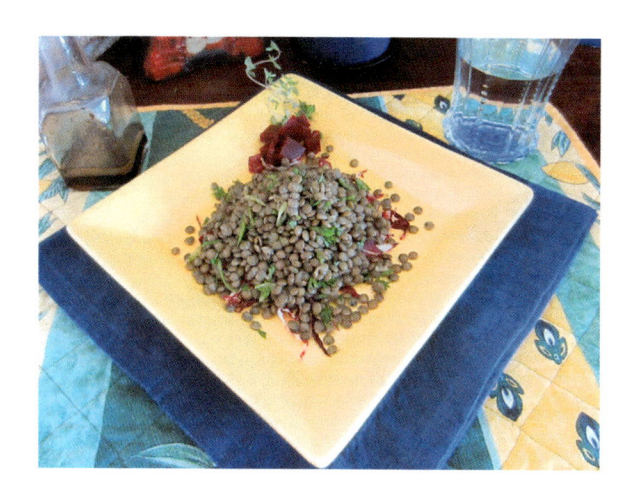

❀ French Lentil Salad with Lemon Vinaigrette
DF/GF/SF/V
Servings: 2

1 cup French lentils, (or Puy lentils) rinsed
1 bay leaf
3 cups water
1 tablespoon chives, chopped
1 tablespoon parsley, coarsely chopped
1 tablespoon organic lemon peel
1½ teaspoons black pepper, coarsely ground
½ teaspoon Himalayan salt

Lemon Vinaigrette
1 tablespoon sunflower oil
1 tablespoon lemon juice

Combine the lentils, bay leaf and water in a 2½-quart pan and bring to a boil. Reduce heat and simmer uncovered. As the lentils cook, skim off any foam that accumulates on the surface of the water. The lentils are done when they are tender and squish when gently pressed between your fingers. If you overcook these lentils, they will lose their shape and become soggy, but they will still taste OK. The lentils cook quickly and will be done in 15-20 minutes, so keep an eye on them. When done, drain, discard the bay leaf and cool to room temperature.

While the lentils are cooking, prepare the vinaigrette by whisking together the oil and lemon juice. In a 2½-quart mixing bowl, combine the cooked lentils, chives, parsley, lemon peel, pepper, salt and vinaigrette; toss gently. Serve.

SERVING SUGGESTIONS: Serve as a main dish salad with a side of mixed greens (arugula, watercress and Boston lettuce) or *puréed parsnips with thyme* or *rosemary roasted root vegetables* or *creamy corn soup*; as a side dish accompanying poached halibut (or scallops) with *pomegranate orange reduction sauce*.

VPK: This is a very balanced dish that is easy to digest. Vata can add more oil and salt to their serving; kapha may opt to omit the oil in the vinaigrette (i.e., simply squeeze fresh lemon juice on the lentils).

VARIATIONS: Add ½ cup diced raw fennel, celery or carrot; substitute finely chopped scallions for the chives; add a few sprigs of fresh tarragon and mint; add pressed garlic to the vinaigrette.

ABOUT: This salad can be prepared ahead, making it ideal for lunches or to bring to parties.

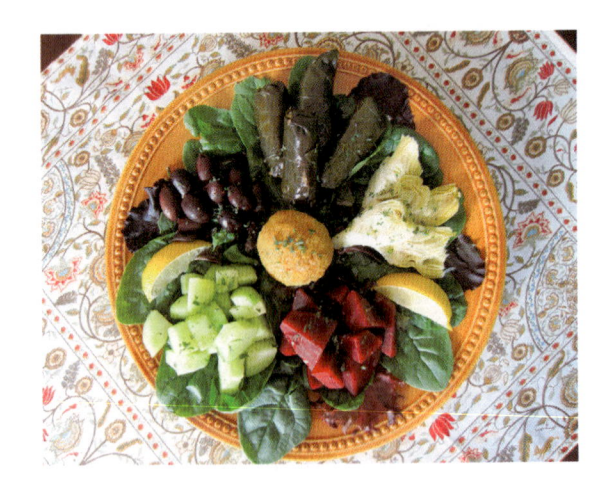

SERVING SUGGESTIONS: Serve with *oregano vinaigrette* and *GF corn bread* or pita bread.

VPK: Vata can top with tahini dressing or *vata lemon cashew cream sauce*. Pitta and kapha may try the *pitta kapha pomegranate vinaigrette*.

VARIATIONS: Add stuffed grape leaves, tabbouleh salad, hummus, chickpeas, *zucchini hummus* or white couscous with lemon for a heartier dish.

❁ Tri-doshic Mediterranean Salad Plate
DF/GF/SF/V
Servings: 2

1 cup red leaf lettuce
1 cup spinach
4 *baked falafel balls*
½ cup cucumbers, peeled, seeded, chopped
½ cup tomatoes, peeled, seeded, chopped
4 kalamata olives
½ cup beets, peeled, cut into ½-inch cubes, boiled
½ cup artichoke hearts, quartered

❁ Oregano Vinaigrette
Yield: ⅔ cup

6 tablespoons avocado oil (or olive)
2 tablespoons lemon juice
1 teaspoon apple cider vinegar
½ teaspoon oregano (dried)
½ teaspoon honey
½ teaspoon Himalayan salt
¼ teaspoon ground black pepper

Whisk all ingredients together; refrigerate and store in a glass container for up to 1 week.

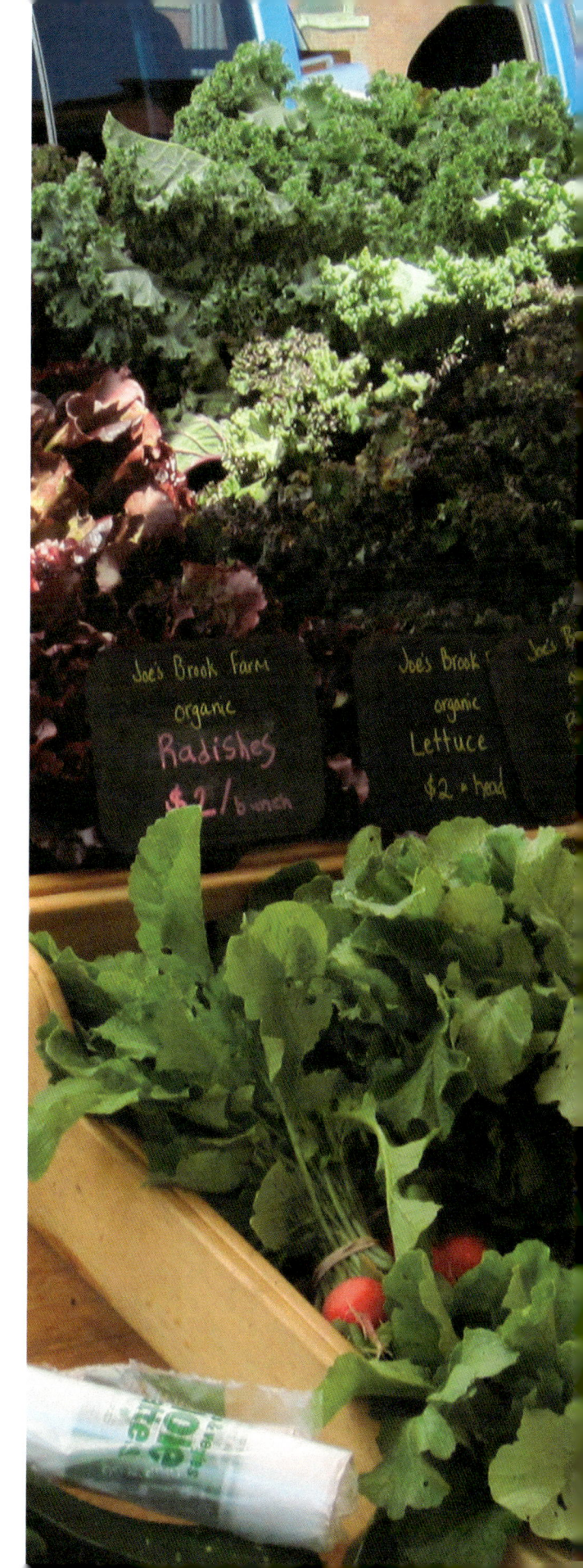

❁ Mizuna Mixed Greens Salad
DF/GF/SF/V
Servings: 3

2 cups mizuna, rinsed, dried, chopped
1 cup chicory (frisee), rinsed, dried, chopped
1 cup red leaf lettuce, rinsed, dried, chopped

In a 2½-quart mixing bowl, combine all the ingredients. Toss with *tri-doshic Asian tamari dressing*.

SERVING SUGGESTIONS: Serve with *broiled lime-ginger shrimp* (or tofu) and *dashi puy lentil soup*.

VPK: This is tri-doshic.

ABOUT: Mizuna is mildly heating with a peppery taste; it is well tolerated by all three doshas. It can be purchased at Asian markets and larger grocery stores.

🍽 Build Your Own Salad
DF/GF/SF/V

This cook book includes recipes for some great tri-doshic salads and dressings. If you want to experiment with a dosha-specific salad, you can use this chart as a reference to build your own salad.

	Vata	Pitta	Kapha
Greens	baby arugula, baby spinach, chicory (endive/frisee), mizuna, mustard greens	green lettuce, kale, spinach, chicory (endive/frisee), dandelion greens, mizuna, radicchio	arugula, chicory (endive/frisee), dandelion greens, kale, mizuna, mustard greens, radicchio
Vegetables	beets, cilantro, cucumbers, fennel, asparagus	artichokes, celery, cilantro, cucumber, fennel, jicama	artichokes, beets, celery, cilantro, corn, fennel, mushrooms, onions, chilies
Fruits	dried apricots, avocado	avocado, dried dates, dried figs, raisins	dried apricots, dried cranberries
Condiments	black olives, paneer, umeboshi plums	sprouts, paneer	chives, daikon, paneer, radish, scallions, sprouts, wasabi
Dressing	lemon tahini, *vata tamarind honey dressing*	lime juice, *pitta kapha pomegranate vinaigrette*	lime juice, *pitta kapha pomegranate vinaigrette, kapha wasabi dressing*

❀ Basic Vinaigrette
DF/GF/SF/V
Yield: ¼ cup (about 2-3 servings)

Most of the recipes in this book have been paired with complimentary vinaigrettes. But for those who want to venture on their own, I have prepared the chart on the following page to help you create your own unique dressing.

A basic vinaigrette can be made by blending together: oil, vinegar and a pinch of salt and black pepper. Select the dosha from the top row, then decide which oil and vinegar you would like to use. Select the optional seasonings. Combine all the ingredients in a clean, dry, 8-ounce glass jar; close the lid tightly and shake until well combined; store in the refrigerator for up to a week.

🍽 Basic Vinaigrette

	Quantity	Vata	Pitta	Kapha	Tri-doshic
Oil	3 tablespoons	• almond • avocado • olive • sesame • sunflower	• avocado • olive • soy • sunflower	• sunflower • corn • mustard	• sunflower
Vinegar	1 tablespoon	• apple cider • white balsamic • rice	• apple cider • white balsamic • rice	• apple cider	• apple cider
Citrus juice *(select 1)*	1 teaspoon	• lemon • lime • orange • grapefruit • tamarind or umeboshi paste (¼ teaspoon)	• lime • orange	• lime	• lime
Sweetner *(select 1)*	½ teaspoon	• honey • coconut sugar • rice syrup	• coconut sugar • maple sugar • rice syrup • pomegranate syrup	• honey • apple or pear juice concentrate • pomegranate syrup	• coconut sugar
Herbs, dry *(select 1)*	¼ teaspoon	• cumin powder • cayenne (a pinch) • oregano • parsley • tarragon	• cumin • tarragon	• cumin powder • cayenne (a pinch) • oregano • mustard	• cumin • dill • fennel
Herbs, fresh *(select 1)*	¾ teaspoon	• garlic • chives • mint • parsley • scallions	• cilantro • dill • mint • tarragon	• chives • garlic • parsley • rosemary • scallions	• mint

❀ Tri-Doshic Asian Lime Vinaigrette
DF/GF/V
Yield: ¼ cup

1½ teaspoons apple cider vinegar
1 tablespoon lime juice
1 tablespoon sunflower oil
1 tablespoon sesame oil
1 tablespoon honey
2¼ teaspoons tamari
⅛ teaspoon cayenne powder

Whisk all ingredients together in a non-metallic bowl. Set for 15 minutes then pour over the salad.

SERVING SUGGESTIONS: Serve over *Asian vegetables* or *mizuna mixed greens salad*.

❀ Tri-Doshic Lime-Cumin Vinaigrette
DF/GF/SF/V
Yield: ½ cup

2 tablespoons lime juice
6 tablespoons sunflower oil
1 tablespoon honey (substitute coconut sugar if using for a marinade)
½ teaspoon Himalayan salt
½ teaspoon cumin powder
½ teaspoon cumin seeds, lightly crushed
½ teaspoon coriander powder
½ teaspoon crushed black pepper

Whisk all ingredients together in a non-metallic bowl; let set for 15 minutes. Serve with *black bean avocado salad*, over a salad of mixed greens or use as a tri-doshic marinade for fish.

❀ Tri-doshic Asian Tamari Dressing
DF/GF/V
Yield: ¼ cup

1 tablespoon rice vinegar
2 tablespoons sunflower oil
2 teaspoons sesame oil
2 teaspoons honey
4 teaspoons tamari
¼ teaspoon cayenne powder

Whisk all ingredients together in a non-metallic bowl. Set for 15 minutes then serve.

SERVING SUGGESTIONS: Serve with *wakame daikon salad* or *barley sauté with sweet potato, asparagus & burdock root*.

❀ Tri-doshic White Balsamic Vinaigrette
DF/GF/SF/V
Yield: ½ cup

2 tablespoons white balsamic vinegar
6 tablespoons sunflower oil
1 teaspoon honey
⅛ teaspoon Himalayan salt
⅛ teaspoon crushed black pepper

Whisk all the ingredients together and serve.

ABOUT: White balsamic vinegar is made from white grapes. It is milder (less sour) and less heating than regular balsamic vinegar.

❁ Vata Tamarind Honey Dressing
DF/GF/SF/V
Yield: ½ cup

4 tablespoons water
4 tablespoons sunflower oil
1 tablespoon raw honey
2 teaspoons lime juice
2½ teaspoons seedless tamarind sauce (Neera's®)
⅛ teaspoon Himalayan salt

Whisk all ingredients together in a non-metallic bowl. Serve over salads. To use as a marinade, replace the honey with coconut sugar. Store in an airtight container in the refrigerator for up to a week.

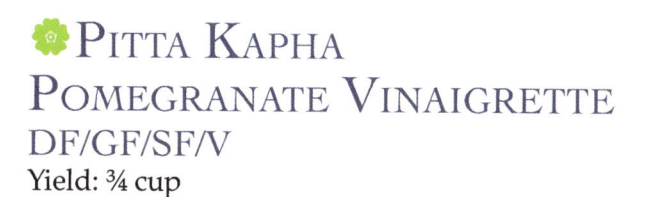

❁ Pitta Kapha Pomegranate Vinaigrette
DF/GF/SF/V
Yield: ¾ cup

6 tablespoons sunflower oil
1 tablespoon apple cider vinegar
2 tablespoons pomegranate molasses
1 tablespoon lime juice
¼ teaspoon grated lime rind (or orange or lemon)

Whisk all ingredients together in a non-metallic bowl. Serve over salads; use as a marinade for seafood or chicken. Store in an airtight container in the refrigerator for up to a week.

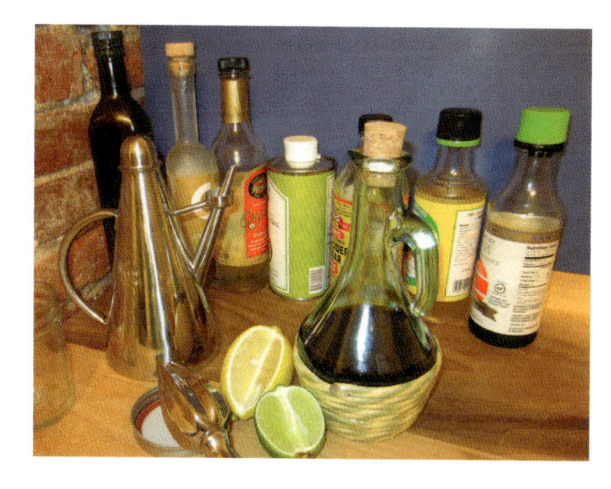

❁ Kapha Wasabi Dressing
DF/GF/V
Yield: ½ cup

2 teaspoons water
4 teaspoons wasabi powder
4 teaspoons rice vinegar
4 tablespoons sesame oil
2 teaspoons ginger, GRATED
2 teaspoons honey
2 teaspoons tamari
2 teaspoons lemon juice
a pinch of cayenne (optional)

Mix the water and wasabi powder to form a thick paste. Whisk in the remaining ingredients then let stand for 20 minutes to allow the flavors to blend. Serve over salads, rice or broiled fish; serve with ginger salmon temaki roll. Store in an airtight container in the refrigerator for up to a week.

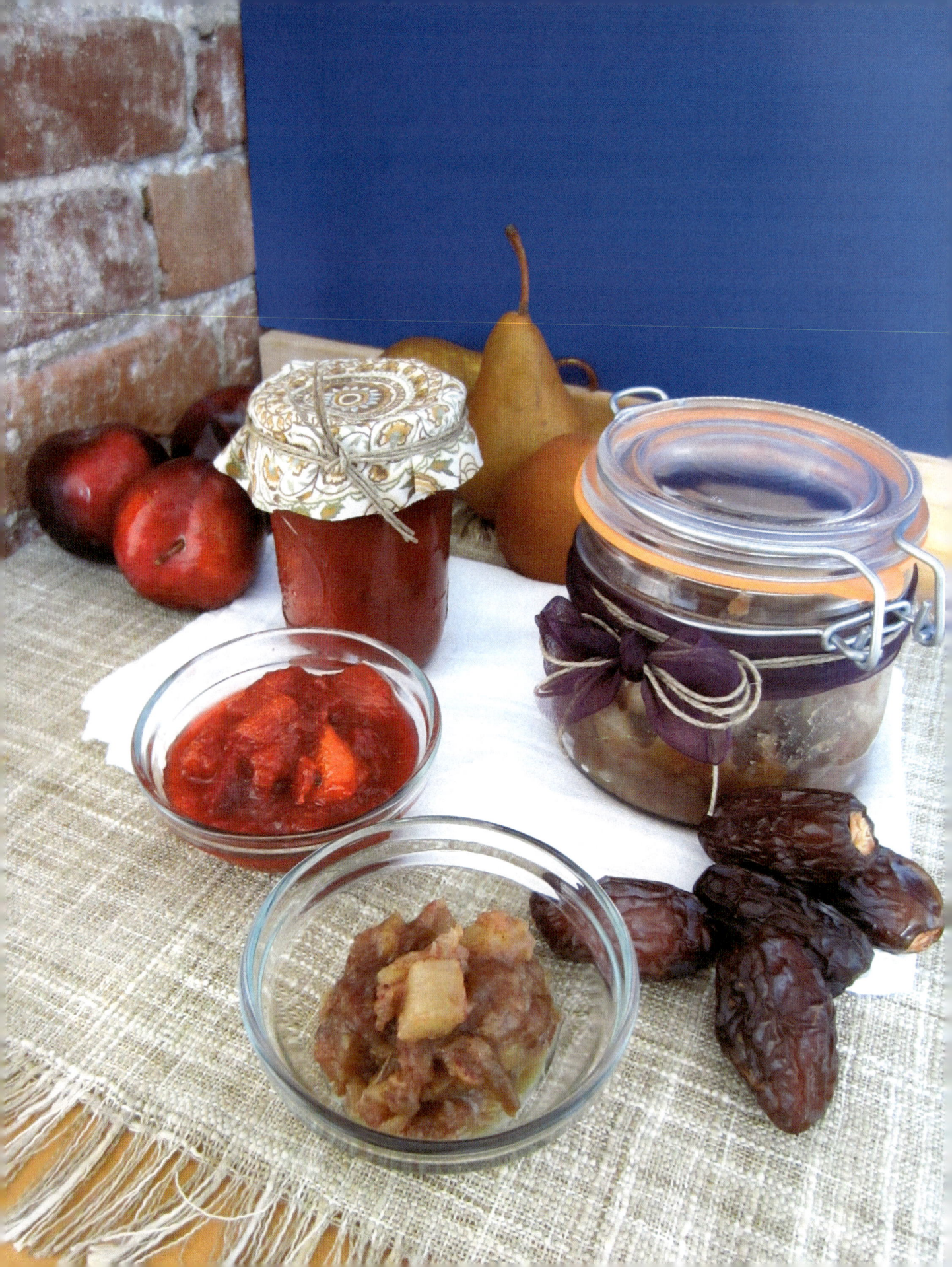

Chapter 14: Sauces, Chutneys & Churnas

The recipes in this chapter are generally designed to be dosha-specific; the sauces, dressings and chutneys have been tailored to be balancing specifically to vata, pitta or kapha. You can use this chapter when you want to target a specific dosha. For instance, if you feel like you need to reduce the fire element (pitta) in your body, look for sauces, chutneys or churnas that are specifically balancing for pitta.

I have included a basic recipe for making a nut butter which can be used for any type of nut, seed or combination of nuts and seeds. Nut butters can be purchased at most grocery stores but they are often quite expensive and contain unnecessary salt and preservatives. Making your own nut butter is a low-cost, healthy, dairy-free answer for tailoring recipes to suit your individual needs. Nut butters should be stored in a glass container with an air-tight lid in the refrigerator; be sure to use clean dry utensils when scooping out the butter to avoid contamination and potential bacterial growth; if the recipe is comprised of solely nuts and oil (i.e., no fresh herbs, garlic, lemon juice, etc.), the nut butter will last for a few months in the refrigerator.

Cashew nut butter and almond nut butter can be substituted in many baking recipes calling for butter. You can make creamy sauces by whisking together ¼ cup nut butter with 1 cup of water, then season to taste with tamari, cayenne, cinnamon, allspice, fresh mint, fresh thyme, fresh savory, grated orange peel, grated lemon peel, etc. Nuts are generally heavy and oily and most suited for vata, but on occasion, in moderation and properly spiced, nut butters can be enjoyed by all.

Churnas are dosha-specific combinations of spices to aid digestion and provide balancing energetics. I have included three basic churnas. You can pre-mix a small jar of these spices and keep them handy to add to your meals; sprinkle ¼ - ½ teaspoon onto your food and enjoy!

If making churnas is too much effort, you may alternatively chew a few fennel seeds (or ajwain seeds) at the end of a meal to aid digestion. Keep some in a Ziploc® baggie at work or in your car for whenever you are eating on-the-go.

ॐ

ॐ Recipes - Sauces, Chutneys & Churnas

- BASIC NUT BUTTER/SEED BUTTER
- BASIC TAHINI
- TZATZIKI (CUCUMBER DILL SAUCE)
- VATA LEMON CASHEW CREAM SAUCE
- ARTICHOKE LEMON CREAM SAUCE
- TANGY TAMARIND SAUCE
- MOROCCAN SPICE BLEND
- TRI-DOSHIC SOUTHWEST PUMPKIN SEED CITRUS DRESSING
- TRI-DOSHIC POMEGRANATE ORANGE REDUCTION SAUCE
- VATA PLUM COMPOTE
- VATA SWEET ONION CHUTNEY
- PITTA COOLING DATE CHUTNEY
- COOL COCONUT CHUTNEY
- KAPHA SPICY PEAR CHUTNEY
- KAPHA HOT ONION CHUTNEY
- DOSHA SPECIFIC CHURNAS

❁ Basic Nut Butter/Seed Butter
DF/GF/SF/V
Yield: ½ cup nut butter

**1 cup nuts, peeled, unsalted
(or seeds, raw, unsalted)
1-2 tablespoons sunflower oil**

Toast the nuts in a 10-inch non-stick fry pan over medium heat for 5 minutes, tossing the nuts frequently with a wooden spatula. Do not allow to brown. Cool for 20 minutes. Transfer the toasted nuts into a food processor and add 1 tablespoon of oil. Blend until you have the consistency of a nut-butter (like peanut butter), scraping the sides of the bowl as needed and adding additional oil to smooth out the consistency; store in a glass jar in the refrigerator.

SERVING SUGGESTIONS: Use to replace peanut butter in sandwiches; use to replace butter in baking recipes; use as a base for sauces for salads and vegetables by adding lemon juice and/or water and spices.

VPK: Nuts are generally balancing for vata, but not the other doshas. Almonds, when they are peeled and blanched, are considered tri-doshic. Refer to the dosha diet aids in the Appendix for dosha-specific nut and seed recommendations.

VARIATIONS: You may sweeten with 1 teaspoon of raw honey or add a pinch of salt if desired.

❁ Basic Tahini
DF/GF/SF/V
Yield: ½ cup

**1 cup unhulled, raw sesame seeds
¼ cup sunflower oil**

Toast sesame seeds in a 10-inch non-stick skillet over medium heat for 5 minutes, tossing the seeds frequently with a wooden spatula; do not allow to brown. Cool for 20 minutes. Transfer the toasted sesame seeds into a food processor and add oil. Blend for 2 minutes until you have the consistency of a nut-butter (like peanut butter) – this is basic tahini. Store in a glass jar in the refrigerator.

SERVING SUGGESTIONS: Use to replace peanut butter in sandwiches; use to replace butter in baking recipes (be aware that it will impart a sesame flavor); use as a base for salad dressings and sauces for vegetables.

VPK: Sesame seeds are heating, oily and heavy. They are ideal for vata. Pitta can use in moderation or with cooling spices such as cilantro or mint; kapha is best to avoid tahini, unless it is thinned in a sauce and accompanied by a dish that is very drying, such as millet.

VARIATIONS: As a sauce for salads or vegetables add ½ teaspoon lemon juice to 1 tablespoon tahini and add water to desired consistency. Combine with ½ cup cooked chickpeas and 1 tablespoon lemon juice to make traditional hummus.

🌸 Tzatziki (Cucumber Dill Sauce)
GF/SF/V
Yield: 1 cup

1 cup plain, whole fat yogurt, strained
½ cup cucumber, peeled, seeded
¼ -½ teaspoon fresh dill
¼ teaspoon garlic, pressed
½ teaspoon lemon juice
½ teaspoon grated lemon rind
⅛ teaspoon Himalayan salt

Combine all ingredients in a food processor and purée until smooth. Chill for 1 hour; serve.

SERVING SUGGESTIONS: Serve with *Marinela's Dolmathakia* (stuffed grape leaves) or mung dal.

VPK: Best for vata and pitta; kapha can eat in moderation if the yogurt is fresh (not more than 3 days old).

VARIATIONS: Substitute mint leaves for the dill.

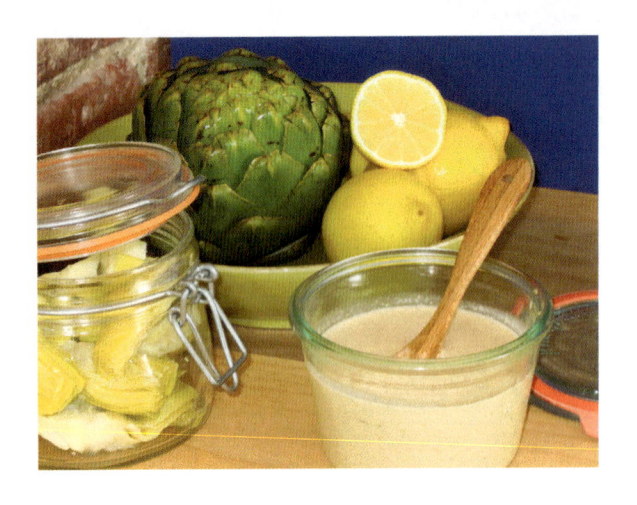

🌸 Vata Lemon Cashew Cream Sauce
DF/GF/SF/V
Yield: ½ cup

¼ cup cashew nut butter (see nut butter recipe)
¼ cup water
1 tablespoon lemon juice
½ teaspoon grated lemon rind
½ teaspoon Himalayan salt
1 tablespoon parsley

Combine all ingredients in a food processor and mix until it becomes smooth and creamy. If you desire a thinner consistency, add more water.

SERVING SUGGESTIONS: Season with ½ teaspoon ground cinnamon and serve over millet, couscous or polenta; use as a base to create artichoke lemon cream sauce for pasta and gluten-free pasta dishes.

VPK: This is sweet, a little sour, heavy and warming – ideal for grounding vata.

VARIATIONS: You can vary the seasonings by adding one or two of the following: tamari (1 teaspoon), cayenne (a pinch), cinnamon (⅛ teaspoon), allspice (a pinch), fresh mint (1 teaspoon), fresh thyme (½ teaspoon), fresh savory (½ teaspoon), grated orange peel (½ teaspoon), grated lemon peel (½ teaspoon), etc.

❁ Artichoke Lemon Cream Sauce
DF/GF/SF/V
Yield: ¾ cup

¼ cup cashew butter
½ cup artichoke hearts (canned, packed in water, no salt)
½ cup water
¼ teaspoon Himalayan salt (omit if the artichokes were packed with salt)
⅛ teaspoon pepper
1 tablespoon lemon juice

Combine all ingredients in a food processor and pulse until it becomes a smooth, sauce consistency.

SERVING SUGGESTIONS: Serve over *zucchini pasta*, wheat pasta or steamed vegetables; serve as a dipping sauce for *baked falafel balls*.

VPK: The artichokes are astringent, light and warm and the cashews are sweet, heavy and warm. This is ideal for vata; a little warm for pitta and a little heavy for kapha, but OK in moderation. This sauce will balance dry, light dishes such as with *zucchini pasta* or *baked falafel balls*.

VARIATIONS: Try substituting arugula or zucchini for the artichoke hearts.

❁ Tangy Tamarind Sauce
DF/GF/SF/V
Yield: ¾ cup

½ cup water
6 tablespoons honey
2 tablespoons tamarind paste

Whisk ingredients together in a small bowl.

SERVING SUGGESTIONS: Drizzle over *Moroccan veggie burgers* or *fennel crusted paneer*.

VPK: The moist, heavy, sweet and sour qualities of this dressing are ideal for vata. It can be used on any dish that needs grounding. Pitta and kapha can use in moderation with a cold, light dish.

❁ Moroccan Spice Blend
DF/GF/SF/V

2 teaspoons ground coriander
2 teaspoons ground cumin
1½ teaspoons ground cinnamon
1 teaspoon ground ginger
½ teaspoon paprika
½ teaspoon Himalayan salt
¼ teaspoon ground nutmeg
¼ teaspoon turmeric
¼ teaspoon allspice
¼ teaspoon oregano

Combine all ingredients together in a 4-ounce glass jar or airtight container.

SERVING SUGGESTIONS: You can use this spice blend as a "rub" on fish or meat; or use to season any dish when you want a taste of Morocco. This mixture is used in the *Moroccan lamb meatballs*, *baked falafel balls* and *Moroccan veggie burger* recipes.

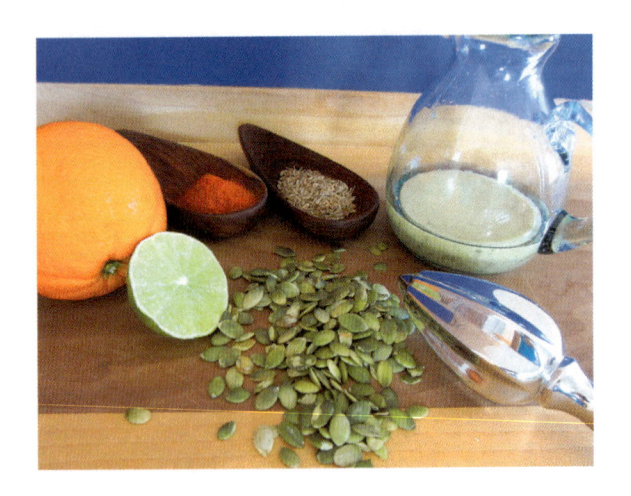

❀Tri-doshic Southwest Pumpkin Seed Citrus Dressing
DF/GF/SF/V
Yield: ½ cup

⅓ cup pumpkin seeds
1 tablespoon sunflower oil
1 teaspoon grated orange rind
¼ cup orange juice
¾ teaspoon honey
1 tablespoon lime juice
½ teaspoon chili powder
½ teaspoon coriander powder
½ teaspoon cumin
½ teaspoon cinnamon
⅛ teaspoon salt
pinch of cayenne pepper
1-3 tablespoon water, to desired consistency

Place all the ingredients, except the water, in a food processor; pulse until the pumpkin seeds are coarsely chopped. Add water to desired consistency. Transfer to a non-metallic container and let set for 20 minutes before serving.

SERVING SUGGESTIONS: With *summer Israeli couscous salad* or *black bean avocado salad*.

Variations: Add 1 tablespoon of chopped fresh mint and/or cilantro.

❀Tri-doshic Pomegranate Orange Reduction Sauce
DF/GF/SF/V
Makes ¾ cup

¾ cup water
3 tablespoons pomegranate syrup
1 tablespoon lemon juice
2 tablespoons white balsamic vinegar
6 tablespoons orange juice
¼ teaspoon orange rind

Wisk together all the ingredients in a 1-quart saucepan; bring to a boil then reduce heat to simmer. Continue whisking until the sauce thickens and reduces by half (about 15-20 minutes).

SERVING SUGGESTIONS: Serve drizzled over *fennel crusted paneer*, grilled halibut, scallops, chicken breast or venison.

VARIATIONS: Try adding ¼ teaspoon of fresh herbs after the sauce is reduced (i.e., mint, tarragon, basil, rosemary) to complement your dish.

ABOUT: Pomegranate is astringent and is best for balancing pitta and kapha. The sourness of the vinegar and the sweetness of the orange juice round out the flavors and provide balance for vata.

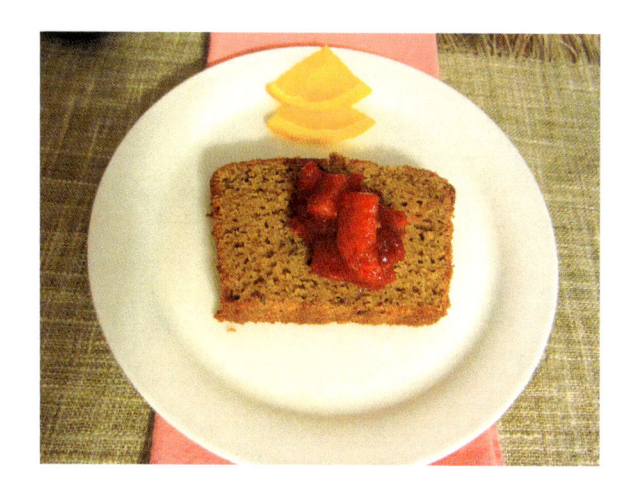

❁ Vata Plum Compote
DF/GF/SF/V

Yield: ½ cup

1½ cups plums, pitted and quartered
¼ cup water
1 tablespoon coconut sugar (or maple syrup)
1 teaspoon grated orange peel
¼ teaspoon powdered cloves
2 teaspoons lemon juice
½ teaspoon Himalayan salt

Combine all ingredients in a 1½-quart sauce pan. Bring to a boil, then reduce heat to low and simmer for 20 minutes or until the plums dissolve into a thick sauce.

SERVING SUGGESTIONS: Serve on the side with fluffy *cinnamon currant millet*, couscous, quinoa or rice.

❁ Vata Sweet Onion Chutney
DF/GF/SF/V

Yield: 1 cup

½ tablespoon sunflower oil
½ teaspoon thin green chili peppers, seeded, chopped fine
1 cup onion, chopped
½ teaspoon garlic, pressed
¼ teaspoon tamarind paste
5 curry leaves
¼ - ½ cups water
2 tablespoons sunflower oil
1 teaspoon urad dal
1 teaspoon mustard seeds
1 teaspoon tomato paste
½ teaspoon Himalayan salt

In a 10-inch fry pan, heat ½ tablespoon sunflower oil over medium heat. Add the chilies, onion and garlic and stir fry for one minute until golden brown. Reduce heat to low and add the tamarind paste and curry leaves, stirring to combine; cook for another minute then remove from heat. Transfer the contents to a mini food processor and add ¼ cup water; pulse to combine. It should be a thick consistency.

Heat 2 tablespoons sunflower oil in the 10-inch fry pan over medium heat. Add the urad dal and sauté until they are golden brown. Add the mustard seeds and sauté until you hear the seeds pop (about 30 seconds). Add the onion mixture, the tomato paste and the salt to the pan. Stir to combine all the ingredients well. If the mixture is sticking to the pan, you can add a few teaspoons of water. Continue cooking until the chutney thickens. Allow to cool and store in an air-tight glass jar for up to a week.

SERVING SUGGESTIONS: Serve with *Moroccan veggie burgers*.

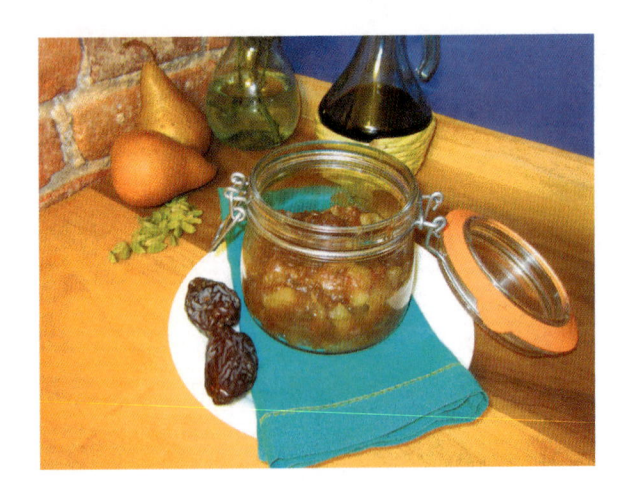

Pitta Cooling Date Chutney
DF/GF/SF/V
Yield: 1 cup

⅔ cup medjool dates, pitted, coarsely chopped
¼ cup onion, finely chopped
½ cup Bartlett pear (or red apple), peeled and coarsely chopped
⅛ teaspoon cardamom
1 cup water
¼ teaspoon balsamic vinegar

Combine all ingredients in a 1½-quart sauce pan and bring to a boil. Reduce heat to low and simmer, uncovered, stirring occasionally; the moisture will reduce and it will become a chunky consistency after about 15 minutes. Remove from heat and mash the pears a little bit with the back of a fork.

SERVING SUGGESTIONS: Serve alongside dishes with a warming energetic such as *polenta with minted shitake sauce* or a spicy dal.

VPK: This is sweet, heavy and cool - balancing for pitta; vata can eat in moderation; kapha should avoid as it is too sweet.

Cool Coconut Chutney
DF/GF/SF/V
Yield: ⅔ cup

½ tablespoon ghee (or sunflower oil)
½ tablespoon urad dal
¼ cup onion, coarsely chopped
2 teaspoons fresh ginger, peeled, finely chopped
4 curry leaves
½ teaspoon Neera's® tamarind paste
½ cup fresh or frozen shredded coconut, unsweetened [do not use dried coconut]
¼ teaspoon thin green chili, seeded, sliced
¼ teaspoon Himalayan salt
1½ teaspoons lime juice
6 tablespoons water
2 teaspoons cilantro, leaves only, chopped

In a 1-quart saucepan over medium heat, melt the ghee. When ghee is hot, but not smoking, add the urad dal; stir fry until the urad dal starts to brown. Then add the onion, ginger, curry leaves and tamarind paste; stir until well combined. Continue cooking for about 3 minutes. Add the coconut, chili and salt; stir fry for an additional 3 minutes until all the flavors have combined. Remove from heat and transfer to a mini food processor. Add the lime juice and 6 tablespoons of water. Pulse until it becomes a thick, smooth paste. If necessary, add more water to achieve desired consistency.

SERVING SUGGESTIONS: Serve with *urad dal with tamarind*, *Kerala inspired tur dal* or *Bangalore tur dal sambhar*.

ABOUT: The chili pepper will give this a mildly spicy taste, but the coconut will provide an overall cooling energetic. You can reduce or omit the chili if you prefer a sweeter taste.

❀ Kapha Spicy Pear Chutney

DF/GF/SF/V
Yield: 1½ cups

2 cups Bartlett pears (or red apple), peeled, seeded, chopped
½ cup water
1 teaspoon coconut sugar (or maple syrup or pomegranate syrup)
1 teaspoon grated orange rind
¼ teaspoon cloves
⅛ -¼ teaspoon cayenne
½ teaspoon apple cider vinegar
¼ teaspoon salt

Combine all ingredients in a 1½-quart sauce pan. Bring to a boil then reduce heat to low; cover and simmer for 20 minutes or until the pears are soft; mash with a fork to create a chunky chutney.

SERVING SUGGESTIONS: Serve warm as an accompaniment to rice dishes, meat (*bison meatloaf*), *baked falafel balls*, etc.

❀ Kapha Hot Onion Chutney

DF/GF/SF/V
Yield: ½ cup

1 teaspoon tomato paste
1 teaspoon water
¼ teaspoon honey
1 teaspoon apple cider vinegar
¼ - ½ teaspoon cayenne pepper
½ teaspoon garlic
½ cup raw onions, minced
1 teaspoon cilantro (or parsley), coarsely chopped

In a 1-quart non-metallic bowl, whisk the tomato paste with water to make a thick sauce. Whisk in the honey, apple cider vinegar, cayenne and garlic. Add the onions and cilantro and stir to evenly coat the onions with the seasonings. Let set for 15 minutes to allow the flavors to blend.

SERVING SUGGESTIONS: Serve with rice dishes, heavy dals such as *urad dal with tamarind*, and meat dishes such as *bison meatloaf*; a little goes a long way – one or two tablespoons is all you need.

VPK: This is balancing for kapha.

🌸 Dosha-Specific Churnas

DF/GF/SF/V
Yield: 5 teaspoons

Vata

2 teaspoons cumin powder
2 teaspoons ginger powder
1 teaspoon cardamom powder
½ teaspoon Himalayan salt
¼ teaspoon turmeric

Combine ingredients and store in an airtight container for up to 2 months. Sprinkle over food to provide warming and grounding energetics.

Pitta

2 teaspoons coriander powder
2 teaspoons cumin powder
1 teaspoon licorice powder*
1 teaspoon dried, fine shred coconut
¼ teaspoon turmeric powder
⅛ teaspoon Himalayan salt

Combine ingredients and store in an airtight container for up to 2 months. Sprinkle on food to provide cooling and calming energetics. *If you have high blood pressure, omit the licorice; substitute fennel powder.

Kapha

1 teaspoon ginger powder
1 teaspoon cumin powder
1 teaspoon black pepper
1 teaspoon fennel powder
¼ teaspoon turmeric powder
⅛ teaspoon Himalayan salt

Combine ingredients and store in an airtight container for up to 2 months. Sprinkle over food to provide warming and stimulating energetics.

ABOUT: "Churna" means powder in Sanskrit. The churnas that I have created here are designed to balance individual doshas. They contain all the tastes except for sour. You can make a batch and store it in an airtight container/Ziploc® baggie. Sprinkle (i.e., ¼ - ½ teaspoon) on your meals; keep some at work or in your briefcase/laptop bag so you always have it handy.

The recipes above yield a small amount. If you find them to be of benefit, then you can double or triple the recipe so you have enough to last you for a month at a time.

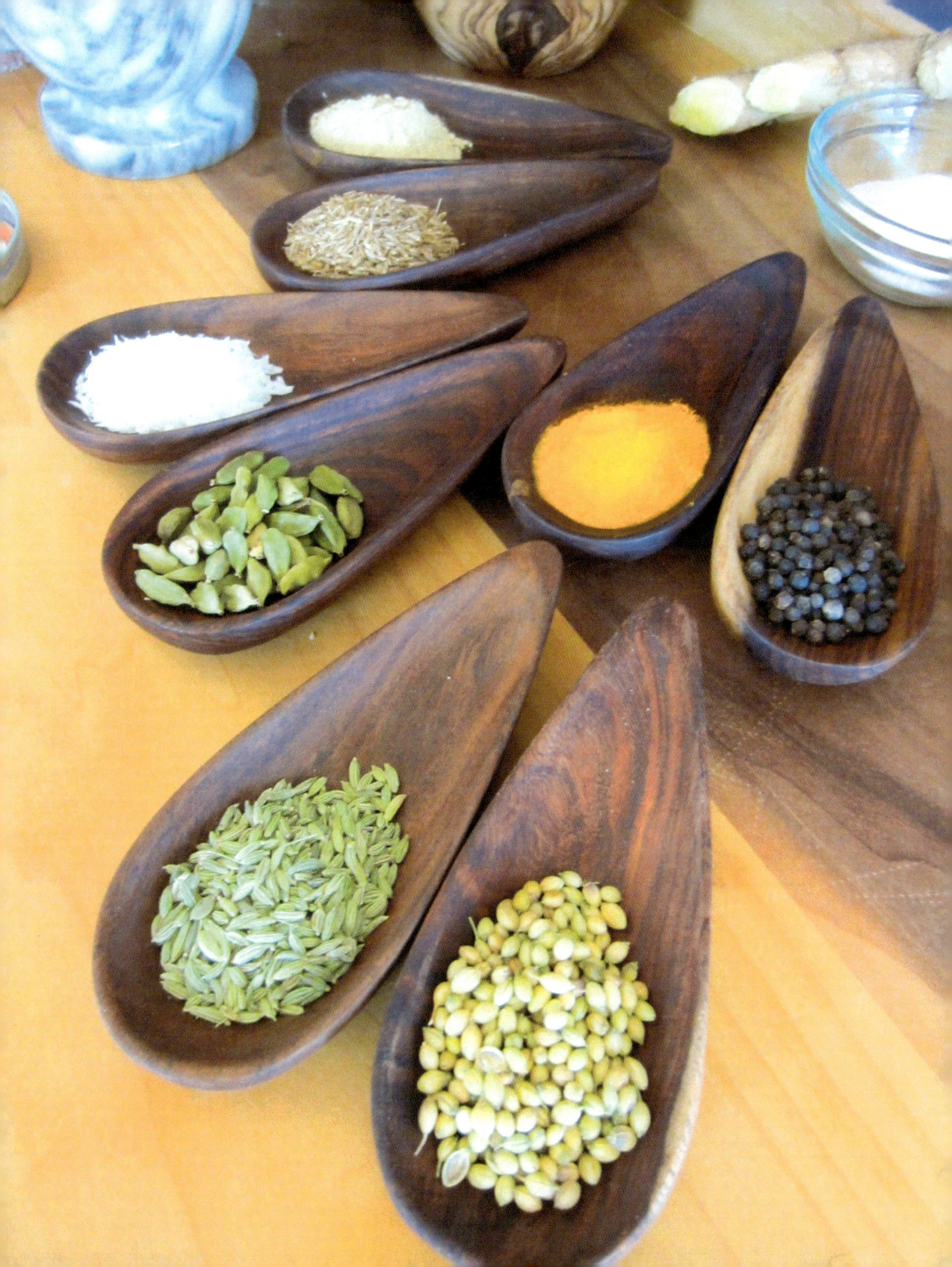

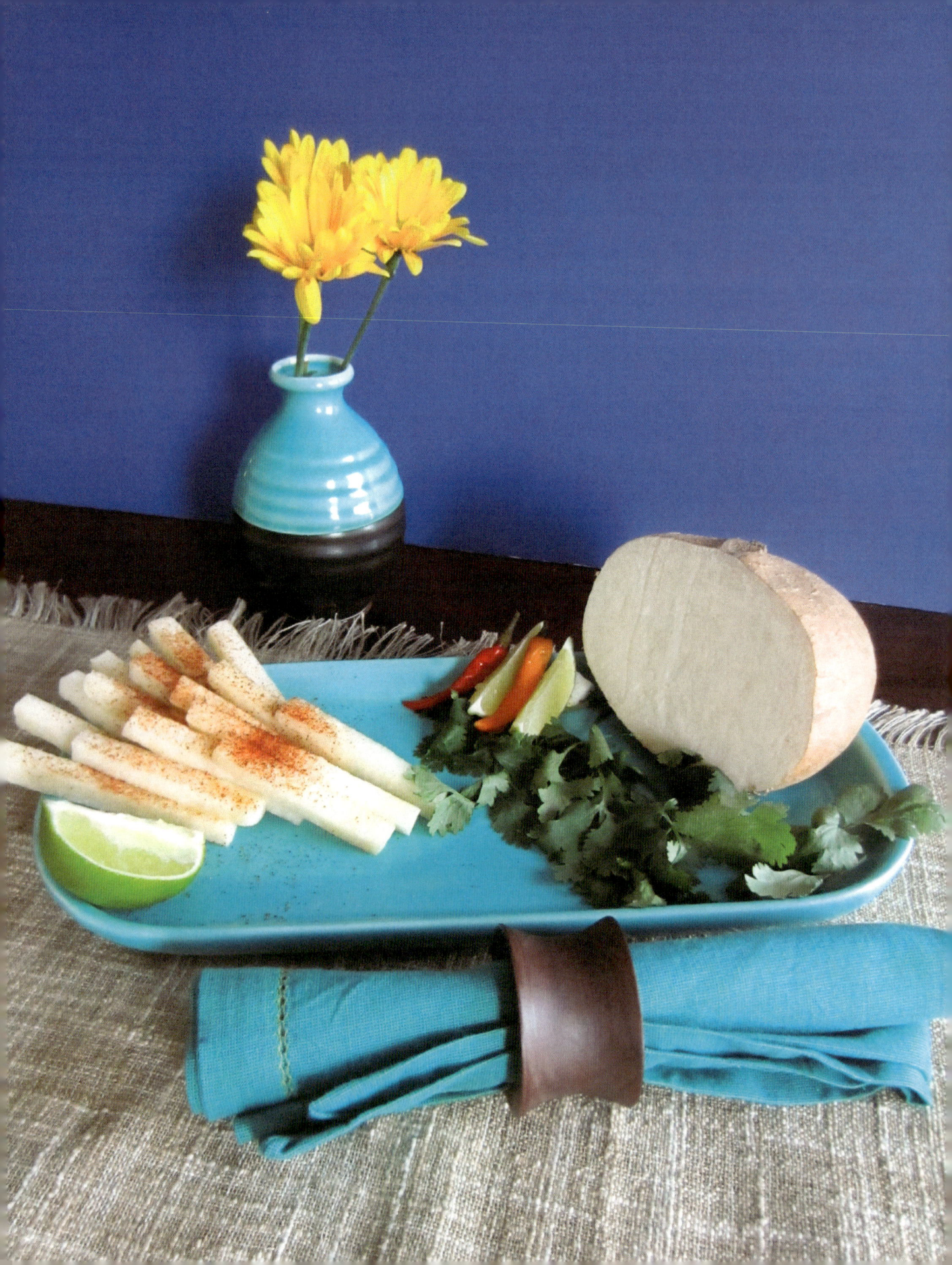

Chapter 15: Snacks and Dips

Ayurveda does not recommend snacks. The rationale is that we should give our system adequate time in between meals to process and assimilate nutrients from the last meal. If one is eating well balanced, meals at regular intervals there should not be a need for snacking.

But today, meals tend to be haphazard in terms of timing and generally not balanced as per an ayurvedic definition. As such, I feel there is a need for some healthy snacks that can be eaten on the go (in the car, on the train, at your office, etc.). Now you may be recalling that eating "on the go" violates one of one of the TOP 10 rules – eating mindfully. True. But if the alternative is consuming fast-food laden with sodium, sugar, fat and/or grease, then I feel that eating a healthy snack is a preferable alternative and is taking a step in the right direction.

This chapter includes many dips and spreads (*lemony cannellini bean spread*, *tri-doshic red lentil hummus*, *tri-doshic carrot (with a kick) spread*, and *tri-doshic zucchini hummus*) which are quick to prepare, can be made ahead and will keep in the refrigerator for several days. They can be used as a spread for a sandwich or a wrap, a base topping for a bruschetta, served with a salad, eaten with organic corn chips and much more. Dips and spreads are best stored in glass jars, tightly sealed in the refrigerator. Use a clean, dry utensil when scooping out the contents to avoid contamination and potential bacteria growth.

In the heat of the summer, minted fruit (grapefruit, blueberries, watermelon, apricots, papaya or peaches) can provide a refreshing burst of energy. This can be prepared ahead and stored in an airtight container in the refrigerator for consumption later in the day; consider bringing fruit to the airport when you travel as a healthy snack. When I was in India I used to bring my Rubbermaid® container filled with pomegranate seeds and snack on them in the airport waiting for my flight…it kept me from the temptations of the fried snacks and candy.

Trail mix is another option for pitta and vata. Combine goji berries, toasted almonds, pumpkin seeds and sunflower seeds in equal quantity in a large Ziploc® baggie stored in the refrigerator. Portion out a 1-cup serving size to keep handy for on the go refueling; this is another healthy snack for airplane, train or car travel. Sprinkle over organic yogurt (fresh or frozen) for more of a substantial snack.

ॐ

ॐ Recipes - Snacks & Dips

- **TRI-DOSHIC ARTICHOKE PESTO**
- **LEMONY CANNELLINI BEAN SPREAD**
- **TRI-DOSHIC ZUCCHINI HUMMUS**
- **MEXICAN BLACK BEAN SPREAD**
- **TRADITIONAL MEXICAN SALSA**
- **TRI-DOSHIC RED LENTIL HUMMUS**
- **MUSHROOM ALMOND PÂTÉ**
- **TRI-DOSHIC CARROT (WITH A KICK) SPREAD**
- **MARINELA'S DOLMATHAKIA (STUFFED GRAPE LEAVES)**
- **ENDIVE HONEY GOAT CHEESE**
- **JICAMA LIME STICKS**

❀ Tri-doshic Artichoke Pesto
DF/GF/SF/V
Yield: ½ cup

1⅓ cup basil leaves, rinsed, dried, leaves removed from stems
⅔ cup canned artichoke hearts, packed in water, rinsed
4 tablespoons almonds, blanched, peeled
1½ teaspoons lemon juice
¼ teaspoon garlic, pressed
⅛ teaspoon Himalayan salt
⅛ teaspoon crushed black pepper
4-6 teaspoons avocado oil (vata can add the higher amount of oil)

Combine the basil, artichokes, almonds, lemon juice, garlic, salt and pepper in a food processor and turn the motor on; slowly drizzle the oil into the mixing bowl as the motor continues to chop. The slower you pour the oil, the smoother the texture will be and the less likely the sauce will separate later. Since this is a low oil version of pesto, the texture will be a light paste consistency.

Scoop into a glass jar and pour a layer of oil on top to act as a preservative.

SERVING SUGGESTIONS: Spread over toast or crackers or serve as a dip with raw vegetables; use as a base in a veggie sandwich or wrap (add lettuce, tomatoes, sprouts, cucumbers).

VPK: The artichokes are astringent, heating and sweet; they are most suitable for pitta and kapha. The sweet basil and warm oil brings the balance to the spread for vata.

VARIATIONS: Add ⅓ cup arugula for an earthier flavor. To make a pesto sauce, add equal parts of water (plus some cream to achieve desired consistency) and purée with immersion blender; warm over low heat and serve over pasta, vegetables or couscous.

ABOUT: A nice tri-doshic alternative to traditional pesto. It will keep for a week or longer if you are diligent about keeping the pesto covered with the oil and not contaminating the jar with water or other food. It's so versatile you can eat it all week in various combinations.

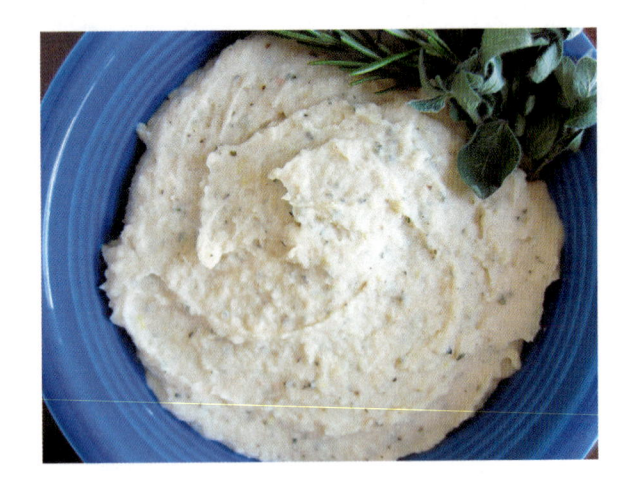

❦ Lemony Cannellini Bean Spread
DF/GF/SF/V
Yield: 1½ cups

15-ounce can of cannellini beans*, rinsed and drained
½ teaspoon garlic, pressed sautéed in 1 tablespoon olive oil (or ½ teaspoon garlic, pressed, raw)
1½ tablespoons olive oil
⅛ cup lemon juice and 1 teaspoon grated lemon rind
1 teaspoon fresh oregano, chopped (½ teaspoon dried)
¾ teaspoon fresh basil, chopped (¼ teaspoon dried)
¾ teaspoon fresh rosemary, chopped (¼ teaspoon dried)
½ teaspoon Himalayan salt
¼ teaspoon crushed black pepper

*If using raw, dried beans: soak overnight and cook until soft (about 1 hour). Combine all ingredients in food processor and pulse until smooth and creamy.

SERVING SUGGESTIONS: Serve on bruschetta (use the spread as the base layer then top with fresh chopped tomatoes tossed in olive oil and oregano); as a spread for a sandwich or wrap with cucumbers, lettuce, tomatoes and shredded fennel.

VPK: Vata can eat this in moderation, but may need to increase the oil and lemon. Kapha can add a bit of cayenne and use the raw garlic; pitta should used the cooked garlic or omit the garlic completely.

❦ Tri-doshic Zucchini Hummus
DF/GF/SF/V
Yield: 2 cups

3 cups zucchini, washed, ends removed, chopped
⅛ cup tahini
⅛ cup lemon juice
½ teaspoon grated lemon rind
½ teaspoon paprika
⅛ teaspoon cayenne
½ teaspoon Himalayan salt
⅛ teaspoon crushed black pepper

Place all ingredients in a food processor and blend until smooth.

SERVING SUGGESTIONS: As a dip serve with carrots, radishes or celery; spoon onto leaves of Belgium endive; wrap in radicchio leaves. Serve with: minted grilled vegetables, *purple coconut rice* with roasted pecans, bulgur salad with cucumber scallions and lemon vinaigrette.

ABOUT: This is much lighter version of hummus than the traditional recipe made with sesame seeds and chickpeas.

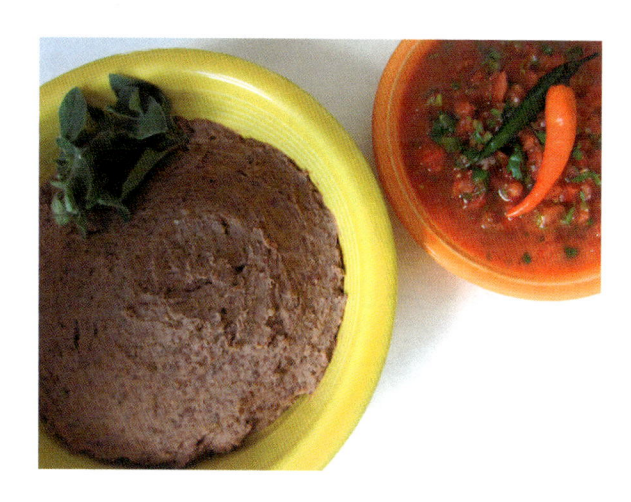

🌸 Mexican Black Bean Spread
DF/GF/SF/V
Yield: 1½ cups

15-ounce can of black beans*, rinsed and drained
½ teaspoon chili powder
½ teaspoon cumin powder
⅛ teaspoon cayenne powder
2 tablespoons avocado oil (or sunflower oil)
5 teaspoons lime juice
½ teaspoon Himalayan salt
¼ teaspoon crushed black pepper
⅛ teaspoon oregano, dried
2 tablespoons cilantro, chopped

*If using raw, dried beans: soak overnight and cook until soft (about 1 hour). Combine beans, chili powder, cumin, cayenne, oil, lime juice, salt and pepper in a food processor and pulse until smooth and creamy. Add cilantro and pulse until combined.

SERVING SUGGESTIONS: Spread on bruschetta then top with *traditional Mexican salsa* and oregano; spread on a sandwich or wrap with avocado and lettuce or endive.

VPK: Vata can eat in moderation; this is well balanced for pitta and kapha.

🌸 Traditional Mexican Salsa
DF/GF/SF/V
Yield: 1 cup

1 cup red ripe tomatoes, peeled, seeded, chopped
½ teaspoon jalapeño, seeded, finely chopped
1 teaspoon olive oil
1 tablespoon lime juice
¼ teaspoon Himalayan salt
¼ teaspoon pepper
2 tablespoons scallion, sliced thin
1 tablespoons cilantro, coarsely chopped

Combine all ingredients in a bowl and mix gently with a wooden spoon. Set in the refrigerator for a half hour before serving.

SERVING SUGGESTIONS: Serve with *Mexican black bean spread* and broiled chicken (or red snapper or halibut) marinated in a *Tri-doshic lime-cumin vinaigrette* and *Mexican rice*.

VPK: This is balancing for kapha; vata can eat in moderation; pitta can eat in moderation with the addition of extra cilantro and lime.

ABOUT: This recipe is from my friend from LA who preferred the simple salsa that he ate growing up in Guanajuato, Mexico. I've modified the recipe (less salt and less jalapeño) to make it more balancing for pitta.

❀Tri-doshic Red Lentil Hummus

GF/SF/V
Yield: 2 cups

3 cups water
½ cup red lentils
1 tablespoon sunflower oil
1 teaspoon butter
1 cup onion, peeled, chopped
2 cups crimini (baby bella) mushroom caps, peeled and chopped
½ teaspoon garlic, pressed

Spice Mix (COMBINE IN A SMALL BOWL):
- ½ teaspoon chili powder
- ¼ teaspoon coriander powder
- ¼ teaspoon cumin powder
- ⅛ teaspoon cayenne powder
- ⅛ teaspoon turmeric powder
- ½ teaspoon Himalayan salt
- ¼ teaspoon crushed black pepper

¼ cup orange juice
1 teaspoon grated orange zest
2 tablespoons honey
½ teaspoon Himalayan salt
¼ teaspoon crushed black pepper

In a 1½-quart sauce pan, boil the lentils in 3 cups of water until tender (about 10 minutes). Strain through a mesh sieve and remove excess water by pressing the lentils with the back of a spoon into the strainer; set aside.

In a 2-quart sauté pan, warm the sunflower oil and butter over medium heat. Add the onions, mushrooms and garlic and sauté for 5 minutes, stirring continually. Add the spice mix and cook until fragrant (about 1 minute). Add the orange juice and orange zest and deglaze the pan, scraping up all the bits of brown from the bottom of the pan. Add the cooked lentils and stir until the liquid has evaporated. Allow to cool to room temperature, then transfer to a food processor. Add the honey, salt and pepper; purée to a smooth spread. This will thicken as it cools.

SERVING SUGGESTIONS: Serve as a dip with crudités, crackers or pita bread; spread on sandwiches with mint, shredded carrots and shredded beets.

VARIATIONS: Add ¼ cup fresh *paneer* when blending for a richer tasting spread.

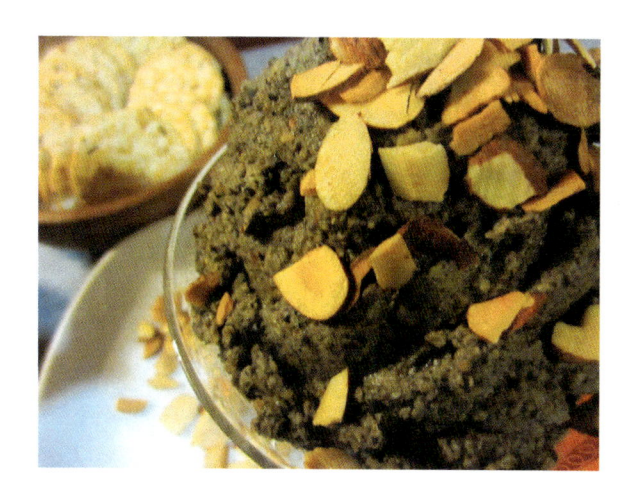

Mushroom Almond Pâté
DF/GF/SF/V
Yield 1½ cups

⅓ cup french lentils, boiled in 3 cups of water until they are over done (about 20 minutes)
4 ounce dried shiitake (rehydrated in 1 cup water; stems removed, soaking water reserved)
1 tablespoon butter (or sunflower oil)

Spice Mix (combine in a small bowl):
- ¾ teaspoon thyme
- ½ teaspoon paprika
- ⅛ teaspoon allspice
- ¼ teaspoon Himalayan salt
- ½ teaspoon crushed black pepper

½ cup onion, peeled, coarsely chopped
¼ cup toasted almonds (or cashews if for vata only)
3 tablespoons lemon juice
½ teaspoon grated lemon rind
2 tablespoons fresh parsley, coarsely chopped

Drain the lentils in a mesh sieve; squeeze out extra liquid by pressing the back of a spoon to the lentils. **Prepare Shiitake**: Coarsely chop mushroom caps. In a 3-quart sauté pan over medium heat, melt the butter. Add the spice mix and gently stir. Add onions and mushrooms; cook and stir until onions are soft and mushrooms are golden brown (about 5-10 minutes). Remove from heat and cool. Transfer mushroom mix to a food processor. Add the lentils, nuts, lemon juice and lemon rind and process until smooth. Add parsley and pulse briefly to combine. Transfer to a mold or serving dish; cover and chill for 1 hour to allow the flavors to assimilate.

SERVING SUGGESTIONS: Serve with crackers, crudités or serve as part of a "salad" plate.

VPK: This is relatively balanced for all three doshas; the heavy and oily qualities of the nuts are balanced by the light, dry qualities of the lentils and shiitake.

VARIATIONS: Add ½ teaspoon chopped mint to lighten the dish. Substituting Portobello mushrooms will change the texture and taste (it will be more watery and heavy).

ABOUT: Ayurveda typically designates mushrooms as being heavy, dull and depressing – the opposite qualities of the recommended ayurveda diet. As such, mushrooms were not typically used in cooking, but were occasionally recommended for medicinal purposes or used where grounding was required. However, the Portobello (and shiitake in Asian medicine) is regarded as a nutritive tonic and aphrodisiac; it is cooling, moistening, invigorating and gives strength and vitality. It can help improve immunity. In excess, mushrooms may increase ama (toxins) in the body and blood; ayurveda says they should be avoided when there is fever or infection.

❀ Tri-doshic Carrot (with a Kick) Spread
DF/GF/SF/V
Yield: 1½ cups

1½ cups carrots, washed and chopped
½ cup Yukon potato, peeled and chopped
4 cups water
1 tablespoon sunflower oil
1 tablespoon lemon Juice
½ teaspoon garlic, pressed
½ tablespoon cumin powder
¼ teaspoon cayenne
1 tablespoon coriander
¼ teaspoon Himalayan salt
⅛ teaspoon crushed black pepper

In a 2½-quart pan, combine the carrots, potatoes and water and bring to a boil. Continue cooking until the carrots and potato are tender (about 20 minutes). Drain and transfer to a food processor. Add remaining ingredients and process until smooth.

SERVING SUGGESTIONS: Serve as a dip on roasted garlic spelt chips, wheat crackers, toasted baguette or with crudités. As a wrap on pita bread serve with sprouts, lettuce, tomato, avocado and pumpkin seeds.

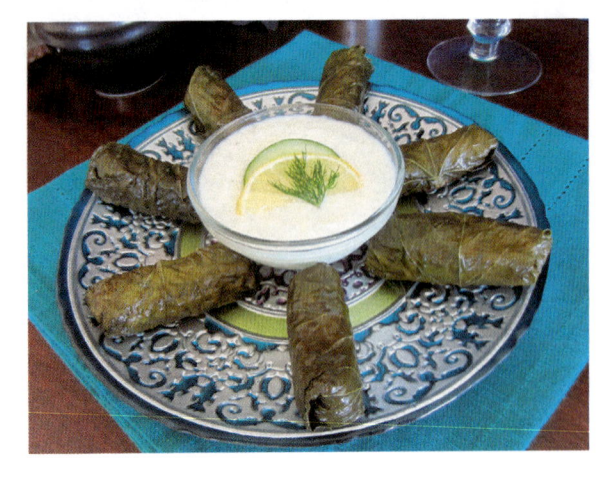

❀ Marinela's Dolmathakia (Stuffed Grape Leaves)
DF/GF/SF/V
Yield: about 20 stuffed leaves

**30 grapes leaves (packed in water), rinsed, drained, patted dry, stems removed
1 cup Arborio rice, soaked for 1 hour, then rinsed under cold water
6 tablespoons lemon juice,** *divided*
**1 teaspoon lemon rind
1 cup onion, finely chopped
1 cup scallions, finely chopped
⅓ cup tomato pulp, slice tomato in half then grate with box grater to make a pulp
1 cup water
¼ cup olive oil,** *divided*

Herb mix (combine in a small bowl):
- ¾ cup parsley, finely chopped
- ¼ cup fresh dill, finely chopped
- 1 tablespoon dried basil (or 3 tablespoons fresh)
- ¼ cup fresh mint
- ¾ teaspoon Himalayan salt
- ¼ teaspoon crushed black pepper

Transfer the rice to a 2 ½-quart mixing bowl; combine with 2 tablespoons of the lemon juice. Set aside. In a 3-quart sauté pan, add 2 tablespoons oil and warm over medium high heat. Add the onions and scallions and sauté (stir constantly) until the onions are translucent (about 3-4 minutes).

Add the rice and mix to combine. Add the water and tomato pulp; simmer uncovered until the water is absorbed (about 7-10 minutes; the rice will be half-cooked). Remove from heat and add the herb mix, 2 tablespoons of lemon juice and lemon rind; cool for 10 minutes. Sort through the leaves selecting medium-size leaves that are well shaped, without any holes; stack them in a pile: shiny (smooth or top) side down, vein (bumpy or bottom) side up. Use the discarded leaves to line the bottom of a heavy 3-quart pan; make a "bed" of several layers.

ROLL THE DOLMATHAKIA: Place a leaf with the base (stem-end) towards you on a flat surface. The bottom (bumpy/vein) side of the leaf should be face up. Place a tablespoon of filling at the center of the base end of the leaf. Fold the bottom section up to cover the filling. Fold the right and left sides in towards the center, then continue rolling the packet up towards the top of the leaf (similar to rolling a burrito or spring roll). **Do not roll too tightly** or the leaves will burst open as the rice expands during cooking. Repeat until all the rice is used.

Place the rolls, seam side down, in the pan on top of the bed of grape leaves arranging in a circular layer. Pack them in snugly (this helps keep the leaves intact as they cook); add another layer on top until all the stuffed leaves are in the pan. Pour remaining ⅛ cup olive oil and 2 tablespoons lemon juice over the dolmathakia; add enough water to cover them by a half-inch. Place a heatproof plate on top of the rolls to keep them submerged during cooking. Heat the pan until the water just begins to bubble; reduce heat and simmer, covered until done. The leaves will be fork tender and rice will be chewy (about 30-40 minutes).

SERVING SUGGESTIONS: Serve with *Mediterranean Salad Plate*, *tzatziki sauce* or tahini sauce.

VPK: Grape leaves are cool and astringent; combined with the rice and spices, they are tri-doshic.

ABOUT: This recipe comes from my neighbor Marinela and was handed down from her mom in Greece. We have reduced the oil by half. You can add ½ cup cooked ground beef or lamb for non-vegetarian. These will keep in the refrigerator for 5 days, wrapped tightly in plastic wrap.

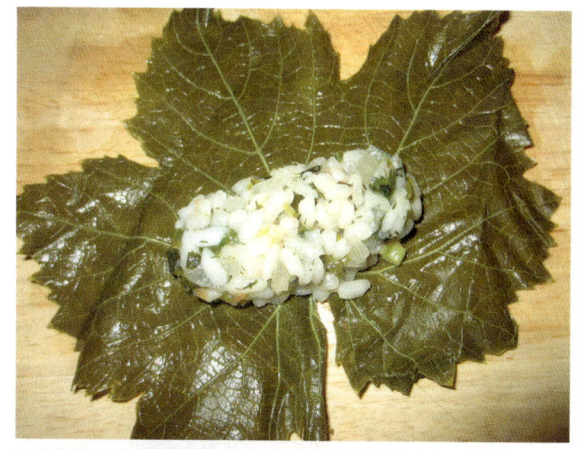

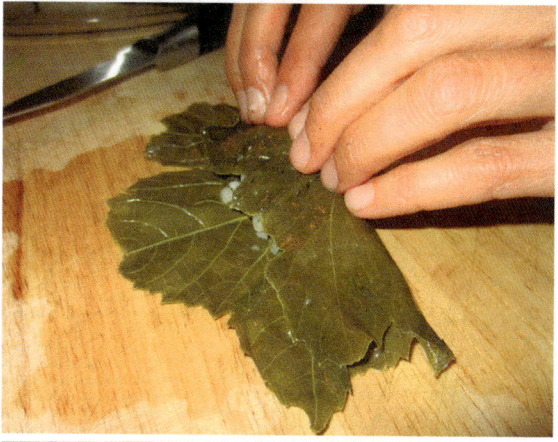

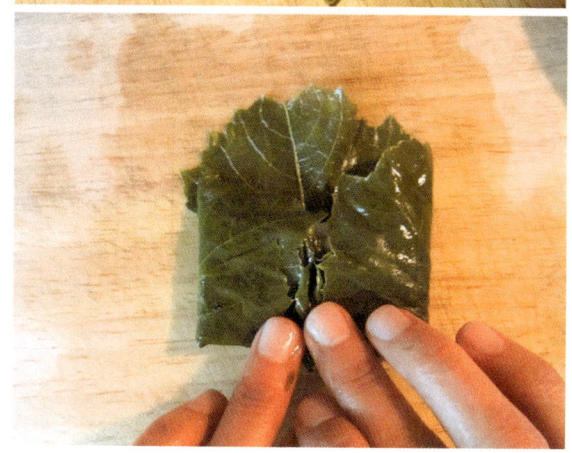

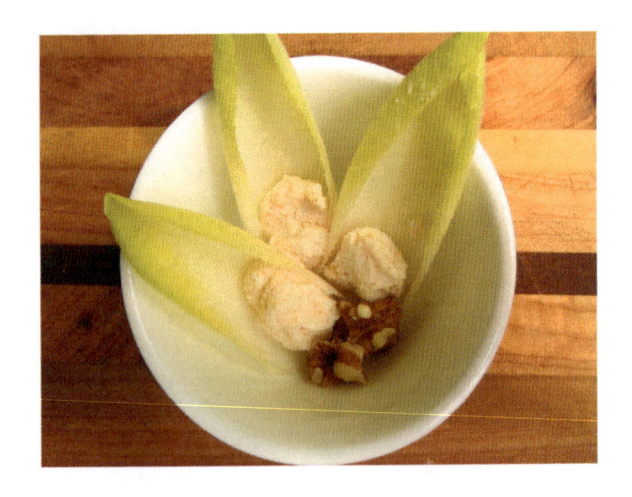

🌸 Endive Honey Goat Cheese
GF/SF/V
Servings: 2

4 tablespoons goat cheese (or paneer)
1 teaspoon raw honey
⅛ teaspoon cayenne
8 Belgian endive* leaves (or radicchio)
toasted walnuts or almonds (optional garnish)

In a 1-cup mixing bowl, combine the cheese with honey and cayenne using a fork; mix thoroughly. Divide the cheese mixture into eight and place in each endive leave. Garnish with nuts if desired.

VPK: This is best for vata and pitta; if made with fresh paneer, this is tri-doshic.

VARIATIONS: Replace cayenne with ½ teaspoon grated lemon or orange rind.

ABOUT: The honey and cayenne are heating and add lightness to the cheese while balancing the taste with the addition of spicy and sweet. Pairing cold, heavy cheese with the slightly bitter, cool, light endive makes for a compatible food combination.

*Belgian endive is also called: French endive, witloof and chicory; the leaves are slightly bitter and are moist and crunchy; the heads with green tips are more bitter than the yellow tips. If you cannot find endive, radicchio is a good substitute, but tends to be more bitter (cooling).

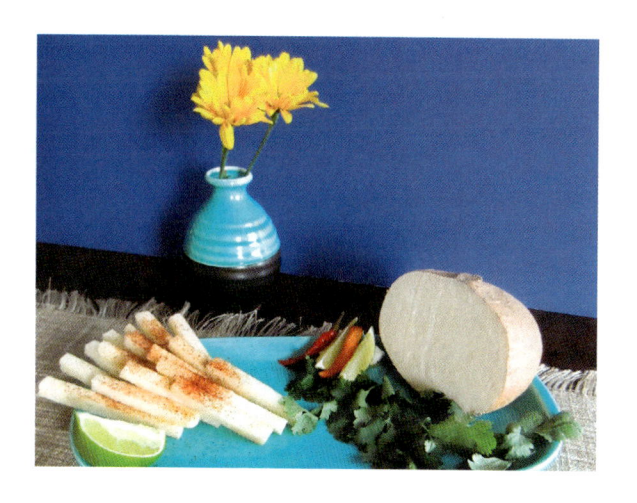

❁ Jicama Lime Sticks
DF/GF/SF/V
Servings: 4

4 cups jicama
3 tablespoons lime juice
¼ teaspoon Himalayan salt
½ teaspoon crushed black pepper
2 tablespoons cilantro, chopped
¼ teaspoon chili powder
⅛- ¼ teaspoon cayenne (optional)

Peel the jicama and cut into 3-inch strips (about ¼ inch thick). Put in a 2 quart bowl and toss with the lime, salt and cilantro (and cayenne if using). Arrange on a plate and serve. This can be stored in an air tight container in refrigerator for up to 4 days.

SERVING SUGGESTIONS: This is a cooling snack, great in the summer or anytime for pitta. Kapha and vata must add the cayenne to warm it up. Serve with a side of guacamole for vata and pitta; serve with *traditional Mexican salsa* for kapha. Add jicama to a crudités platter.

VPK: Best for reducing pitta, but tolerated by all doshas on a hot summer day as a snack.

VARIATIONS: Add jicama to salads (mixed greens, quinoa, couscous, rice, etc.) for a crunchy surprise.

ABOUT: Jicama is a cool, sweet, crunchy and moist tuberous root with a neutral flavor. It is ideal for pitta, but is also tolerated (with appropriate heating spices) by vata and kapha in the summer season.

You can find them in the produce section of most supermarkets. I first had jicama at a restaurant on a scorching beach in Mexico – it was very refreshing! Jicama is a dietary staple in Latin American cultures. Other names for Jicama include: the Mexican potato, Mexican yam bean, ahipa, saa got, Chinese turnip, lo bok, and the Chinese potato.

Jicama looks like a giant, round potato. Its skin is thin and can be gray, tan, or brown in color; the inside is a white flesh. When purchasing jicama, select tubers that are firm and dry. The skin is typically peeled before eating it raw. Jicama has a neutral, sweet flavor so it combines well with other dishes. It does not discolor when exposed to air so you can use it on vegetable platters. Jicama has a high amount of vitamin C and dietary fiber, is low in sodium, and has no fat.

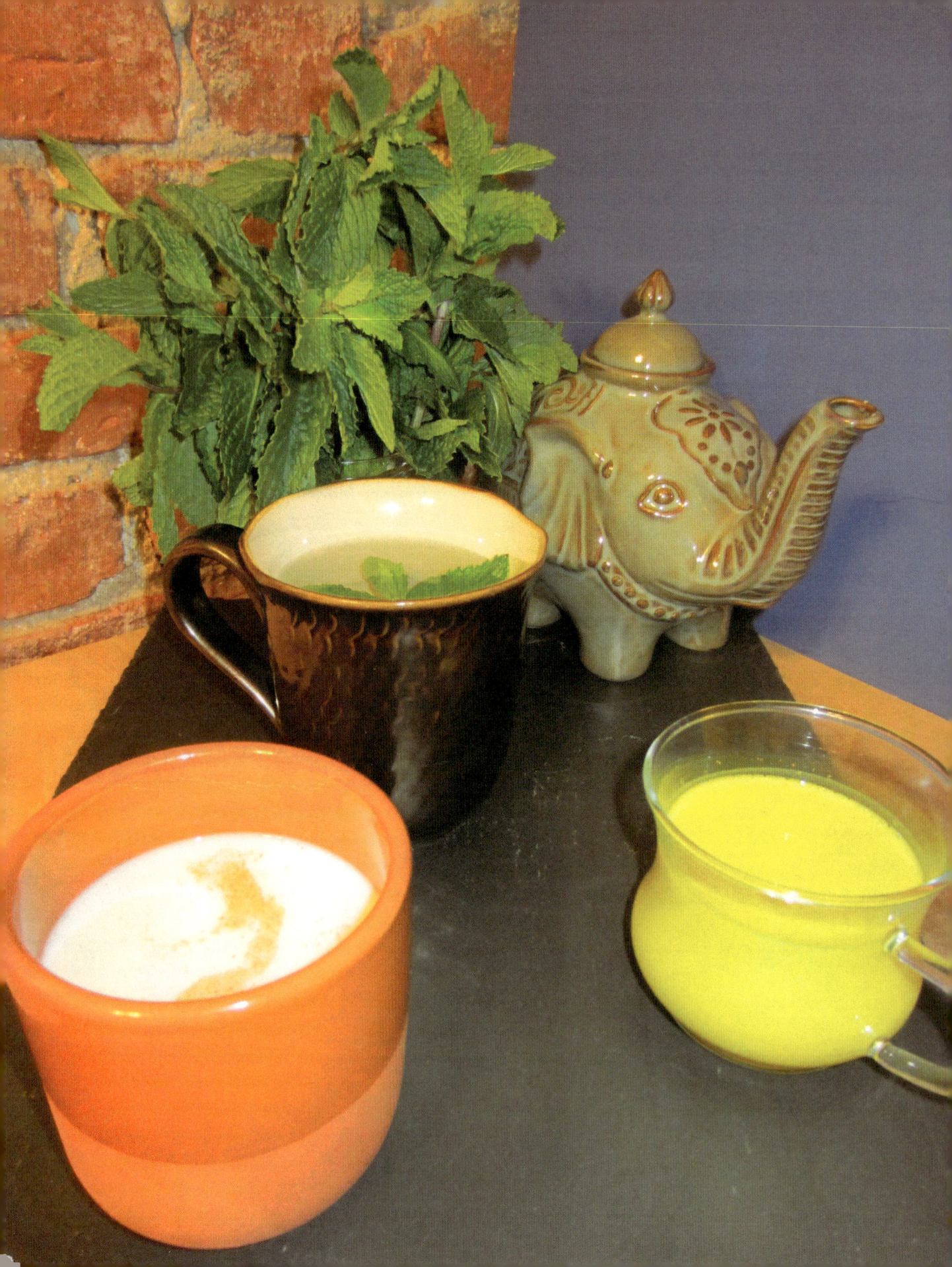

Chapter 16: Drinks

Ayurveda considers clean, pure water served warm or at room temperature to be the ideal drink. The recommended daily intake is determined by several factors including: your constitution (kapha needs the least); your lifestyle (if you sweat a lot, you need to drink more water); your diet (if you eat a lot of salty foods or dry foods you will need to drink more water); and the climate (a dry or hot climate will require that you drink more water). Ayurveda recommends avoiding iced drinks.

Alcohol is occasionally recommended in small amounts (i.e., 4 tablespoons of wine diluted with equal parts of water) to stimulate digestion prior to eating a meal; but in general, alcohol causes imbalance and is best avoided.

Likewise, coffee is best avoided as caffeine stresses the adrenal glands. An ayurvedic antidote to minimize the impact on the adrenals is to add a pinch of cardamom or cinnamon to your coffee. If you are interested in reducing your caffeine intake, try substituting with an herbal coffee such as Teeccino®. Teeccino® is astringent and bitter, making it well-balanced for kapha or pitta; vata will need to add some steamed milk (or non-dairy alternative) and honey to balance it out.

ॐ Recipes - Drinks

- DOSHA SPECIFIC DRINKS & JUICES
- PITTA SOOTHING MINT ROSEWATER DRINK
- PITTA COOLING CORIANDER MILK
- PITTA REFRESHING ALOE LIME DRINK
- TRI-DOSHIC MINT TEA
- GO TO SLEEP NUTMEG MILK
- KAPHA GINGER TEA
- VATA PITTA GINGER TEA
- VATA PITTA COCONUT CHAI SHAKE
- TURMERIC MILK
- VATA PITTA VITALITY DRINK

Dosha Specific Drinks & Juices
DF/GF/SF/V

In ayurveda clean, warm water is the drink of choice. But herbal teas and milks are often used for balancing doshas. The following table outlines some drinks that are used to ground vata, cool down pitta and get kapha moving. Recipes are included on the following pages for the drinks that are highlighted.

	Vata	Pitta	Kapha
Drinks	*vata pitta ginger tea*	*pitta soothing mint rosewater*	*kapha ginger tea*
	masala tea (i.e., masala chai)	*pitta refreshing aloe lime*	
	vata pitta coconut chai shake	*pitta cooling coriander milk*	
	go to sleep nutmeg milk	*go to sleep nutmeg milk*	
	vata pitta vitality drink	*vata pitta ginger tea*	
		vata pitta vitality drink	
		vata pitta coconut chai shake	

The following are dosha specific juice combinations; kapha should dilute their fruit juices 50% with water so as to minimize their sugar intake. Some ayurvedic doctors advise that the juice of fruits not be combined with the juice of vegetables. So I have followed that advice in preparing this table.

	Vata	Pitta	Kapha
Juices*	carrot-ginger-beet	apple-cranberry	apple-lemon
	orange-lime	apple-lime	kale-carrot-parsley
		coconut water	pomegranate-lime-ginger-apple
		carrot-kale	
		watermelon	
Spices (optional)	fresh ginger, mint	cilantro, mint	fresh ginger, cayenne, mint

*no sweetners added

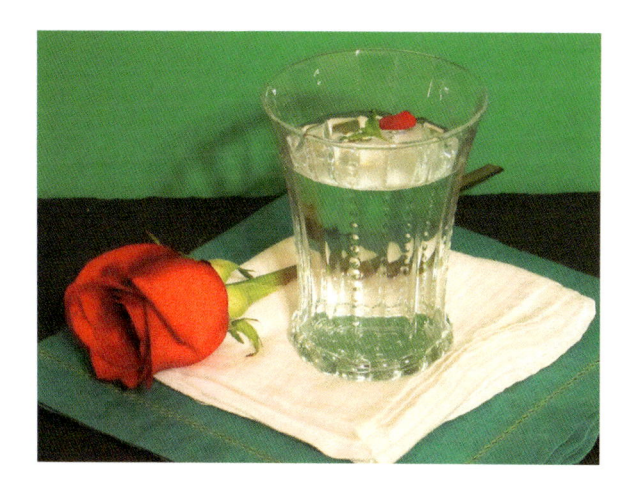

❁ Pitta Soothing Mint Rosewater Drink
DF/GF/SF/V
Servings: 1

1 cup water
¼ teaspoon rosewater
1 teaspoon chopped mint
½ teaspoon maple syrup

Combine all ingredients in a jar with a lid. Shake and serve.

ABOUT: Mint calms pitta; combined with cooling rosewater and the sweet maple syrup, this makes a deliciously soothing drink.

❁ Pitta Cooling Coriander Milk
DF/GF/SF/V
Servings: 1

1 cup organic milk (cow, soy, almond, coconut)
1 teaspoon coriander seed, coarsely crushed

In a 1-quart sauce pan, heat the milk and coriander seed until it just begins to boil. Remove from heat and cool for 5 minutes before serving.

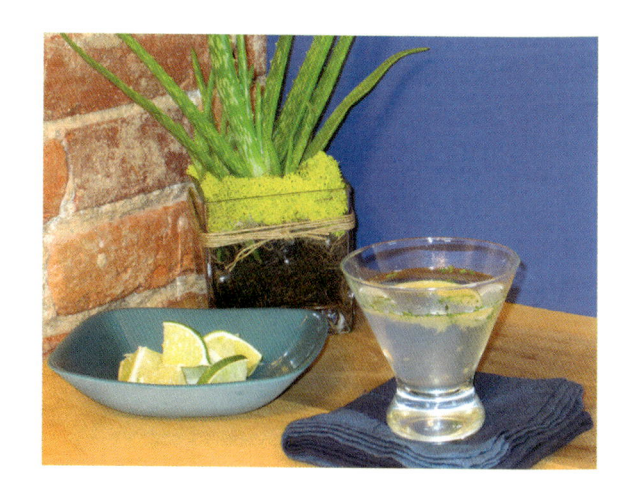

❁ Pitta Refreshing Aloe Lime Drink
DF/GF/SF/V
Servings: 1

½ cup water
1 teaspoon coconut sugar
¼ cup aloe vera juice
1 teaspoon lime juice
1 teaspoon chopped cilantro

In a 1-quart sauce pan, heat the water and coconut sugar over medium heat until sugar dissolves. Allow to cool to room temperature. Pour into a glass and add the aloe vera, lime juice and cilantro.

ABOUT: Coconut sugar is cooling and the ancients say that aloe vera juice is good for the liver. The cilantro is cooling and helps to pacify feelings of anger.

❁ Tri-doshic Mint Tea
DF/GF/SF/V
Servings: 1

1 cup boiling water
2 tablespoons fresh mint leaves

Steep leaves in water for 3 minutes; serve.

❀ Go to Sleep Nutmeg Milk
DF/GF/SF/V
Servings: 1

1 cup organic raw milk (or almond, coconut)
1 pinch of nutmeg

A half-hour before bed, prepare the drink: boil milk in a 1-quart sauce pan; add the nutmeg - just a pinch; simmer for 5 minutes. Transfer to your favorite mug and drink slowly.

VPK: Ideal for vata or pitta….kapha probably doesn't need this.

❀ Kapha Ginger Tea
DF/GF/SF/V
Servings: 1

1 cup boiling water
½ teaspoon ginger powder

Combine all ingredients in a 1-quart sauce pan and bring to a boil. Reduce heat and simmer for 3 minutes. Sweeten with honey if desired.

❀ Vata Pitta Ginger Tea
DF/GF/SF/V
Servings: 1

1 cup boiling water
½ teaspoon ginger, peeled, chopped

Combine ingredients in a 1-quart sauce pan and bring to a boil. Reduce heat and simmer for 3 minutes. Sweeten if desired (honey for vata; maple syrup for pitta).

ABOUT: Fresh ginger is mildly heating and is said to cleanse the blood; this is a nice alternative to a caffeinated tea.

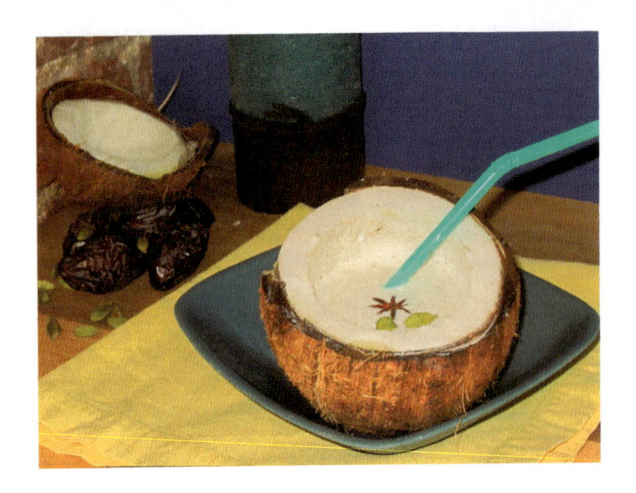

❀ Vata Pitta Coconut Chai Shake
DF/GF/SF/V
Servings: 1

8 ounces coconut milk
¼ teaspoon cinnamon powder
¼ teaspoon cardamom powder
¼ teaspoon ginger powder
1 bay leaf
1 star anise
1 pinch of powdered cloves
1 teaspoon coconut sugar

Combine all ingredients in a 1-quart sauce pan and simmer for 5 minutes until the spices blend into the milk. Cool. Transfer to glass jar and refrigerate for an hour. Shake and serve.

SERVING SUGGESTIONS: Sprinkle chopped mint over the top before serving. Sweeten with minced medjool dates.

VPK: Best for vata and pitta, kapha can dilute with 2 ounces of water and omit the coconut sugar.

ABOUT: Leftover coconut milk can be used to make *Thai Lemongrass Vermicelli Soup*.

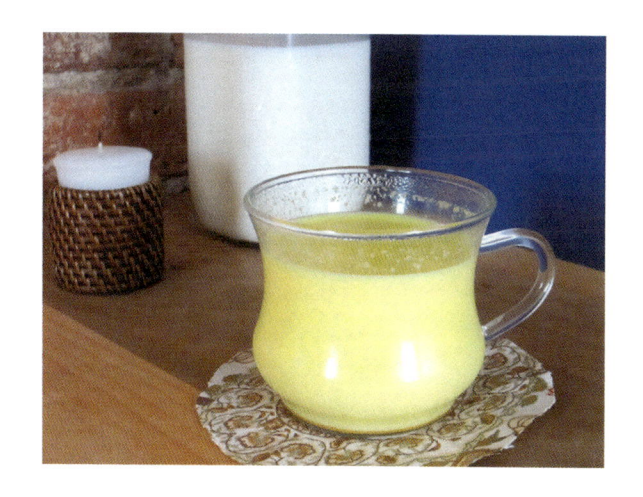

❋ Turmeric Milk
DF/GF/SF/V
Servings: 1

1 cup organic raw milk (cow, almond, coconut)
¼ teaspoon turmeric

A half hour before bed, prepare the drink: bring the milk to a boil in a 1-quart sauce pan; reduce heat to low and add the turmeric; simmer for 5 minutes. Transfer to a cup and serve.

VPK: Tri-doshic if with cow or almond milk.

VARIATIONS: Add a pinch of saffron.

ABOUT: Warm milk makes you sleepy and the benefits of turmeric in ayurveda are seemingly endless. It's generally good for the immune system and turmeric milk is recommended daily before bed for preventative health measures.

The ancients say that turmeric was antispasmodic, anti-inflammatory and antihelminthic (i.e., it expels parasites, bacteria, virus and fungus); they used it for treating dandruff, menstrual cramps, skin blemishes (discoloration, scars and spots) and general immunity. Turmeric is bitter, pungent, astringent and heating. It is dry, light and good for digestion as it stimulates production of bile in the liver, improving the body's ability to break down fats. It is considered tri-doshic.

Modern medicine has identified curcumin (the active ingredient in turmeric), to be an antioxidant (effective for cancer prevention) and to have therapeutic potential against H. pylori, herpes simplex, hepatitis B, salmonella and Candida infections; it has been shown to regulate blood sugar levels which helps prevent Type-2 Diabetes[20].

❋ Vata Pitta Vitality Drink
DF/GF/SF/V
Servings: 1

1 cup milk (cow or almond)
3 fresh dates (soaked overnight in water, pitted, chopped)
8 almonds (blanched, peeled, crushed into small pieces with mortar and pestle)
⅛ teaspoon cardamom powder
2 threads of saffron

Combine all ingredients in a 1½-quart saucepan and bring to a boil. Reduce heat and simmer for 3 minutes. Remove from heat, cool and serve. The dates and almonds don't stay blended with the milk; I typically eat this with a spoon.

SERVING SUGGESTIONS: Drink in a calm, peaceful environment before sunrise.

VPK: Grounding and replenishing to vata; cooling and restorative to pitta.

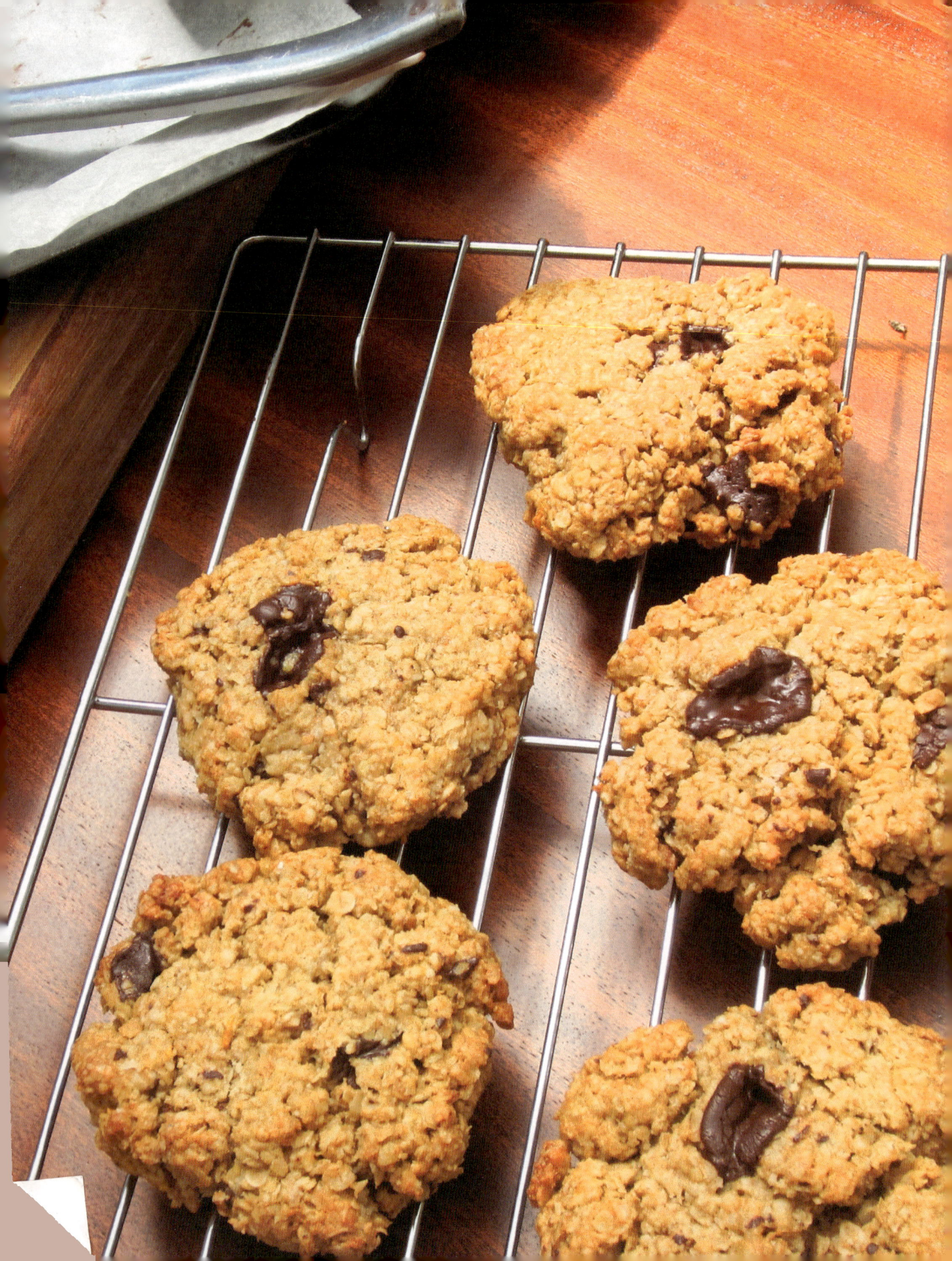

Chapter 17: Not too Sweet Desserts & Gluten Free Options

This chapter is perhaps stretching the limits as to what should be included in an ayurvedic wellness cookbook. However, if the alternative is purchasing a candy bar containing refined sugar, chemical preservatives and additives, I feel a home-made sweet will be a better choice.

My sweetener preference is coconut sugar. It is low Glycemic Index (releases glucose slowly and steadily into the blood) and minimally refined (it is high in minerals and vitamins). It is cooling, sweet and heavy making it ideal for vata and pitta. I find it to be sweeter than cane sugar and I generally use about 25% less than I normally would in recipes, which makes it "less unbalancing" to kapha. It costs more than refined cane sugar, but since you are using less, your true cost is comparable.

Much to the chagrin of my family members, the sweets I bake now are much lower in sugar than the sweets from my pre-ayurveda days. Likewise, the recipes I have created here have less sugar than traditional western sweets. In some instances, the recipes will have a range for the sugar amount (i.e., ½-¾ cup). In these recipes, prepare the batter with the lesser amount of sugar and taste; if it doesn't seem sweet enough, add the additional sugar to the batter. For best results, do not reduce the sugar any further, especially in the gluten-free recipes. Sugar provides moisture and texture as does the gluten. So you need to be mindful of these properties when reducing and/or omitting sugar and gluten. I see many gluten-free recipes where the quantity of sugar has been significantly increased to replace the moisture loss from the gluten. While this solution retains the texture, the added sugar is too sweet for my taste.

Honey is the best sweetener for kapha, due to its heating energetic. I have included a recipe for *Turkish halva* made from toasted sesame seeds and raw honey; suitable for kapha…in moderation.

ॐ

ॐ Recipes - Not too Sweet: Desserts & Gluten Free Options

- TURKISH HALVA
- TRUFFLES
- GF CHOCOLATE ALMOND ROSE CAKE WITH GANACHE & MINTED WHIP CREAM
- GF POMEGRANATE ORANGE CHIP BARS
- ADUKI BEAN SQUARES
- CARDAMOM ALMOND BALLS
- LAVENDER ESSENCE TEA BREAD
- GF CORN BREAD
- GF MACADAMIA PIE CRUST

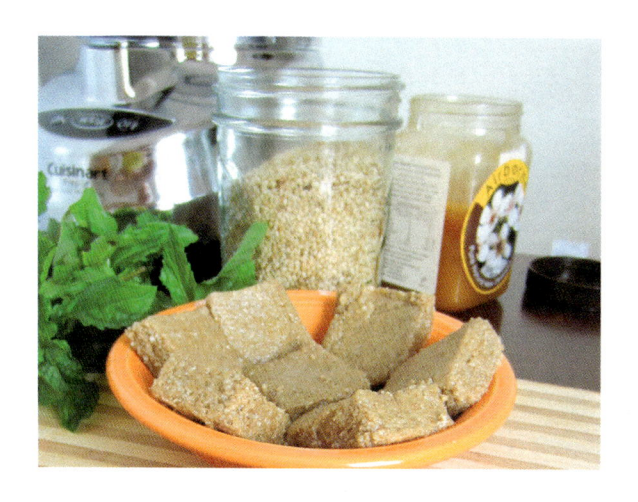

Turkish Halva
DF/GF/SF/V

Yield: one 8x8-inch pan

¾ cup unhulled raw sesame seeds
1 cup basic tahini
2 tablespoons raw honey
¼ teaspoon cardamom powder
1 teaspoon rose water

In a food processor, grind ¾ cup of raw sesame seeds to a coarse consistency (about 2 minutes). Add the tahini, honey, cardamom powder and rose water and pulse until combined. Transfer to an 8x8-inch pan, smoothing the top by pressing with the back of a metal spoon. Cover and refrigerate for 1 hour. Slice into squares; this will keep in the refrigerator in an air-tight container for up to a month.

SERVING SUGGESTIONS: Great for pujas (Hindu worshipping ceremonies requiring vegan sweets), holiday gatherings and snacks for work.

VPK: These are heating and oily so they are best for vata; pitta can substitute cooling maple syrup for the honey; kapha could try the coffee flavoring (see variations). All doshas should eat in moderation and share with friends.

VARIATIONS: You may add any of the following ingredients in place of the cardamom powder: 1 teaspoon vanilla extract; ½ teaspoon instant coffee dissolved in ½ teaspoon boiled water; ½ teaspoon orange oil; 1 teaspoon cocoa powder; 1½ tablespoons pistachios (chopped); 1½ tablespoons almonds (blanched, peeled, chopped).

ABOUT: This version of halva has reduced honey; the honey isn't cooked so we receive all its natural goodness.

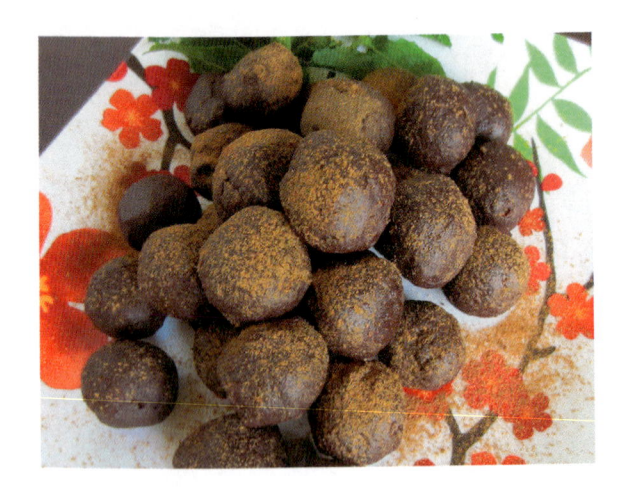

❀ TRUFFLES
GF/SF/V
Yield: 30 teaspoon size balls

Basic Recipe - Dark Chocolate
3½ ounces organic cream
5 teaspoons unsalted butter
7 ounces dark chocolate (Green & Black® 85%)
1 tablespoon honey

TOPPINGS
- cocoa powder (sifted) (P/ K)
- shredded coconut (V / P)
- toasted ground nuts (almonds, hazelnut, cashews, pecans) (V)

In a 1½-quart saucepan, heat the cream and butter over medium low heat, stirring constantly. When the mixture reaches just below boiling (you will see tiny bubbles beginning to form), remove from heat and add the chocolate. Stir with a flexible spatula until the chocolate is completely melted and the texture is smooth. When the mixture has cooled to room temperature, stir in the honey. Cover with plastic wrap and place in the refrigerator to chill (1 – 2 hours) until the ganache is firm enough to roll into balls. Remove from refrigerator; place the desired topping on a plate.

Scoop out one teaspoon of the ganache and mold into a small ball using the palm of your hand; roll in the topping, then place in a single row in an air-tight container. If the ganache gets too warm, it will start to melt and stick to your hands. You can put the ganache in the freezer for 5 or 10 minutes to let the ganache firm up, then continue with making the balls. Rinsing your hands with cold water will also help. The truffles will keep for 1 week in the refrigerator in an air-tight container; they may be frozen for up to 1 month.

SERVING SUGGESTIONS: Eat in moderation and share with friends.

VARIATIONS: Mayan Gold: reduce Green & Black® 85% dark chocolate to 5 ounces; add 2 ounces Green & Black Mayan Gold® chocolate.

ABOUT: Cocoa is bitter, astringent, acidic and contains caffeine; minimize these treats, especially in the evening. The quality of the chocolate is important; Green & Black® 85% dark chocolate is gluten free and dairy free (as of this writing); it has a creamy, smooth texture due to the addition of vanilla. Note that the Green & Black Mayan Gold® chocolate is not dairy free as it has a milk chocolate base.

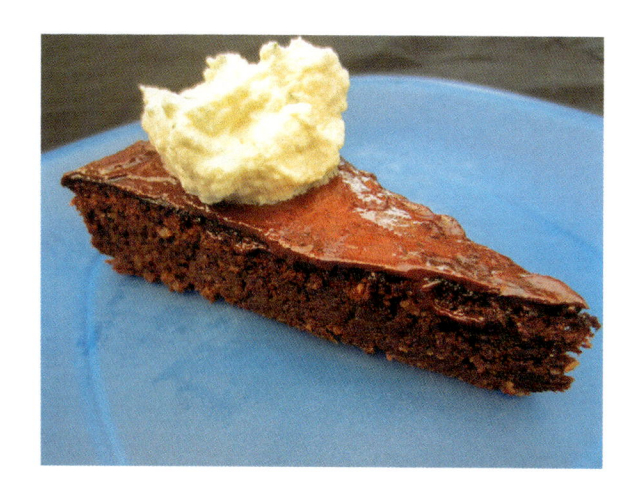

GF Chocolate Almond Rose Cake with Ganach & Minted Whip Cream
GF / SF / V
Yield: one 8-inch cake

1⅛ cup Green & Black® dark chocolate 85%
8½ tablespoons unsalted butter
⅔ - ¾ cup coconut sugar
4 egg yolks
½ teaspoon rose water
1½ cups almond flour
4 egg whites
1 teaspoon coconut sugar
¼ teaspoon Himalayan salt

Preheat oven to 350°F. Grease an 8-inch spring form cake pan and line the bottom with wax paper. Melt the chocolate in the top of a double boiler; remove from heat and cool. In a 2½-quart mixing bowl, cream the butter and sugar. Add the melted chocolate, egg yolks and rose water, beating until well combined; fold in the almond flour and salt.

In a 2½-quart mixing bowl, use a hand mixer to whip the egg whites; when froth begins to form, add the teaspoon of coconut sugar. Continue beating until soft peaks form. Gently stir half of the egg whites into the chocolate mixture; fold in the rest of the egg whites.

Pour batter into prepared pan and bake for 30-35 minutes; begin checking for doneness after 25 minutes. **You will know the cake is done when**: the edges of the cake start to pull away from the sides of the pan; a toothpick inserted into the center of the cake comes out clean with just a few crumbs; and the center of the cake bounces back after lightly touching (but no fingerprints should remain on the surface). Remove from oven and cool on a wire rack for 10 minutes; remove the cake from pan by inverting the pan onto the rack. The cake will keep for 3-4 days in an air-tight container, stored in a cool, dark place.

Ganache Topping:
8 ½ ounces Green & Black® dark chocolate, room temperature, chopped into ½-inch pieces
5 ounces cream

In a 1½-quart sauce pan, bring the cream to a boil then immediately remove from heat. Add the chocolate to the cream. Whisk until the chocolate melts and the texture is smooth. Allow to cool for 10 minutes; then spread a smooth layer on the top and sides of the cake.

Minted Whipped Cream
1¼ cups cream
¼ teaspoon rose water
1 tablespoon coconut sugar
1 tablespoon fresh mint leaves, minced

Combine cream and rose water in 2½-quart mixing bowl. Beat with hand blender until frothy. Add the sugar and mint leaves. Beat until soft peaks form. Spoon the whipped cream onto the cake.

ABOUT: This recipe is adapted from "Otto Lenghi - The Cookbook" by Yotam Ottolenghi and Sami Tamimi. One of the marvelous books I read while cat-sitting for Oreo and creating recipes at the Goldblatt's residence in Wellington, New Zealand.

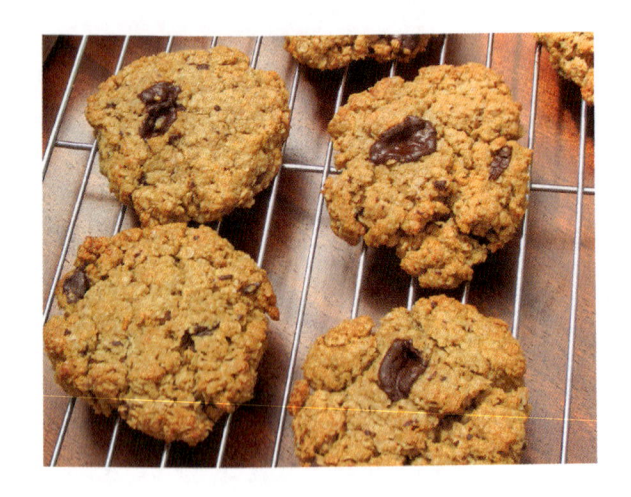

❀GF Pomegranate Orange Chip Bars (or Cookies)

GF/SF/V
Yield: one 8x8-inch pan

4 tablespoons butter
½ cup coconut sugar
¾ cup almond butter
1 tablespoon pomegranate syrup
½ teaspoon cinnamon
1 teaspoon grated orange zest
¼ teaspoon Himalayan salt
1 large egg
⅝ teaspoon baking soda
1½ cups quick oats
¼ cup dark chocolate chunks

Preheat oven to 350°F. Cream together the butter, sugar, almond butter, pomegranate syrup, cinnamon, orange zest and salt. Add the egg and mix. The batter will be very thick and oily. Stir in the baking soda. Add the oats and chocolate chips stirring until mixed well. Transfer to an 8x8-inch non-stick pan and bake for 20-22 minutes until the edges just start to brown. If the entire top is brown, then they are overcooked and will be very dry. The dough should be soft coming out of the oven. Place the pan on a wire rack and cool for 10 minutes; slice into bars and transfer to the rack to completely cool. Store in an airtight container.

VPK: Eat in moderation and share with friends.

VARIATIONS: Try substituting white chocolate chips in place of the dark chocolate; substitute lemon rind in place of the orange rind.

ABOUT: This was adapted from Trader Joe's chocolate oat cookie recipe. You can use this same batter to make cookies. They should be cooked for 7-8 minutes and will be soft coming out of the oven. Allow to cool on a wire rack where they will firm up. Yield: one dozen cookies.

The raw batter can be refrigerated for up to a week, so you can make individual fresh baked cookies whenever you like.

❁ Aduki Bean Squares

SF/V

Yield: one 8x8-inch pan

For filling:
15-ounce can aduki beans, rinsed and drained
½-¾ cup coconut sugar
1 tablespoon maple syrup
½ teaspoon cardamom powder
¼ teaspoon Himalayan salt

For dough:
8 ounces butter (2 sticks), cut into ½ inch cubes
1½ cups almond meal (or flour)
1 cup white flour
1 cup rice flour
½ cup coconut sugar
1 teaspoon almond extract

Preheat oven to 350°F. Grease an 8x8-inch pan and line the bottom with parchment paper (or wax paper). Place all the "filling" ingredients in a 1½-quart sauce pan. Cook over low heat, stirring constantly until the sugar dissolves and filling becomes thick. Remove from heat and cool.

Place dough ingredients in a food processor with the dough blade. Pulse until the mixture looks like moist crumbs. Place half the dough mixture into the bottom of the greased pan, pressing with the back of a metal spoon to level the surface. Spread the aduki filling on top of the bottom crust layer. Sprinkle the remaining dough crumbs on top. Bake for 25-30 minutes until the top layer is golden. Allow to cool in the pan then cut into squares. Carefully remove individual squares from the pan; the topping mixture tends to crumble (because the rice flour is dry).

VPK: Eat in moderation.

ABOUT: This recipe was adapted from "The Many Little Meals of Rose Bakery" cookbook, by Rose Carrarini.

Cardamom Almond Balls

SF/V

Yeild: 30+ balls

½ cup whole wheat pastry flour
½ cup unbleached wheat flour
¾ teaspoon baking powder
¼ teaspoon baking soda
½ teaspoon Himalayan salt
½ cup butter (1 stick), softened
⅓ cup coconut sugar
1 large egg
1 teaspoon vanilla extract
2 teaspoons lemon peel
1½ cups blanched slivered almonds, (coarsely ground)
1 tablespoon ground cardamom
3 tablespoons flax seeds, coarsely ground
powdered sugar for topping

Preheat the oven to 350°F. In a 1½-quart mixing bowl, sift together the flours, baking powder, baking soda and salt. In a 2½-quart mixing bowl, cream together the butter and sugar. Add the egg, vanilla and lemon peel, and beat until light and fluffy. Add the almonds, cardamom and flax seeds, stirring until well combined. Add the flour mixture to the cream mixture, combining thoroughly (the dough will be oily from the almonds). Using about 1½ teaspoons of dough, roll into balls and place on an ungreased baking sheet about one inch apart. Bake for 8 minutes, until cookies are just beginning to brown slightly on the bottom. Be careful, as they will quickly burn and dry out if left in the oven for too long.

Remove cookies from oven and place on a cooling rack. Put some powdered sugar in a sieve. Hold the sieve above the cookies and gently tap the sieve to allow a fine powder to flow onto the cookies.

ABOUT: While attending ayurveda school in Albuquerque, New Mexico I would frequent Anupurna's World Vegetarian Café for healthy ayurvedic meals, a cup of chai, and their amazing sweets. This recipe was inspired by their cardamom cookies.

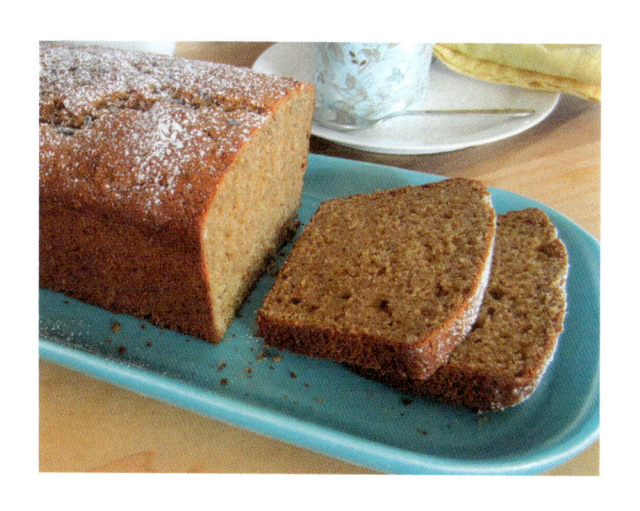

❇ Lavender Essence Tea Bread

GF/SF/V

Yeild: one 8-inch loaf

¾ -1 cup coconut sugar
5 tablespoon butter
1½ teaspoons organic lavender leaves, lightly crushed with a mortar & pestle
1 teaspoon vanilla
2 eggs
1¼ cup wheat pastry flour
½ cup almond flour
1 tablespoon flax seeds
1 teaspoon baking powder
¼ teaspoon baking soda
¼ teaspoon Himalayan salt
1 cup yogurt, plain
2 tablespoon confectioners' sugar (to dust top)
½ teaspoon grated lemon rind (garnish on top)

Preheat oven to 350°F. Grease an 8-inch loaf pan and line the bottom with wax paper (or parchment paper). All ingredients should be at room temperature prior to preparation.

In a 3-quart mixing bowl, beat the butter and sugar until creamy. Stir in the crushed lavender and vanilla. Add the eggs; beat well with an electric whisk (or hand blender). In a 2-quart mixing bowl, whisk together the pastry flour, almond flour, flax seeds, baking powder, baking soda and salt.

Gently fold ⅓ of the flour mixture into the sugar cream mixture. Fold in half the yogurt. Repeat the alternating pattern of flour and yogurt until all the ingredients are blended together.

Transfer the batter into the prepared pan. Bake until done, about 45 minutes. Test for doneness after 40 minutes. The bread is done when a wooden toothpick inserted in the middle comes out clean and the bread starts to separate from the edges of the pan. Cool in the pan for 20 minutes on a wire rack; then turn out onto the rack to cool completely.

VPK: This is a reduced sugar tea cake that can be eaten in moderation by all doshas.

ABOUT: Lavender is calming; this cake will be soothing to pitta and vata – in moderation. The addition of the flax seeds is helpful to kapha. You can freeze this for up to 1 month wrapped in freezer wrap and a freezer baggie; but do not dust with the confectioners' powder prior to freezing. When ready to use, unwrap and thaw at room temperature for 2 hours before serving. Dust with confectioners' powder.

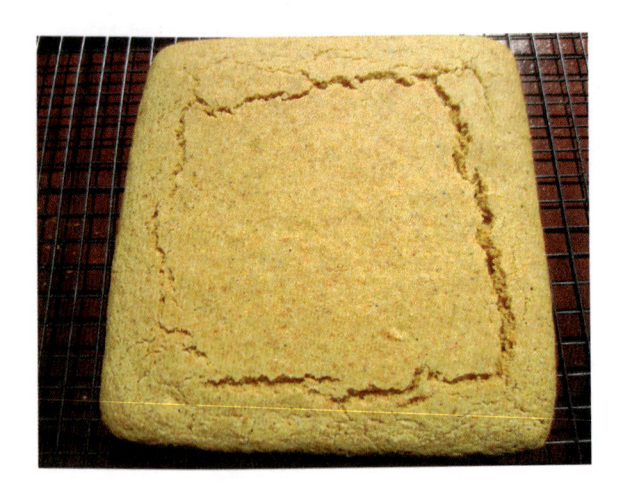

❀GF Corn Bread
GF/SF/V
Yield: one 8x8-inch pan

1 cup coconut milk
1 tablespoon lime juice
2 cups yellow cornmeal
¼ cup glutinous rice flour*
⅛ cup arrowroot flour
1 teaspoon double acting baking powder
¼ teaspoon baking soda
½ teaspoon Himalayan salt
1 large egg
2 tablespoons maple syrup
3 tablespoons butter, melted

Preheat oven to 425°F. Combine the coconut milk with the lime juice in a small bowl and let sit for 10 minutes while you prepare the other ingredients. In a 2½-quart mixing bowl, whisk together the cornmeal, glutinous rice flour, arrowroot flour, baking powder, baking soda and salt. In a 1½-quart mixing bowl, whisk the egg. Add the maple syrup, butter and milk/lime mixutre, whisking until well combined. Slowly add the wet ingredients to the dry ingredients and swiftly combine with a wooden spoon. Do not over mix. Pour into an 8x8-inch non-stick pan. Bake for 15-18 minutes or until done. The bread is done when a toothpick inserted in center comes out clean and the sides of the bread start to separate from the pan edges. Remove from the oven and place on a cooling rack; cool in the pan for 10 minutes. Invert to remove from the pan and cool to room temperature on the cooling rack.

SERVING SUGGESTIONS: Serve with *Caribbean aduki bean stew* or *lime ginger tofu* or *French lentil soup with pork* and a salad.

VPK: Corn is heating and dry – ideal for kapha. The coconut milk and maple syrup cool and moisten the bread. The coconut milk does not impart a coconut flavor to this bread. This bread is best paired with lentils, beans and salads. Vata should apply liberal amounts of butter or ghee.

ABOUT: * Glutinous rice flour (or sweet rice flour) is ground from short-grain glutinous rice (also known as sticky rice which is used in making sushi). It has a much higher starch content than other types of rice, but it does not contain gluten. It can be purchased at Asian grocery stores usually under the brand name "Erawan" (about $3 for a pound).

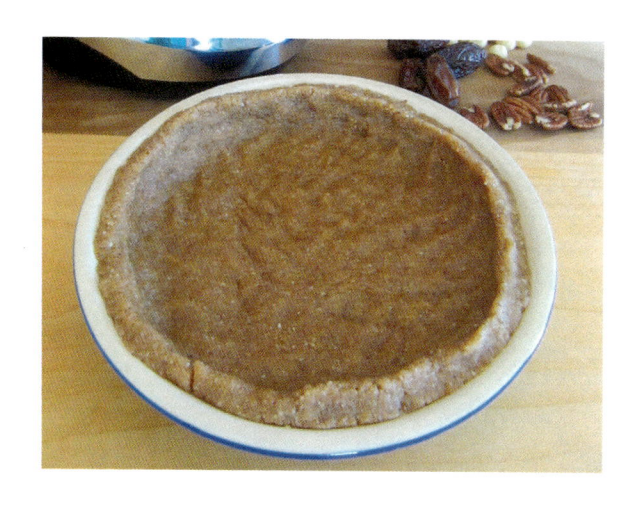

❀GF Macadamia Nut Pie Crust

DF/GF/SF/V
Yield: one 9-inch pie crust

⅜ cup coconut, shredded, unsweetened
2 teaspoons coconut oil
½ cup medjool dates, pitted
1½ cups macadamia nuts, toasted
1 cup pecans, toasted
½ teaspoon Himalayan salt

Place the coconut and coconut oil into a food processor. Blend until it is transformed into nut butter (about 5 minutes). Add the dates and pulse about 8-10 times until they are finely chopped. Add the macadamia nuts and pulse about 8 times. Add the pecans and salt; pulse until all the ingredients are well combined and chopped (about 1 minute). The consistency will be a thick paste.

Press the batter into the bottom and sides of a non-stick 9-inch pie pan; about ¼-inch in thickness. If you spread the batter too thin, it will break apart when you slice the pie. Add desired filling and bake at 325°F for 25 minutes. The crust must be cooked on low heat or the exposed edges will burn.

SERVING SUGGESTIONS: Serve as the crust for *ginger almond squash pie*; or fill with *purée parsnips with thyme*. This crust pairs well with chocolate pudding, coconut cream, key lime, or pomegranate lemon mascarpone.

VPK: This is ideal for vata or pitta as the dish is moist and grounding for vata while also being cooling for pitta; the heavy, oily nuts are least beneficial for kapha, so kapha should avoid or eat only on special occasions.

VARIATIONS: Add 1 teaspoon grated orange rind or lemon rind.

ABOUT: This recipe was adapted from a recipe I found online by Rhonda Malkmus.

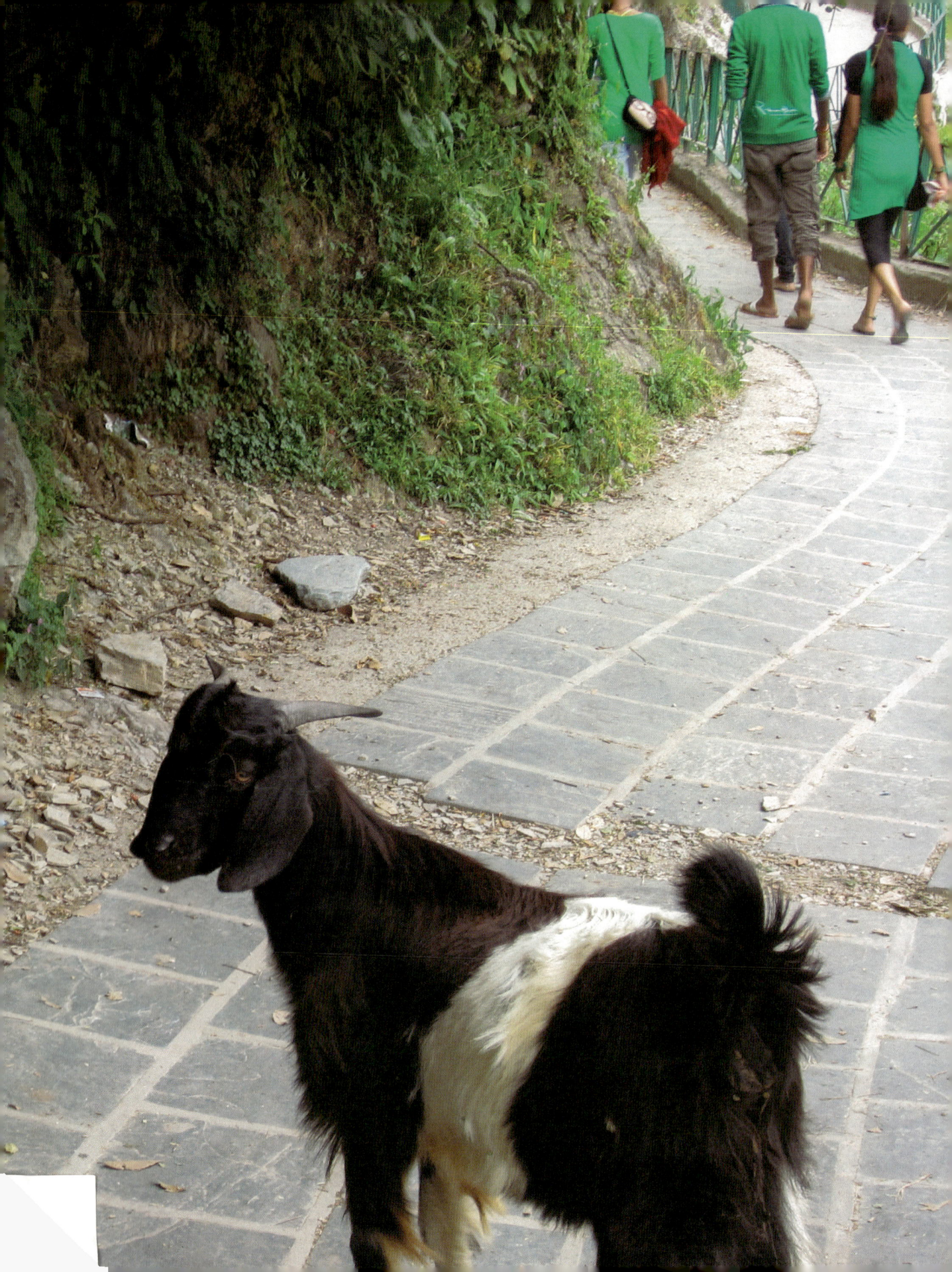

Chapter 18: Leftovers

Ayurveda recommends eating fresh foods and is not a proponent of leftovers. However, in our western culture where most people are working 40+ hours per week and do not have someone at home cooking their meals, eating leftovers is a healthier alternative than eating most comercially prepared foods. Here are some tips on how to prepare common leftovers, so you can move from one day to the next without wasting a lot of food or time.

Leftover Food	Transformation
Rice (white or brown)	• warm in a sauté pan with a few tablespoons of water; cover and gently steam over low heat for lunch or dinner the next day • add to sauté pan and stir-fry with a tablespoon of oil, sliced ginger, a pressed garlic clove and some fresh sliced vegetables and/or meat • *baked falafel balls*
Risotto Rice	• combine with an egg and bread crumbs then form into patties and fry; serve with salad for a lunch or with a poached egg for breakfast.
Millet	• combine with an egg and a mashed yam to make *breakfast millet patties*; serve with salad and avocado for a lunch or with a poached egg for breakfast. • *bison meatloaf*
Quinoa or Amaranth	• *Moroccan veggie burgers* • add to soup • combine with lentils in a salad • add to quick breads or cookies as a substitute for nuts
Meat	• add to soup • slice and serve on a corn tortilla or wrap for lunch • dice and add to a grain or vegetable salad for lunch
Dips	• make a creamy dressing; combine with a few tablespoons of oil, some lemon (or lime or apple cider vinegar) and some water to achieve desired consistency
Coconut Milk	• *Thai lemongrass vermicelli soup* • *vata pitta coconut chai shake* or add to smoothies • add to hot chai
Cabbage	• *borsht lentil soup* • *Asian vegetables*
Artichokes (canned)	• broil, grill or lightly sauté and add to a salad of greens or cannellini beans • purée into an artichoke dip with some basil or arugula and lemon juice • dilute the above artichoke dip with water or cream and use as a topping for pasta, such as in *artichoke lemon cream sauce*
Fennel (fresh)	• chop and add to salad of greens, lentils or beans • add to soups
Purée yam or parsnip	• substitute for tomatoes in a soup when you're looking for something to cool pitta
Barley	• add to *miso soup* or vegetable soup

Appendix A: Elements and the Twenty Qualities

Ayurveda explains that each of the five elements is comprised of energies or qualities (i.e., fire has the qualities of hot, sharp, penetrating, etc.). Ayurveda summarizes the qualities of all the elements into a group of 10 with their corresponding opposites (so twenty qualities in total). The table below lists those qualities, paired with their opposites. Referring to the table below, we can see that the quality of "hot" has a balancing quality of cool or cold; we can see that the quality of sharp or penetrating has the balancing quality of slow or dull.

These qualities are present in everything, but in varying quantities; and typically a few of the qualities will dominate. For instance, the ether element has all twenty qualities, but the dominant qualities are clear, subtle and light; the earth element has all 20 qualities, but the dominant qualities are heavy, hard, dense and static, etc.

Let's look at the twenty qualities listed in the table below. Most of the "pairs of opposites" are intuitive, but a few are not. For instance, the opposite of dry is oily (not wet). So if one is experiencing symptoms of dryness (dry skin, constipation), the opposite quality to bring in would be something oily (oil massage, consumption of foods that are high in oil content) and to avoid dry foods (such as beans). If we apply this principle to cooking, then we can see that it is important to add liberal amounts of ghee or oil to bean dishes – to balance the dryness and reduce likelihood of digestive disturbance (gas and bloating). The opposite of slimy (or smooth) is rough. Rough can be thought of as a more extreme version of dry. It can manifest in the physical body as chapped or cracked skin (think of your heels, elbows or fingertips), or a hoarse throat; it could also manifest as a rough personality (i.e., one who is not refined). Honey would be soothing to that hoarse throat.

To recap, just as all the elements are present in everything, all the qualities are present in everything, but in differing amounts. Further, some qualities will express themselves more strongly than others. Ayurveda has given us the tools to determine the dominant energetic (i.e., in our food, in our body, in our emotions) so we may discriminate between foods that will bring balance versus imbalance.

To reinforce your understanding of the opposite qualities, you can try this exercise: review the table below and identify examples of emotions or physical manifestations of each quality.

Twenty Qualities - Paired with Opposites	
Heavy	Light
Slow/Dull	Sharp/Penetrating
Cold/Cool	Hot
Oily	Dry
Slimy/Smooth	Rough
Dense	Liquid
Soft	Hard
Static	Mobile/Spreading
Subtle	Gross
Clear	Cloudy/Sticky

Appendix B: Dosha Evaluation[21]

To determine your prakruti (your state of balance), review each characteristic in the left most column and place a check mark in one of the three columns to the right that BEST describes you. When making your selection, consider how the characteristic has applied over the course of your life in general with emphasis on how that characteristic displayed itself as a child. It may be helpful to get unbiased input from people who have known you for a long time (family members or long-time friends) as you complete this survey. Compare their observations to yours and try to be completely honest. When you have completed each section, tally the check marks in each column to see which dosha predominates. To determine your vikruti (your current energetic state), you should review the characteristics in the evaluation form a second time; but this time make your choice based on how the characteristic applies to you today. Again, it is helpful to get someone who knows you well (i.e., a close friend or co-worker) to complete the survey with you (or on your behalf) to achieve the most unbiased results. Tally the columns. Compare your prakruti to your vikruti to determine which doshas are out of balance.

Characteristic	Column 1-Vata	Column 2-Pitta	Column 3-Kapha
Frame Size/ Body	☐ small, thin, small bones ☐ delicate or lanky	☐ medium, average ☐ athletic build, develops muscles easily	☐ large, heavy, large bones ☐ well-developed chest, a curvaceous or round body
Skin	☐ thin (you can easily see your veins), dry, rough, chapped (tendency for cracked heels, finger tips, elbows) ☐ rashes tend to be dry and itchy ☐ sometimes blackheads	☐ hot, oily (tendency toward hives and eczema) ☐ rashes tend to be red and burning ☐ sometimes red pimples	☐ thick, smooth, cool, clammy ☐ rashes tend to be wet and oozing ☐ sometimes white pimples
Skin Tone*	☐ dark, brown	☐ red, yellow, freckles	☐ white, marble like
Nails	☐ dry, brittle, cracked	☐ shiny, pink	☐ shiny, thick, white
Hair*	☐ dark, wiry, dry	☐ shiny, thin, oily ☐ red, auburn highlights ☐ premature grey, bald	☐ wavy, thick, lustrous
Face	☐ angular, thin, sunken cheeks ☐ non-symmetrical features, crowded teeth ☐ thin lips	☐ heart-shaped ☐ straight, pointy nose and chin	☐ round shape ☐ broad nose ☐ large white teeth ☐ full lips
Eyes*	☐ small ☐ dark ☐ darting	☐ medium, almond-shaped, ☐ hazel color ☐ sensitive to light and bright light	☐ large, round ☐ sometimes blue ☐ thick eyelashes

Appetite	☐ varies (sometimes you feel very hungry, but when you sit to eat, your appetite is satiated after a few bites) ☐ often forgets to eat ☐ becomes light-headed or cranky when meals are missed	☐ voracious appetite; can become angry if food is not available when hunger strikes ☐ rarely skips meals	☐ emotional eating ☐ tends to eat large amounts even when not hungry ☐ if skips a meal does not experience discomfort
Digestion	☐ flatulence, bloating, abdominal distention after eating	☐ heartburn, acid reflux, sour stomach after eating	☐ heavy, sleepy feeling after eating
Elimination	☐ irregular ☐ tends toward constipation, dry stools, small "rabbit pellet" shaped, at times may have to strain and "push" to eliminate	☐ hot, oily stools, may be loosely shaped like a "cow patty" ☐ tends toward diarrhea; at times stools may burn	☐ well-formed banana shaped stool ☐ sometimes constipation
Weight	☐ difficult to gain weight	☐ weight is moderate	☐ difficult to lose weight and tendency to carry a few extra pounds
Circulation	☐ cold hands and feet	☐ hot body temperature	☐ cold hands and feet but warm at the core
Perspiration	☐ scanty	☐ fleshy smell	☐ profuse
Mind	☐ learn quickly but forget quickly	☐ intelligent, brilliant	☐ slow to learn, but never forget
Disposition – In Balance	☐ joy, happiness, friendly ☐ flexible views ☐ free-spirit	☐ leader ☐ great orator ☐ passionate ☐ brave, courageous	☐ team player ☐ loving, compassionate ☐ stable, dependable
Disposition – Out of Balance	☐ fear ☐ loneliness ☐ forgetfullness, scattered thoughts ☐ afraid of the dark	☐ anger ☐ cut-throat competitiveness ☐ judgmental, critical, sarcastic ☐ suicidal thoughts	☐ depression ☐ moody, feeling sorry for oneself ☐ slow to change (mind and habits), stubborn ☐ greedy ☐ attached (tendency to stay in relationships even if they are ill serving)
Perception	☐ subtle, almost clairvoyant, perceives feelings of others ☐ may absorb the energy of people/situations	☐ understands feelings of others using logical analysis	☐ subtleties are elusive, may be unaware of feelings of others
Relationships	☐ loner ☐ short-term relationships	☐ likes prestigious friends and status symbols ☐ may abruptly terminate a relationship that is not serving him/her	☐ desire to be liked by everyone ☐ keeps friends for a long time ☐ has difficulty terminating relationships (even if they are ill serving) ☐ prefers doing things with a partner/friend (i.e., exercise, travel, etc.)

Energy Levels	☐ tires easily ☐ suited for artistic, creative job	☐ tends to work beyond physical capacity ☐ best suited for intellectual job	☐ strong as an ox ☐ good laborer
Attire	☐ eclectic, trendy fashion	☐ designer, polished fashion	☐ not worried about fashion, loose fitting and relaxed clothing that they never discard
Monetary Attitudes	☐ money comes and goes ☐ inconsistent savings	☐ tends to save ☐ spends on luxury items	☐ consistent saver ☐ frugal spending habits; thrifty
Speech	☐ high pitch, fast, clipped, stuttering ☐ off topic, run-on sentences ☐ chatty	☐ quick-witted ☐ clear, precise speech ☐ sarcastic	☐ deep, slow, dull speech ☐ mono-syllabic answers to questions ☐ melodious singing voice
Organization	☐ non-linear, creative	☐ organized, logical and methodical	☐ untidy, "packrat" saves everything, but can find everything
Reaction To High Stress	☐ anxiety, worries, fear	☐ ulcer, acid stomach	☐ calm and cool, plodder, no worries
Environmental Influences	☐ does not tolerate cold weather; prefers sun	☐ prefers cool weather and shade	☐ likes moderate weather
Sleep	☐ light sleeper, easily awoken; has difficulty getting back to sleep ☐ tendency for nightmares	☐ moderate sleeper, likes to read before bed ☐ easy to rise in the morning	☐ sound sleeper; can sleep anywhere, tendency for dreams about/with water ☐ slow to rise in the morning
Disease Proneness	☐ dehydration, constipation ☐ anxiety, breathlessness, heart palpitations, wheezing ☐ fatigue ☐ insomnia ☐ sciatic pain, low back pain ☐ dry, itchy external hemorrhoids	☐ heart-burn, indigestion, inflammation ("itis" diseases), ulcers ☐ rashes, hives, acne ☐ depression ☐ dizziness, nausea, migraines ☐ fever ☐ diarrhea ☐ sour taste in mouth ☐ bleeding disorders (i.e., in rectum, gums, blood-shot eyes, internal hemorrhoids)	☐ cold, congestion, cough, phlegm, mucus ☐ swelling/water retention, excess salivation, drooling ☐ lethargy ☐ diabetes, high cholesterol, obesity ☐ lipomas, cysts, tumors
Total: Prakruti			
Total: Vikruti			

*The questions on skin tone, hair color and eyes need to be considered relative to others within your ethnic background. For instance, Asians generally have dark skin, dark hair and dark eyes. So Asians should compare their skin tone to other Asians (i.e., is your skin fair or dark in comparison?); and compare your skin texture (i.e., is your skin smooth and marble-like without flaws? That would be a kapha complexion; if your skin is thin and darker than others in your ethnic background, then it is vata.) If you are still unsure, simply leave that box unchecked. You will be able to get a good approximation of your prakruti and vikruti by answering the remaining questions in this evaluation. Of course, the best results are obtained from a consultation with a qualified ayurveda practitioner.

Appendix C: Dosha Diet and Aid for Vata

Vata	Balancing	Unbalancing
Tastes	sweet, sour, salty	pungent, bitter, astringent
Qualities	warm, heavy, oily, smooth, stable, gross, cloudy	cold, light, dry, rough, mobile, subtle, clear, astringent
Snacks	nuts, guacamole, tahini dip, *vata breakfast banana, zucchini trail bread, vata pitta vitality drink, carrot (with a kick) spread, zucchini hummus, endive honey goat cheese, go to sleep nutmeg milk, vata pitta coconut chai shake*	potato chips, rice cakes, corn chips, energy bars, crackers, chocolate, sweets with refined white sugar or high-glycemic index
Meals	soups, stews, pasta with pesto (basil or arugula), meat broth soups (beef, buffalo, dark chicken), *beet sweet potato soup, mung dal cilantro soup, dashi clear broth soups, thai lemongrass vermicelli soup, urad dal with tamarind, Guajarati wedding dal, Marco's porcini risotto, broiled salmon in maple lime marinade, Spanish chicken, fennel crusted paneer, bison meat loaf*	beans, salads, raw dishes, heavy combinations
Exercise & Lifestyle	Exercise should be short duration, low intensity (minimal, if any, sweating) and mindful: walking; easy bike rides; gentle yoga combined with ujjayi pranayama (standing poses and forward bends are most grounding), alternate nostril pranayama and meditation*. Lifestyles that help ground vata include: slowing down; staying hydrated; keeping to a routine; getting plenty of rest; morning self-massage with sesame oil (leave on for 15-20 minutes and follow with warm shower).	Exercise and lifestyles that will aggravate vata include: high intensity (heavy sweating), depleting, exercises; running; salsa dancing; tennis. [If you partake in these exercises, replenish/balance vata by having adequate rest, grounding oily foods, water and *vata pitta vitality drink*]; avoid caffeine (too much stimulation) and alcohol (too much ether/air quality).

* CAUTION: to avoid injury, seek guidance of a qualified yoga instructor.

Vata Imbalance	
Signs & Symptoms	constipation, forgetfulness (i.e., "space cadet"), fear, loneliness, insecurity, nervousness, anxiety, dry skin, cracked heels, popping joints, difficulty with speech (i.e., stuttering), emaciation, black circles under eyes, gas, bloating, vague abdominal pain and distention, neuromuscular disorders (tremors, spasms, numbness, tingling), osteoporosis, inability to concentrate/racing thoughts, nightmares, sciatic pain, heart palpitations, breathlessness, hiccups, wheezing, asthma, fatigue, insomnia
Causes	excess cold (food, drink, environment), excess talking, running, jumping, travel, windy days, excess dry (food, environment), bitter, pungent, astringent food, leftover foods, staying up late, suppressing natural urges (burping, defecation, urination, flatulence, etc.)

Vata Foods[22]		
Fruits	avocado, apricots, bananas, blueberries, cantaloupe, cherries, coconut, dates, figs, grapes, grapefruit, kiwi, lemon, lime, mango, melons, oranges, papaya, peaches, pineapple, plums, prunes (soaked), raisins (soaked), rhubarb, umeboshi plums	apples, cranberries, pears, persimmons, pomegranate, raisins (un-soaked), strawberries, watermelon
Vegetables	asparagus, beets, carrots (cooked), chilies, chicory (endive, frisee), chives, cilantro, cucumber, green beans, fennel, leeks (cooked), mizuna, mustard greens, okra, olives (black), onions (cooked), parsnip, potato (sweet), rutabaga, spinach, zucchini	artichokes, beet greens, bitter melon, burdock root, cabbage family†, carrots (raw), celery, corn, dandelion greens, kale, kohlrabi, lettuce, mushrooms, nightshades‡, onion (raw), peas, radish, sprouts, squash (winter), turnips
Grains	amaranth, durham flour, oats (cooked), quinoa, rice (basmati, brown, white), seitan, wheat	barley, buckwheat, corn, millet, oat bran, pasta (wheat), rice cakes, rye, sago, soy flour (and powder), spelt, tapioca
Beans, Lentils	kidney beans, miso, mung beans, soy (cheese, sauce), tur dal, urad dal	beans (aduki, navy, pinto, white, soy), black eyed peas, garbanzo (chickpeas), lentils (brown, puy, red), tempeh, tofu
Sweetener	barley malt, date sugar, fructose, honey, jaggary/palm sugar, maple syrup, molasses, rice syrup, sucanat, turbinado, unrefined, low-glycemic	white sugar
Dairy	butter, buttermilk, cheese (hard and soft), milk (cow, goat), ghee, sour cream, yogurt (fresh or store bought)	
Animal	beef, buffalo, chicken (dark meat), duck, eggs, fish (freshwater, salmon, sea, shrimp, tuna), turkey (dark)	chicken (white meat), lamb, mutton, pork, rabbit, turkey (white), venison
Nuts	almonds, brazil, cashew, charole, coconut, hazelnut, macadamia, peanut, pecan, pine nut, pistachio, walnut	
Seeds	psyllium, poppy, pumpkin, safflower, sesame, sunflower	popcorn
Oils	almond, avocado, castor, ghee, mustard, olive, peanut, safflower, sesame, sunflower	corn, soy
Spices	ajwan, allspice, anise, basil, bay leaf, black pepper, caraway, cardamom, cayenne, cinnamon, clove, coriander, cumin, dill, fennel, fenugreek, garlic, ginger (dry and fresh), horseradish, hing, mace, marjoram, mint, mustard, nutmeg, oregano, paprika, parsley, rosemary, rosewater, rock salt, sea salt, saffron, savory, tarragon, turmeric, vanilla	chocolate, neem

†cabbage family – broccoli, Brussels sprouts, cabbage, cauliflower
‡nightshades – tomatoes, potatoes, eggplant, peppers

Appendix D: Dosha Diet Aid for Pitta

Pitta	Balancing	Unbalancing
Tastes	sweet, bitter, astringent	sour, salty, pungent
Qualities	dry, slow/dull, cold, heavy, dense	oily, penetrating, hot, light, fleshy smell, spreading, liquid, pungent, sour
Snacks	artichoke dip, *zucchini hummus*, spirulina energy bars, sweet fruits, almonds (peeled/soaked), ice cream, coconut water, artichoke pesto, *lemony cannellini bean spread, Mexican black bean spread, endive honey goat cheese, jicama lime sticks, go to sleep nutmeg milk, coconut chai shake, mint rosewater, aloe lime drink, coriander milk*	nuts (except almonds and charole), corn chips and salsa, bananas, potato chips, popcorn, chocolate (due to acidic quality), buffalo wings, aged-cheddar cheese, salt & vinegar chips
Meals	salads, steamed green leafy vegetables, puy lentils, egg white omelets with cilantro & fennel, turkey meatloaf, *Moroccan veggie burgers, baked falafel balls, cannellini kale & artichoke sauté, red quinoa with endive & cranberries, barley sauté with sweet potato asparagus & burdock, fennel crusted paneer, roasted turkey breast with fennel cream sauce, rabbit coconut fenugreek stew, Brazilian black bean stew, Caribbean aduki bean stew, pitta kapha barley kale soup, mung dal cilantro soup, dashi clear broth, French lentil soup with pork*	spicy Mexican/Asian foods, fried foods, chilies, tomato-based dishes; instant soup and packaged foods (due to high sodium), sauerkraut, pasta with tomato sauce
Exercise & Lifestyle	Exercise should be cooling and moderate in duration/intensity: swimming; yoga asana (slow flowing postures that emphasize the stomach, forward bends and twists); pranayama (alternate nostril breathing, shitali)*. Lifestyles that help cool pitta include: spending time in nature especially around calm water and with mellow friends; getting to bed before 10pm; meditating; "chilling out"; morning self-massage with coconut oil (leave on for 15 minutes then shower with warm water).	Exercise and lifestyles that will aggravate pitta include: running; excessive hours at the office; excessive debating/arguing; excessive time in the hot sun. Pitta should avoid coffee due to its stimulating, acid qualities (otherwise add a pinch of cardamom or cinnamon to offset some of the effects; try Teechino® mixed with coffee as a substitute). The anti-dote to burning the mid-night oil is *pitta cooling coriander milk*.

* CAUTION: to avoid injury, seek guidance of a qualified yoga instructor.

Pitta Imbalance

Signs & symptoms	heartburn, indigestion, inflammation, ulcers, rashes, jaundice, depression, suicidal thoughts, dizziness, nausea, fever, diarrhea, migraines, sour taste in mouth, bleeding disorders (i.e., in rectum, gums, blood-shot eyes, bleeding internal hemorrhoids), anger, hate, judgmental and critical, mistrusting, controlling, fiercely competitive
Causes	excess hot, spicy, oily foods; excess external heat (summertime, sunshine) and running; repressed anger; inflated ego (sense of self); prolonged fasting; sour, salty and fermented foods

Pitta-Foods[23]		
Fruits	apples, avocados, sweet berries, cherries (sweet), coconuts, dates, figs, grapes (red), lime, melons, pears, pomegranate, prunes (soaked), raisins, watermelon	apricots, sour berries, bananas, cherries (sour), cranberries, grapes (green), grapefruit, kiwi, lemon, papaya, peaches, persimmon, pineapple, plums, rhubarb, tamarind
Vegetables	arugula, asparagus, beet greens, bitter melon, cabbage family†, carrots (cooked), celery, chicory (endive, frisee), cilantro, cucumber, dandelion endive, greens, fennel, green beans, jicama, kale, leeks (cooked), lettuce, mizuna, parsnip, peppers, potatoes (sweet and white), radicchio, rutabaga, spinach (raw), sprouts, squash (winter and summer), zucchini	beets, burdock root, carrots (raw), chilies, corn, eggplant, kohlrabi, mustard greens, olives (black), onions (raw), radish, spinach (cooked), tomato, turnips
Grains	amaranth, barley, durham flour, oat bran, oats, pasta (wheat), quinoa, rice (basmati, rice cakes, white), sago, seitan, soy flour and powder, spelt, tapioca, wheat	buckwheat, corn, millet, rice (brown), rye
Beans, Lentils	beans (aduki, kidney, mung, navy, pinto, soy, white), black eyed peas, garbanzo (chickpeas), lentils (brown, red), tempeh, tofu	miso, soy (cheese, sauce, sausage), tur dal, urad dal
Sweetner	barley malt, date sugar, fructose, maple syrup, rice syrup, sucanat, sugar (white), turbinado	honey, jaggary/palm sugar, molasses
Dairy	butter, soft cheese, cottage cheese, cow's milk, ghee, goat's milk, yogurt (fresh/not store bought)	cheese (hard), sour cream, yogurt (store bought)
Animal	buffalo, chicken (white meat), eggs (white), rabbit, shrimp, turkey (white), venison	beef, chicken (dark meat), duck, eggs, egg (yolk), fish (freshwater, salmon, sea, tuna), lamb, mutton, pork, turkey (dark)
Nuts	almonds (soaked and peeled), charole, coconut	almonds (with skin), brazil, cashew, hazelnut, macadamia, peanut, pecan, pine nut, pistachio, walnut
Seeds	popcorn, psyllium, safflower, sunflower	pumpkin, sesame
Oils	avocado, castor, coconut, ghee, olive, soy, sunflower	almond, corn, mustard, peanut, safflower, sesame
Spices	coriander, cumin, dill, fennel, mint, rosewater, saffron, salt (rock), tarragon, turmeric, vanilla	ajwan, allspice, anise, basil, bay leaf, black pepper, caraway, cayenne, clove, fenugreek, dry ginger, horseradish, hing, mace, marjoram, mustard, nutmeg, oregano, paprika, poppy seed, rosemary, salt (sea)

†cabbage family – broccoli, Brussels sprouts, cabbage, cauliflower

Appendix E: Dosha Diet Aid for Kapha

Kapha	Balancing	Unbalancing
Tastes	pungent, bitter, astringent	sweet, sour, salty
Qualities	light, mobile, sharp, warm	heavy, slow, cool, oily, slimy, thick, soft, stable, liquid, sweet, salty
Snacks	apples, sweet berries, plain popcorn, corn chips & salsa, rice cakes with pesto, *lemony cannellini bean spread, Mexican black bean spread, mushroom almond pâté, traditional Mexican salsa*	bananas, candy, cheese, chocolate, ice cream, nuts
Meals	*Moroccan veggie burger, baked falafel balls, pitta kapha cannellini kale & artichoke sauté, red quinoa with endive & cranberries, cinnamon currant millet, polenta with shitake sauce, barley sauté with sweet potato asparagus & burdock, roasted turkey breast, rabbit fenugreek stew, lemon garbanzo soup, barley kale soup, creamy corn soup, borscht lentil soup, mushroom tarragon puree, French lentil salad*	beef bean and cheese burrito, cheese tortillas, grilled cheese sandwich, meatloaf and mashed potatoes, peanut butter sandwiches, Philly cheese-steak sub, pizza, steak with hollandaise sauce
Exercise & Lifestyle	Exercise should be daily: vigorous, sweaty, long duration workouts; running (unless overweight due to impact on knees); cycling; swimming; salsa dancing; vinyasa yoga (sun salutations, abdominals, twists, arm balances and back bending); pranayama (bhastrika, kapalabhati)*. Lifestyles that keep kapha from stagnating include: lots of group activities; new adventures and varying daily routine.	Exercise and lifestyles that will aggravate kapha include: day napping; unvaried routine; lack of variety in life; lack of a social network; lack of love/close frienships.

* CAUTION: to avoid injury, seek guidance of a qualified yoga instructor.

Kapha Imbalance	
Signs & Symptoms	cold, congestion, phlegm, mucus, swelling/water retention, excess salivation, lethargy, diabetes, lipomas (benign tumors composed of fatty tissue), cysts, tumors, high cholesterol, obesity, stubbornness, selfishness, moodiness, depression, greed, attachment (to possessions and relationships), weight gain (from emotional eating)
Causes	rich, heavy, oily foods; eating for pleasure (without hunger); lack of feeling loved; cold drinks; hydrophilic substances; winter and spring; day sleeping; not enough variation in routine; inadequate vigorous physical activity

Kapha Foods[24]		
Fruits	apples, apricots, berries, cherries, cranberries, peaches, pears, persimmon, pomegranate, prunes (soaked), raisins, raspberries, strawberries	avocado, bananas, cantaloupe, coconut, dates, figs, grapes (green), grapefruit, kiwi, lemon, lime, melons, plums, rhubarb, tamarind, watermelon
Vegetables	arugula, artichokes, asparagus, beets, beet greens, bitter melon, burdock root, cabbage family**, carrots, celery, chicory (endive, frisee), chilies, chives, cilantro, corn, dandelion greens, eggplant, fennel, green beans, kale, kohlrabi, leeks (cooked), lettuce, mushrooms, mizuna, mustard greens, okra, onion, peas, peppers, potato (white), radicchio, radish, rutabaga, scallions, spinach, sprouts, squash (winter), turnips, wasabi	cucumber, black olives, parsnip, potato (sweet), tomato
Grains	amaranth, barley, buckwheat, corn, millet, oat bran, oats (dry), quinoa, rice (basmati), rice cakes, rye, sago, seitan, tapioca	durham flour, oats (cooked), pasta (wheat), rice (brown, white), soy flour, soy powder, spelt, wheat
Beans, Lentils	beans (aduki, navy, pinto, white), black eyed peas, garbanzo (chickpeas), lentils (brown, puy, red, tur dal), miso, tempeh	kidney beans, soy beans (cheese and sausage), urad dal
Sweetner	honey (heating and scrapes fat)	barley malt, date sugar, fructose, jaggary/palm sugar, maple syrup, molasses, rice syrup, sucanat, sugar (white), turbinado
Dairy	cottage cheese (paneer), ghee, goats milk	butter, buttermilk, cheese, sour cream, yogurt (fresh or store bought)
Animal	chicken (white meat), egg whites, rabbit, shrimp, turkey (white), venison	beef, buffalo, chicken (dark meat), duck, egg (yolk), fish (freshwater), fish (salmon, sea, tuna), lamb, mutton, pork, turkey (dark)
Nuts	charole	almonds, brazil, cashew, coconut, hazelnut, macadamia, peanut, pecan, pine nut, pistachio, walnut
Seeds	flax, mustard, popcorn, psyllium, pumpkin, safflower, sunflower	sesame
Oils	corn, ghee, mustard, sunflower	almond, avocado, castor, coconut, olive, peanut, safflower, sesame, soy
Spices	ajwan, allspice, anise, basil, bay leaf, black pepper, caraway, cardamom, cayenne, cinnamon, clove, coriander, cumin, dill, fennel, fenugreek, garlic, ginger, horseradish, hing, mace, marjoram, mint, mustard, neem, nutmeg, oregano, paprika, parsley, poppy seed, rosemary, rose water, rock salt, saffron, turmeric, vanilla	chocolate, sea salt, savory, tarragon

**cabbage family – broccoli, Brussels sprouts, cabbage, cauliflower

Appendix F: Ama

In modern science, we know that ingested food is broken down into a form that is available for the cells, providing the vitamins, minerals and nourishment for normal activity. In ayurveda, the energetic result of digestion is that food is transformed into vital life energy. If food is not properly processed during digestion, the food does not transform into vital life energy and instead becomes "ama". "Ama" is a Sanskrit word that can be translated to mean 'toxic, morbid waste product'; it can result from undigested food or unprocessed emotions (i.e., unresolved anger, fear, depression, insecurity or traumatic events). Ama clogs the channels of circulation in the body. It can prevent nutrients from flowing to the cells, organs and brain. Ama may also block the channels that carry waste from the cells and tissues, resulting in a toxic build-up.

Signs that indicate you may have "ama":
- your tongue has a white, black or brown coating
- your urine, feces and/or sweat (i.e., armpits) has a foul smell
- your breath has a bad odor
- your stool is sticky/glue-ey (i.e., it sticks to the toilet bowl)
- you may have fever
- you may have no appetite
- you have a heavy feeling in your body or mind
- your joints are stiff
- you feel pain at your navel
- you feel dull and sleepy after eating
- your mind is foggy
- you have trouble getting out of bed in the morning, even after many hours of sleeping
- the roots of your hair hurt

Health problems that may be caused by prolonged ama:
- diarrhea
- constipation
- joint pain
- sadness and depression
- dullness and lethargy
- lowered immunity
- frequent colds and flu

Ama, if left unchecked, can be a precursor to disease. If you think you have ama, you should consult your ayurvedic practitioner. He/she can look for the root cause(s) and provide guidance on your options for addressing the situation.

1. Gabriel Von Loon, Caraka Samhita, Handbook on Ayurveda Vol.1,Su1 #15-17, 2002-2003
2. Excerpted with permission from Textbook of Ayurveda: A Complete Guide to Clinical Assessment, Volume Two. Copyright 2006. Dr. Vasant Lad and The Ayurvedic Press. All Rights Reserved.
3. Excerpted with permission from Ayurvedic Cooking for Self Healing. Copyright 1994. Dr. Vasant Lad and The Ayurvedic Press. All Rights Reserved.
4. For simplicity, I have omitted the Sanskrit terminology rasa, virya and vipak and then expanded classifications of the energetics (virya). Rasa refers to "taste". It is the first experience when the food hits the tongue; you can intuit the properties of the food from the taste; virya refers to the energetic effect of the food on the dosha and on the digestive fire. Generally, the virya is defined as being heating or cooling, but it could also be heavy, light, slow, sharp, oily or dry. Vipak refers to the post-digestive effect (or the effect of food on the urine, feces and sweat). The sweet and salty tastes generally have a sweet vipak; the sour taste generally has a sour vipak; the pungent, bitter and astringent tastes generally have a pungent vipak.
5. For simplicity, in classifying the energetic affects of tastes that have multiple conflicting energetics, I have categorized them under the taste which displays the most powerful energetic (and added the lesser energetics/tastes in parentheses). So if an herb has a sweet and pungent taste, with a heating virya and a pungent vipak, it would be classified as pungent, not sweet (because the pungent/heating energetic dominates).
6. Westerners will generally not be combining ghee with honey; you will find the combination in traditional Indian sweets. You will not find this combination in my cookbook. I have included the rule in case you happen to be making something with ghee and honey you will have a reference as to the proper combination.
7. Excerpted with permission from Ayurvedic Cooking for Self Healing. Copyright 1994. Dr. Vasant Lad and The Ayurvedic Press. All Rights Reserved.
8. Ivan Pavlov - Nobel Lecture: Physiology of Digestion. Nobelprize.org. 18 Apr 2013 http://www.nobelprize.org/nobel_prizes/medicine/laureates/1904/pavlov-lecture.html
9. Dr. Sarah Myhill, Digestive Enzymes are Necessary to Digest Food, December 2009, http://www.drmyhill.co.uk/wiki/Digestive_enzymes_are_necessary_to_digest_food
10. Environmental Working Group, The Dirty Dozen - Annual Shoppers Guide, http://www.ewg.org/foodnews/summary.php
11. Erik Smith, L. Ac, Dipl. OM, MSN, Choosing Healthy Cookware, September 2007, www.pointsofhealth.org
12. Nicholas D. Kristof, OpEd Columnist NY Times, Cancer from the Kitchen (Mount Sinai School of Medicine Symposium), December 5, 2009
13. A. Annapoorani, K. R. Anilakumar, Farhath Khanum, N. Anjaneya Murthy, and A. S. Bawa, Studies on the physicochemical characteristics of heated honey, honey mixed with ghee and their food consumption pattern by rats, April-June, 2010, http://www.ncbi.nlm.nih.gov/pmc/articles/PMC3215355/
14. Leif Hallberg, Does Calcium Interfere with Iron Absorption?, The American Journal of Clinical Nutrition, 1998, http://ajcn.nutrition.org/content/68/1/3.full.pdf
15. Jonathan Matthews, GM WatchGM Crops, Research Documenting the Limitations, Risks and Alternatives, 2009, www.banGMfood.org.
16. Brian A. Nummer, Ph.D., "Fermenting Yogurt at Home", National Center for Home Food Preservation, October 2002, http://nchfp.uga.edu/publications/nchfp/factsheets/yogurt.html.
17. Dr. Andrew Weil, Cooking With Grains: Millet, http://www.drweil.com/drw/u/ART03185/Cooking-With-Grains-Millet.html.
18. Asthanga Hrydyam, Chapter 6/Ver. 68.
19. Products labeled "Certified Humane Raised and Handled" meet the Humane Farm Animal Care Program standards which includes: Nutritious diet, without antibiotics, animals raised with shelter, resting areas, sufficient space and the ability to engage in natural behaviors.
20. Sharma S, Kulkarni SK, Chopra K., "Curcumin, the active principle of turmeric, ameliorates diabetic nephropathy in rats", Clinical and Experimental Pharmacology & Physiology, October 2006, http://www.ncbi.nlm.nih.gov/pubmed/17002671
21. Excerpted with permission from Ayurvedic Cooking for Self Healing. Copyright 1994. Dr. Vasant Lad and The Ayurvedic Press. All Rights Reserved.
22. Dr. Vasant Lad, MASc and Usha Lad, Ayurvedic Cooking for Self Healing, 2nd ed. The Ayurvedic Press, Albuquerque, NM
23. Ibid.
24. Ibid.

Acknowledgements

Thanks to everyone who has supported me along this journey. Without their advice for food layout, props for photo shoots, feedback on the recipes, cooking supplies, help with proofing, places to stay, moral support and anything else I needed along the way, this book would not have been possible.

- Diana Adams, RN and gourmet
- Shawn Padulo, carpenter, chef and gastronomist
- Jeanie Kane, office manager and resource extraordinaire
- Jerry Kane, engineer by day artisan woodworker by night
- the girls at Pier I in Manchester
- the staff at Jacques Flower in Manchester
- Heather Armishaw, teacher, chorister and foodie
- the cheery staff at A-Market
- Paula Scarborough, ayurveda goddess
- Laure Lacroix
- Erik Smith
- Hannah Goldblatt
- Dan Schmidt
- Iain Grysak
- Hayden Hernandez
- MaryBeth Ball-Nerone
- Shannon McCall
- Sue Duncan

Gratitude to Michael Richard, *Red Door Media* for his creativity and ability to transform a pile of recipes and photos into the story I wanted to share.

INDEX

ama	19, 88, 90, 161, 196
health problems	196
signs & symptoms	196
unprocessed emotions	196
unresolved emotions	196
amaranth	See grains & seeds
animal & dairy	87–99
anemia	87
bison	99, 87
buffalo	See bison
cheese	88, 91, 92, 164
chicken	87, 96
fish	87, 93, 94, 95
ghee	88, 90
lamb	93
milk	88
mutton	87
paneer	See cheese
rabbit	87, 98
sacred cows	88
turkey	87, 97
yogurt	88
Asian noodles	
soba	40
udon	40
ayurveda for the family	29-30
dosha condiment table	30
drinks, juices	30
salad dressings	30
sauces & chutneys	30
barley	See grains & seeds
beans	See legumes
chef candles	37
chewing food	20, 43
churnas	152
coconut milk	40
coconut sugar	123
curry leaves	36
cutting boards	37
dal	See legumes
desserts	See sweets
dips	See snacks & dips
dirty dozen	43
doshas	9-13
dosha evaluation	187-189
dosha times	12
kapha	10,194
diet aid	194
exercise & lifestyle	194
foods (balancing)	195
drinks (balancing)	170, 182
foods (unbalancing)	194
imbalance (causes)	194
imbalance (signs & symptoms)	194
meals	194
qualities	194
snacks	194
tastes	194
pitta	9, 192
diet aid	192
exercise & lifestyle	192
foods (balancing)	193
drinks (balancing)	169, 170, 171
foods (unbalancing)	193
imbalance (causes)	193
imbalance (signs & symptoms)	193
meals	192
qualities	192
snacks	192
tastes	192
prakruti	7, 8, 12, 187
vata	9, 190
diet aid	190
exercise & lifestyle	190
foods (balancing)	191
drinks (balancing)	170, 171
foods (unbalancing)	191
imbalance (causes)	190
imbalance (signs & symptoms)	190
meals	190
qualities	190
snacks	190
tastes	190
vikruti	187
drinks	167-171
alcohol	167
coffee, antidotes for caffeine	167
warm water	25, 167
elements	3-7
air	3
earth	5
ether	3
fire	4
twenty qualities	7, 186
water	4
food combining	19–27
ama	19
cheese	19, 20
digestion	19-21
fruit	19, 20
honey	19, 20
meats	19, 20
night shades	19, 20
ghee	88, 90
grains & seeds	34, 66-68
amaranth	50, 51, 66
barley	67, 84, 114
hulled	67
pearl barley	67
pot barley	67
scotch barley	67
millet	55, 66, 81, 82

quinoa	57, 80, 67	lime (kaffir) leaves	36, 109
rice	67-68	low Glycemic index	123
bhutanese red rice	67, 68	lunch box/Zojirushi®	4
black rice	See forbidden rice	millet	See grains & seeds
brown rice	67, 68	miso	41
forbidden rice	67, 68	mizuna	41
purple rice	See forbidden rice	mid-day main meals	61-99
rice cooking chart	68	vegetarian recipes	70-85
white basmati	67, 68	non-vegetarian recipes	90-99
white rice	67, 68	morning meals	49-59
wild rice	67, 68, 130	morning routine	49
healthy cookware	39	nut butters	See sauces, chutneys & churnas
Himalayan salt/Himalayan pink salt	32	nuts	41
honey	19, 40	alternative to dairy products	41,145, 146, 147
Japanese arrowroot	40	organic	26, 44
Kitchari	26, 70	pitta	See doshas
knives	36, 38	pomegranate molasses	See pomegranate syrup
kuzu root starch	40	pomegranate syrup	42, 141, 148, 178
leftovers	185	quinoa	See grains & seeds
amaranth	185	raw food	127
artichokes	185	rice	See grains & seeds
barley	185	rock salt	See Himalayan salt
cabbage	185	salads & vinaigrettes	127-141
coconut milk	185	salt	42
dips & spreads	185	sauces, chutneys & churnas	143-152
fennel	185	nut butters	143, 145
meat	185	sesame seeds	42
millet	185	shopping/international items	34, 36, 40-42
pureed yam or parsnip	185	shoyu	42
quinoa	185	six tastes	15-17
rice	185	astringent	17
risotto	185	bitter	16
legumes	34, 62–68	exceptions to the rules	17
beans	64-66	pungent	16
aduki/adzuki/red	65, 66, 103, 179	salty	16
black beans/black turtle beans	65, 66, 102, 129, 159	sour	15
cannellini beans/white kidney beans	65, 66, 78, 158	sweet	15
cooking chart	66	snacks & dips	155-165
garbanzo beans/chickpeas	65, 66, 77, 104	storing dips & spreads	155
Italian kidney beans	See cannellini beans	soups & stews	101-115
Mexican beans	See black beans	soy sauce	42
cooking chart	66	spices	35
mung dal/moong dal/yellow dal	64, 66, 70, 110	sweets, desserts	173-183
split hulled black mapte bean	See urad dal	gluten free	173, 175, 176, 177, 178,182, 183
split hulled green gram	See mung dal	tamari	42
split pigeon peas	See tur dal	tamarind paste	42, 74, 141, 147
tur dal/toor dal	64, 66, 71, 72, 73	three doshas	See doshas
urad dal/urid dal/white dal	64, 66, 74	tofu	79
lentils	62-63	tomatoes	43
cooking chart	66	vata	See doshas
french/Puy	62, 66, 75, 113, 135, 161	vegetables	117-124
red	63-66, 73, 76, 160	vegetarian, aspiring	61, 113
lemongrass	36, 108	yogurt	52, 58, 59
lentils	See legumes	about making	59

Made in the USA
Charleston, SC
28 October 2013